Act Thin, Stay Thin

Act Thin, Stay Thin

New Ways to Lose Weight and Keep It Off

Dr. Richard B. Stuart

PSYCHOLOGICAL DIRECTOR

WEIGHT WATCHERS INTERNATIONAL, INC.

Foreword

Jean Nidetch

FOUNDER

WEIGHT WATCHERS INTERNATIONAL, INC.

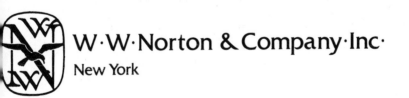

W·W·Norton & Company·Inc·
New York

First Edition

Library of Congress Cataloging in Publication Data

Stuart, Richard B
  Act thin, stay thin.

  New Ways to Lose Weight and Keep It Off
  Includes bibliographical references and index.
  1. Reducing—Psychological aspects. 2. Self-control. 3. Self-perception. 4. Food habits.
I. Title.
RM222.2.S86   1978   613.2'5   77–16198
ISBN 0-393-08805-7

1 2 3 4 5 6 7 8 9 0

Contents

CONTENTS

Foreword

Jean Nidetch
FOUNDER
WEIGHT WATCHERS INTERNATIONAL, INC.

If you are just beginning to lose weight, this book can help you to achieve your goal. If you are making your umpteenth attempt to lose weight, this book can help you to do it right this time. If you have lost weight and are worried about how to maintain your loss, this book can help you to consolidate the changes that brought your eating under your own control.

Many of the ideas expressed in this book have already played a major role in the psychological and medical understanding and treatment of obesity. In his Presidential Address before the American Psychosomatic Medicine Society, Dr. Albert Stunkard referred to Dr. Stuart's early work as a "landmark in obesity research." Dr. Stunkard also introduced Dr. Stuart's first book, *Slim Chance in a Fat World,* as "the best book yet written on the control of obesity." These concepts now used in our classes are regarded by many professional observers as the procedures offering most overweight people their best chance for weight loss.

In this new book, Dr. Stuart has greatly expanded the ideas expressed earlier. He offers a comprehensive program for understanding and controlling not only your eating, but also many aspects of your behavior that bear upon your urge

7

to eat. You will find suggestions for changing those thoughts and feelings that make overeating easy and self-control diffi- cult. You will be shown techniques that can enable you to "reprogram" forces in your environment that trigger your urge to eat too much of the wrong food. You will also learn techniques that you can use successfully to manage hundreds of eating crises and to gain control of your behavior in other areas.

When Dr. Stuart introduced many of these techniques to members of Weight Watchers classes through the Personal Action Plan, members' weight losses improved dramatically —some by as much as *24 percent!* Some of the ideas that Dr. Stuart brought to our members were already in use in our classes: we knew *what* to do although we were not sure of the scientific background. Other ideas were new to our mem- bers. Most of the ideas are presented in the context of the research through which they were derived; knowing where good ideas come from can help us to keep them working for us.

I have learned a great deal from both the modules that Dr. Stuart developed for use by members of Weight Watchers classes and from my careful reading of this book. I have two copies of Dr. Stuart's book. I keep one in my office and the other in the kitchen. I consult the book when I know that certain crises might arise. Each time that I look for an an- swer, an answer is sure to be found.

Selecting this book is a good step in the right direction. When you have the benefit of well-supervised group support and when you have a professionally developed food plan to follow, you will have the elements that can best help you to reach your goal weight. I wish you every success in your efforts to make permanent weight control a reality as you achieve a thin, healthful, and happy life in the years ahead.

Introduction

In this book you will find many new ways to challenge your eating problems by changing aspects of your thoughts, your feelings, your use of your own body, and your social and physical environments. Most of these recommendations have been carefully evaluated in service and research programs in many countries. All of the recommendations will not pay off equally well for you, and some may have to be adapted to your personal needs. To help you in this process, you may wish to consult the research that supports these recommendations. Detailed references to the literature may be found at the back of this book. You may also wish to consult a professional or to join a responsible weight-control group. Either of these steps can help you to develop your personal program for change, and help you to persevere as you meet each new challenge.

Many people have helped to make this book possible. To these people, I would like to offer my sincerest thanks. The book could not have been written were it not for the research of scores of scientists whose efforts provide the basis for the practical program presented here. Albert Lippert, chairman of the board of Weight Watchers International, had the vision and conviction that allowed many of these ideas to be implemented by being offered to hundreds of thousands of members of Weight Watchers classes. Fred Jaroslow, senior vice-president of Weight Watchers International, supported and guided this effort from conception through fruition. The area directors and franchisees of Weight Watchers International contributed their valuable insights all along the way. Fred Jaroslow and Lenore Lippert read early drafts of the manuscript and made invaluable suggestions for its improvement. My editors, Carol Houck Smith and Eric P. Swenson, helped me to transform some useful ideas that were crudely written in several early drafts into a volume that I hope can help a great many people. Luda Holsgrove took each required rewrite in her stride and turned out clear typed copy without so much as a cross look. Finally, Freida, Jesse, Toby, and Gregory all made work on this book easy by drawing closer together and unselfishly permitting me the time to think, to evaluate, and to write.

R.B.S.
June, 1977

Act Thin, Stay Thin

1/ A New Beginning

How many times have you gone out for dinner promising yourself that you would eat neither bread nor dessert —only to eat not one but *two* helpings of both? How often have you resolved not to eat one potato chip during the entire late show or one kernel of popcorn at the movies—only to realize later that you stuffed yourself with junk foods you neither wanted nor enjoyed? How often have you promised yourself to start a new diet on Monday—only to remember on Thursday that Monday is long gone?

If you are like most of the readers of this book, you will have had these and similar experiences time and time again. Like the other readers, you have either been heavy for all or most of your life, you have followed the "yo-yo" cycle of periodically gaining and losing from 5 to 60 pounds, or you manage to hover close to, but a little above, your desired weight by expending boundless energy and worry. Finally, you probably have one more thing in common with your fellow readers: you may have tried repeatedly to make the same weight-control system work for you, but have never been able to maintain your weight loss.

Oh, the details may have been different in your case, but the format was always the same. You talked to friends, perhaps consulted a doctor, or sorted through the dozens of books that promise miraculous weight losses through anything from downing secret formulas to drinking water and holding your breath. Then you selected a diet—perhaps heavy on the steak one time and cabbage or rice the next— and you decided to stick to it come hell or high water. Unfortunately, the high-water mark came early. Whether you followed through for a day, a week, or even a month, the result was always the same: no matter how much weight you lost, you regained it almost as quickly as you took it off.

Most members of the vast army of the weight conscious make the same crucial mistake: when a program fails to bring results they "try and try again." There is a much wiser adage to follow: "If at first you don't succeed, analyze what went wrong and try another approach." This could mean reorganizing your thinking about the method that you choose, or it could mean choosing an entirely different approach.

This book offers a way for you to make that new beginning.

What's Different About This Approach?

On Monday you were a "compulsive eater." You were troubled by constant urges to take a bite of this or a taste of that. Your biting and your tasting added up to quite a bit of food and to extra pounds. Then on Tuesday you decided to turn *everything* around. You would curtail your food intake drastically. Same urges: less food to satisfy them. What could you expect for Wednesday besides a new defeat?

You wouldn't try to light a fire on a windy day without shielding the match. Why would you expect to succeed in changing a lifelong pattern of eating without first reducing your urge to eat? As the wind blows out the match, so your urges to eat stifle your ability to control what you eat.

This book will help you to learn *how to manage your urge to eat* while you learn *what* to eat.

It offers a *rational program* for self-management.

It *stems from research* by hundreds of scientists working in scores of laboratories.

And you will be able to *test its effectiveness* in your eating management efforts every single day.

Its goal is to teach you how to *develop self-control.*

Its promise is the opportunity for you to learn freedom from nagging urges to eat night or day for what may be the first time in your adult life.

Self-Control Is a Skill

What we call "self-control" is our ability to achieve the goals we set for ourselves. We generally refer to self-control when the goals are negative, when we plan to deny ourselves the pleasure of eating a snack, or when we plan to force ourselves to complete some unpleasant task. But self-control is much more than that; it includes, as well, every one of the positive goals that we set for ourselves, whether they be finishing a book, learning to play a new game, or painting a beautiful picture.

Oftentimes when we have trouble meeting a personal objective, we explain our failure as the lack of some basic ingredient of character like "willpower," "backbone," or "grim determination." As we blame our ancestors for not giving us the necessary genes or our childhood experiences for not fortifying our will, we swallow hard and make the same mistakes when we try again to accomplish the feat that we feel both nature and upbringing have placed beyond our reach.

The fact is, however, that self-control is a skill that can be learned—in three phases. First, we need a *clear objective.* Reducers should know how much they have to lose and which behaviors they must change to make this happen. Next, we need a *plan for change in small steps.* Reducers who try to shed pounds too quickly suffer prompt regains. Finally, we need *plans for positive action* rather than resolutions about what to stop doing. Reducers must know what they should do to keep themselves on course. Making resolutions about actions to be avoided confuses matters and often leaves them without a plan.

An illustration can help to make this clear. Alice decided for the 27th time in her adult life to lose the extra weight that gave her that roly-poly look. She knew that her weight had been on the rise since her children entered school. She also knew that while her mealtime eating was under control, she often overate when she was bored and lonely in the afternoons or angry at husband George in the evenings. She borrowed a copy of the 600-calorie diet that her friend had used and she set off on a program that would have put the greatest stoic to the test. Overnight, she planned to eliminate from her diet everything that she enjoyed, permitting herself less to eat than would satisfy her five-year-old daughter, Liz. And those afternoon blues and evening rages? Well, they were just her cross to bear.

The results? You guessed it: Alice lasted on her diet exactly four days. Why? She tried to change her eating while the same events that made her bored and angry still took place. She tried to do too much, too soon. And she concentrated on what she should not do rather than setting her sights on positive change. Clearly, knowledge of a few behavioral basics would have stood Alice in good stead.

Some Behavioral Basics

Behavioral basics are what this book is about. If you understand three basic facts about eating behavior, you will be able to understand the objective of all of the recommendations that follow. You must know about hunger and appetite, about appetite chains, and about the many facets of behavior. Each will be explained in turn.

Hunger and Appetite: What's the Source of Your Urge to Eat?

Most of our eating patterns are learned. In this well-nourished land, we teach ourselves to feel "hungry" in a thousand different ways, but this learned "hunger" is actually appetite. True hunger is motivated by the physical need for food. It usually does not arise for at least six hours after an adequate feeding, it lasts only a short time before disappearing and it brings with it faintness, loss of concentration, and other bodily signs. Most of us have never experienced hunger. Appetite, on the other hand, appears when our minds reach out for food, not when our bodies signal that food is overdue. Appetite is stimulated by our thoughts, our feelings, proximity to food, habits, and virtually anything that we have learned to associate with food. Almost alone in the animal kingdom, we humans have the privilege of eating to satisfy our appetites, when we are not hungry, and this privilege may one day do us in.[1]

Appetite is one response in a long chain of responses that leads to problem eating. For example, a typical sequence might look like this:

1. Alice feels restless with nothing to do;
2. So she turns on the television when only afternoon "soaps" are on;

3. She watches for a while but her boredom deepens;
4. She looks around for something to distract her and finds the pretzel bowl on the coffee table;
5. Vowing to have three and no more, she lets each pretzel melt in her mouth;
6. Now she's hooked and eats on until the bowl is empty.

Looking closely at this chain of events, it is clear that Alice made one choice after another, each bringing her closer to problem eating. She knows that afternoons are a troubled time for her and at (1) she might have planned to pass the time in more interesting, creative, and productive ways. She knows that soap operas bore her; at (2) she might have phoned a friend, undertaken some long-neglected chore, gone for a walk, or picked up a book instead of turning to TV. Once in the grip of TV stupor, she had another choice at (4): some exercise could have provided distraction and it was not too late to turn to some of the activities that would have been better choices in the first place. Now she comes under the control of a poor decision that she had made days before: she should not have left food in convenient places arov·id the house—should not even have had her favorite snack foods in the house. After eating the three test pretzels at (5), she might have put the bowl away, even thrown out the remaining pretzels. Instead, she left them in easy reach and convenience interacted with boredom to bring on another eating disaster.

This and every other eating experience can thus be analyzed as:

A SERIES OF CHOICE POINTS
AT WHICH AT LEAST TWO ACTIONS ARE POSSIBLE:
ONE CONSTRUCTIVE AND ONE DESTRUCTIVE.

Therefore, every eating urge should be analyzed as a link in a chain of decisions, any one of which can be changed with good result.

Breaking the Appetite Chain

Once you understand the choices that lead to your prudent and imprudent eating, you are in a position to plan constructive action. These plans should *always have at least two stages:*

FIRST, PLAN TO BREAK THE APPETITIVE CHAIN
AT THE EARLIEST POSSIBLE LINK.
THEN, BE PREPARED WITH BACKUP ACTIONS
AT LATER POINTS IF THE FIRST PLAN FAILS.

In this way, you give yourself more than one opportunity to rise to the occasion and double your chances of success.

To make the logic of this planning clearer, an analogy may be helpful. Think about the psychologically motivated urge to eat as though it were a river that flows with a definite force. Close to its source, the force of the water is not great but farther downstream it becomes a mighty and irresistible force. It would be a simple matter to cross the river at its source. To do so would probably help you to *avoid* the most serious danger. But something could go amiss during even a simple crossing, so it is a good idea to have a backup plan in mind—a course of action that you can follow should a faster current carry you close to disaster. This would be your way to *escape* the danger that you could not avoid. For example, being ready to scuttle the boat and swim to safety may cost you equipment but not your life.

Deciding where to cross the river and what to do in the event of calamity are moments of truth for the boater. Deciding how to spend her lonely afternoons and what to do to curb her appetite are the moments of truth in Alice's battle for self-control. At a certain point the boater faces a point of no return when all is lost. So, too, does the dieter. Those who succeed in winning their battles with the elements—be they swollen rivers or cresting appetites—plan their first-strike actions carefully and come prepared with backup plans as well. Just knowing the behavioral basic that you should break the chain early and then be ready to act again can start you in the right direction: most of the chapters that follow will help you on your way.

The Need to Take a Broader View

Those who succeed in weight management take action not on one but on many fronts. This was found when a group of 700 former members of Weight Watchers classes were studied to learn the differences between those who did and those who did not maintain their goal weights. All members were offered the same program and all did reach their goal weights. But some maintained their losses and others saw their weights begin to rise. How did the winners differ from the losers in this battle for weight control?

Twice as many maintainers as regainers changed their self-concepts during weight loss: they felt stronger, thought about themselves as "thin at last," and had confidence in their ability to maintain their hard-won losses. The regainers, on the other hand, still thought primarily about their personal weaknesses, considered themselves to be "formerly fat," and doubted their ability to maintain their losses. A different self-concept was therefore one thing that differentiated the winners from the losers.

The maintainers were more likely than the regainers to report that their social life became more active as they lost weight and, as a result, that they considered themselves to be happier. The regainers, on the other hand, were casual in planning meals and in managing their eating environments, two more steps that were squarely in the wrong direction.[2]

In summary, it is a good idea to resist the urge to concentrate all of your energies on a single approach.

Changing the way you *think about yourself* and the challenges that you face is not enough.

Changing the way that you *manage your feelings* is not enough.

Changing the way that you *handle food* in your life space is not enough.

Changing your *interactions with other people* is not enough.

Changing the *way that you use your body* is not enough.

Instead you must do ALL of these and other things as well.

IN A NUTSHELL

Now it's time to sum up. These are the major points in your new beginning.

1. You will have to take an indirect approach, learning to reduce your urge to eat at the same time that you learn new ways of eating.
2. You will have to learn to use your own resources in learning greater skill in self-control.

3. You will have to learn to identify the role of appetite in your urge to eat and then you must learn how to cut that urge.
4. You must learn to identify the choice points in the chain of events that builds your urge to eat.
5. You must learn how to break that chain to avoid some inducement for problem eating and to escape from others that you can't avoid.
6. Finally, be ready to look for opportunities to break the problem-eating chain in many different ways so you can mobilize all of your resources to develop new methods for positive self-control.

If you have attended Weight Watchers classes recently, since I prepared the Personal Action Plan for use by members, you will be familiar with some of the techniques that will be offered. However, for most readers, this approach will be very different from any that you have followed. If you are in the latter group, the fact that you have read this far probably means that your past efforts have not been richly rewarded. Therefore, it is time for you to make a new beginning.

2 / Putting the *Real You* in the Picture

Before you can plan ways to change your eating, you must be able to describe precisely when and how you eat. For example, you must know the hours of the day when your appetite is most likely to get out of hand. You must know the days when your urge to eat is under best control. You must know the times that your self-control is at its peak and the places where your good intentions give way to bad influences. These and dozens of facts like them are essential if you are going to be able to plan successful strategies for controlling what, how much, when, and under what conditions you eat.

The Delusion of the Three Ds

We all share a common frailty: we often confuse what we would have liked to do with what we actually did. For example, we may think that we have followed an eating plan when actually we ate much more than we intended.

Willie, for instance, planned to eat modestly at his sister's Thanksgiving dinner party. He decided in advance that he would pass up sweet potatoes with marshmallows and have fruit instead of pumpkin pie for dessert. Patting himself on the back all the way home, he said, "Oh, what a good boy was I!" But was he? He did have four slices of cranberry bread that he used to soak up that luscious turkey gravy, chestnut stuffing that tasted so good with beans and almonds, and wine to wash down this truly marvelous dinner. The three Ds helped Willy stress what he did right, while allowing him to forget what he did wrong.

The first source of error involves what psychologists call *denial.* Most of us pay much closer attention to those aspects of our own behavior that please us most, and play down our weaknesses. This is all part of a very human process of playing up our positives and playing down our faults.

Denial is a useful defense mechanism because it helps us to maintain a relatively positive image of ourselves. We cannot live happily without it. But when denial becomes excessive, it can lead to self-defeating behavior.[1] So long as Willie denies his eating excesses, how will he ever be able to control them?

Distraction is another source of error. Willie didn't intend to paint his behavior white, but at the dinner party many nice things happened and he was as interested in the warm family feeling that prevailed as in the food that was placed before him. Research has shown that overweight people are more vulnerable to the impact of distraction than those whose weight is normal.[2] And when the distractions are aroused emotions, the effect is all the greater.[3]

The final D that muddles eating recall is *distortion.* Studies have shown that people are more likely to judge their eating intake by what they think they ate than by their eating reality. Expectation reaches out and bends experience out of shape.

When volunteers were fed a liquid diet that they believed

to be nutritionally lacking, they felt dissatisfied. But when the very *same* liquid was fed to them in the belief that it contained everything that they needed to be fully satisfied, satisfaction was truly theirs.[4] The same things happen outside the lab. When you decide in advance that something will please, the food will do the job. When you decide that it will not, large quantities can go down the hatch before you reckon that you have had a bite to eat.

How Written Records Can Help

You can overcome the triple threat of denial, distraction, and distortion if you are willing to keep written records of your urges to eat. These records can help you toward reaching two important goals. First, you can obtain an accurate picture of your own food-related feelings. Second, you can actually make strides in bringing these urges under control just because you are aware that they are taking place.[5]

You doubtless have an awareness of when your fancy turns to food, but like many of the beliefs that we have about our own reactions, these beliefs may not reflect reality. You cannot make sound plans for effective behavior change when you start from where you *think* you'd like to be *instead of where you really are*. You also probably slip into patterns of problem eating without realizing that you have thought about or turned to food. Tracking these urges to eat can put you on your guard and help you to see the opportunity to make some choices that turn you away from food.

What To Do

Records of eating urges are helpful to the extent that they are:

1. Specific;
2. Simple; and
3. Kept *before* the eating has taken place.

In Figure 2.1 you will find a specific, simple record to help you to discover with precision when you are nagged by the urge to eat. Begin by drawing a circle around the hour that you wake up, and at the end of the day circle the hour that you retire. Do this in column 1.

In the second column, make note of the level or intensity of your urge to eat during each hour of the day. As you will recall, Chapter 1 pointed out that many of our thoughts of food are motivated by appetite, a psychologically determined urge to eat. Appetite, in turn, tends to be motivated by feelings such as boredom, frustration, depression, and tension, by simply being too close to tempting food, by social pressure to eat, and by a great many other cues for problem eating. Very often when you are exposed to these cues, you will eat *even though your urge to eat is low.* At these times your eating is under the control of external pressures, not internal pulls.

It is important for you to train yourself to differentiate when your eating is motivated by a need for food, when it results from an internally triggered desire to eat, and when it is a response to totally external events. One way to do this is to learn to monitor the strength of your urge to eat and then to analyze when the urge was high and when it was low.

Keeping track of your urges can also help in another way. Just as self-monitoring in general helps to crystalize the fact

FIGURE 2.1

Urge to Eat Self-Monitoring Chart

Circle Day: Sun. Mon. Tues. Wed. Thurs. Fri. Sat.

(1) Time	(2) Level of Your Urge to Eat	(3) Did You Eat Yes	No	(4) Planned Action		
7:00– 8:00						
8:00– 9:00						
9:00–10:00						
10:00–11:00						
11:00–12:00						
12:00– 1:00						
1:00– 2:00						
2:00– 3:00						
3:00– 4:00						
4:00– 5:00						
5:00– 6:00						
6:00– 7:00						
7:00– 8:00						
8:00– 9:00						
9:00–10:00						
10:00–11:00						
11:00–12:00						
12:00– 1:00						
1:00– 7:00						

that you are making a decision about food, assessing your urges before you eat helps to focus the vital question: "Is this food really necessary?" By asking this question *before* instead of after you eat, you can gain one more valuable assist in your effort to bring your eating under strict control. Therefore, use column 2 to record the level of your urge to eat *whether or not you eat during a particular hour.*

Write "0" if you felt no urge to eat.

Write "1" if you feel hunger and believe that it is a *physically* motivated urge to eat. If you ate prescribed amounts of the recommended foods at the proper times, this is likely to occur *only if you have not eaten for at least four hours.*

Write "2" if you feel an urge to eat which is somewhere between a physically and psychologically motivated urge. This will happen during the "gray" hours—a few hours after your last meal but well before your next time to eat arrives.

Write "3" if you feel a mild urge to eat and know that you are not in physical need of food. This could occur either during or after a normal meal. A good test of this condition is to try to shift your attention away from food: if you can readily change your focus, this category applies; but if your thoughts keep returning to food, then it's the next category that fits.

Write "4" if you feel a strong urge to eat and know that you are not in physical need of food. Here you will think of food, try to put the idea out of your mind but find your thoughts constantly wandering back to something to eat.

To make this step easier, take a few minutes to sit back and reflect upon your recent experience. Can you remember the exact feelings of true hunger—perhaps some stomach contractions, a slight weakness in your limbs, or a lack of mental alertness? Now switch to the feeling which you may sometimes have of knowing that you "must" have something to eat even though you know that you have recently had more than enough to eat. These latter feelings are the villains of weight-management efforts and they will be prime targets in your self-management efforts.

Next, turn to column 3. In this column, you are simply asked to check "Yes" if you did eat anything during this hour, and "No" if you ate nothing during this hour.

Column 4 is set aside for a special purpose. You will use it to keep track of your success in taking the behavior change step that is your current focus. For example, in later chapters you will be asked to use this column to make note of the fact that you did take steps to slow down the rate of your eating, to find alternatives to eating, to change the events that lead to troublesome moods, or to make eating a pure experience, among many, many others. For the present, leave this column blank. In most of the later chapters, you will learn to put it to good use.

What Two People Learned About Their Patterns of Eating

To make clear the use and application of the chart, let's look at the record that Sandra kept of her Tuesday eating and what Paul learned about his between-meal eating all week long.

Sandra is a 37-year-old housewife and she is exactly 37 pounds overweight. If you had asked her to describe her eating patterns on Monday she would have said: "I have trouble all the time. I eat from morning till night and I seem to have *no* control at all." Today, Wednesday, she will give you quite a different answer. Today she will say: "I do very well until three o'clock in the afternoon. Then I feel very hungry and eat a snack. By four, I'm not hungry anymore but I keep on eating anyway. I have got to give some thought to that three o'clock snack and I have to plan steps that will help me to follow my eating plan when my snack satisfies my hunger."

How did Sandra get so smart, so fast? You can easily see from her chart in Figure 2.2 that with the exception of breakfast and lunch at 8:00 and at 12:00 respectively, Sandra ate nothing until 3:00 in the afternoon. At that time she reported very strong ("level 4") appetite so she had a snack. Her urge to eat decreased to a lower ("3") level but she ate nonetheless. She had her dinner at 6:00, and from 7:00 until bedtime she had no urge to eat. Given these observations, Sandra can easily zero in on some eating management planning designed to do two things: she can plan specific snacks for 3:00 and she can work out some interesting activities that will keep her busy and away from food at 4:00 and 5:00. These specific goals will give her a plan of action and they will help to overcome her general feeling of discouragement about the prospects of achieving her self-control objective.

Paul is in his mid-sixties. He has begun to put on extra weight rather rapidly. After charting for one day—he started on Saturday—he did not find anything unusual. He ate three reasonable meals and had little to eat between meals. Denied a clue from a one-day search, he decided to keep track of his eating for seven days to see if he could find a general pattern. To summarize the seven different charts that he used to monitor his eating every day, Paul developed the form shown in Figure 2.3.

Paul sleeps late on Sunday morning so he did not wake up until 9 A.M. that morning. Therefore he simply drew a dash in the 7:00–8:00 and 8:00–9:00 rows under Sunday column. In the other hours for Sunday he wrote the level of his

FIGURE 2.2

Sandra's Self-Monitoring Chart

Circle Day: Sun. Mon. Tues. Wed. Thurs. Fri. Sat.

(1) Time	(2) Level of Your Urge to Eat	(3) Did You Eat		(4) Planned Action
		Yes	No	
7:00– 8:00	0		X	
8:00– 9:00	1	X		
9:00–10:00	0		X	
10:00–11:00	0		X	
11:00–12:00	0		X	
12:00– 1:00	1	X		
1:00– 2:00	0		X	
2:00– 3:00	0		X	
3:00– 4:00	4	X		
4:00– 5:00	4	X		
5:00– 6:00	3		X	
6:00– 7:00	1	X		
7:00– 8:00	0		X	
8:00– 9:00	0		X	
9:00–10:00	0		X	
10:00–11:00	0		X	
11:00–12:00				
12:00– 1:00				
1:00– 7:00				

appetite or hunger for each hour of the day under study. He then filled in blanks for each of the remaining hours.

The summary of his urge-to-eat record tells him when he was and was not strongly preoccupied with food. At the end of each row, he counted up the number of ratings of "2," "3," or "4" he gave himself for each hour of the day throughout the week. At the bottom of each column, he counted up the number of hours during the day that he was plagued by an urge to eat that was at least partly psychologically motivated.

Looking over his chart, can you see where Paul ran into difficulty? Notice that he had no between-meal problems on weekends and almost no problem urges to eat in the evenings. All of his problems seemed to crop up during the day, Monday through Friday. To find an explanation we have to learn a bit more about Paul.

Paul Munson retired from the railroad a little over one year ago. His wife still works in the office and she will not be retiring for another two years. Most of his friends are also still on the job. Therefore he has found himself confronted with idle hours during the day while his wife and friends are at work. He has developed the habit of eating a good deal during these lonely hours, although his eating is under very good control evenings and weekends. To meet the challenge of these idle hours, Paul should make an effort to find activities that will occupy his attention. He could help his wife to run the house. He might clean up his workshop and return to his old hobby of cabinetmaking or he might do volunteer work at a local hospital or school. He could also take advantage of some programs at the public library and might even consider taking a few college courses. Whatever he does, to the extent that he succeeds in constructively and enjoyably occupying his time, he can break the chain which leads to problem eating at a very early link. By knowing exactly when

FIGURE 2.3

Paul's Week-Long Record

	Sun.	Mon.	Tues.	Wed.	Thurs.	Fri.	Sat.	Total
7:00– 8:00	—	0	0	0	0	0	0	0
8:00– 9:00	—	1	1	1	1	1	1	0
9:00–10:00	1	0	0	0	0	0	0	0
10:00–11:00	0	0	2	0	2	0	0	2
11:00–12:00	0	2	0	2	0	0	0	2
12:00– 1:00	0	1	1	1	1	1	1	0
1:00– 2:00	1	0	0	0	0	0	0	0
2:00– 3:00	0	3	2	2	3	2	0	5
3:00– 4:00	0	4	4	2	2	2	0	5
4:00– 5:00	0	2	3	2	4	4	0	5
5:00– 6:00	0	1	0	0	2	0	0	1
6:00– 7:00	1	0	1	1	1	1	1	0
7:00– 8:00	0	0	0	0	0	0	0	0
8:00– 9:00	0	0	0	0	0	0	0	0
9:00–10:00	0	0	0	2	0	0	2	2
10:00–11:00	0	0	0	0	0	0	0	0
11:00–12:00	—	—	—	—	—	—	—	—
Total	0	4	4	5	5	3	1	—

his self-control is put to the severest test, Paul can plan
exactly those actions that will strengthen his control.

In A Nutshell

To be successful in self-control, you will need a good idea
of just when your urge to eat begins to get out of hand.
Unfortunately, your memory of when your thoughts turn to
food is likely to be inaccurate: sometimes you deny your
feelings; sometimes you experience the urge to eat but are
distracted and don't label it as such; and sometimes you
simply distort the realities and label appetitive urges as hunger. Use of the written record that is presented as the Urge-
To-Eat Self-Monitoring Chart can help you to reach the level
of self-discovery that you will need to achieve better self-
control. Through this record, you will learn that there are
some times when you are truly free from the urge to eat and
other times when the urge to eat dominates your life. These
are the times when decisions can be made to help you to
assert your self-management skills. The following chapters
will point the way.

3/ Getting Started with the Right Ideas

Trudy is so far behind in her work she will never be able to catch up. This leads her to feel tense and overwrought. Thinking that she's failed again and is "all washed up," Trudy decides to have a "pick-me-up": for her, this means two cups of coffee and five slices of toast and jelly. Realizing that she has already eaten too much, she thinks she has proven that she is a failure, feels even worse, and eats some more to bolster her faltering ego.

The chain reaction that Trudy just lived through is universal. Our thoughts lead to feelings, our feelings to actions, and our actions to reactions in ourselves and others. For Trudy, a negative thought triggered a negative feeling, and both, in turn, led to negative actions and reactions. If Trudy had thought, instead, that even though she was not finished with her job she had made a good beginning, she might have felt better about herself and worked more instead of turning to food.

Thoughts—feelings—actions—reactions; these are always the links in our chain of behavior; thus, any success that we have in changing one link of the chain can alter its end result. In this chapter and the next we will deal with techniques that can be used to alter thinking so that our action chains can make a strong beginning. Later chapters will deal with techniques for changing feelings, actions, and even the reactions of others.

Six Errors in Thinking That Most Overeaters Make

Because behavior is part of a chain of events, it is fair to assume that a breakdown in one element of the chain is a symptom of flaws in other elements as well. If you sometimes have difficulty in controlling your urge to eat, then the way you think about food is one source of important clues in breaking the chain of eating urges.

The First Mistake: Incorrect Ideas, Arbitrary Inferences

Unfortunately, there is as much falsehood as truth in popular conceptions about food and weight control.[1] For example, many people believe that they must be hungry if they are to be able to lose weight, that toasting bread cuts its calories, that food eaten at night is more fattening than food eaten during the day, that bread is a greater villain in weight control than meat, or that washing spaghetti removes its starch.

The facts are otherwise. Hunger leads to compensatory overeating: an effective weight-control program that you can follow at home must suppress hunger and allow enough food so that eating is well controlled. Toasting bread removes water but not calories. Gram for gram, meat has more calories and more fat than bread. And washing spaghetti removes its vitamins and not its starch. While some of these are small points, they are indicative of the kinds of errors that many people make.

If you are to plan your diet wisely, you must be able to work from food facts, not fancies. To do this, you would be well advised to consult reputable sources for guidance. Your doctor, the nutrition clinic at your local public health center, or a responsible weight-control organization that has a professionally supervised nutritional program, are good sources of information. You can do many things yourself but nutritional planning should not be a do-it-yourself affair.

The Second Mistake: Dichotomous Thinking

Dr. Aaron Beck of the University of Pennsylvania has spent years studying the kinds of thinking that predispose some people to mental illness, others to good health. He has found that one of the most common mistakes that disturbed people make, and that the sound of mind avoid, is the tendency to think in dichotomies, to categorize life events as *either black or white with never a shade of gray.* [2]

Trudy made this mistake. When her work was not completed she felt *all* bad, and when the job was done she felt *all* good: she never felt a *little* bad or a *little* good. When she was all bad she was beyond redemption; when she was all good she could hardly make a mistake.

Like so many dieters, Trudy considered every extra bite or taste to be a clear and present sign of her weak will. Once her will was weakened she felt that all was lost. Every action, therefore, had the potential to become a stepping stone to disaster because there was no way back from the smallest of mistakes. She sometimes thought that she could "never" change because she would "always" be just the same. Shades of gray were hard for her to see.

Think how much better off Trudy would have been if she were willing to regard herself as human and take small mistakes in stride. When Trudy had an extra slice of toast for breakfast, she considered the day a loss. If the day was Tuesday, the rest of the week was "down the tubes." If the week was the third in that particular month, the next week was lost as well. To avoid the terrible trap of dichotomous thinking, Trudy should have considered her extra slice of toast as a minor setback and gone on to plan constructively for the rest of the day.

Be aware of your either/or thinking. "I am lost—you are saved," "This is a completely bad day—everything is going well today," "I have no willpower—I must be in complete control." Whenever you begin to think in terms of either/or, remember that between black and white there are many shades of gray.

The Third Mistake: Magnification of Errors, Disregard of Positives

Many people also have a tendency to recall and *magnify their errors* and to completely *overlook the positives* in their behavior. On the third day of her weight-control program Trudy ate breakfast, lunch, and dinner as planned. She arranged her activities so as to avoid all snacking between breakfast and lunch and between lunch and dinner. But after dinner, while visiting friends, Trudy ate a slice of her hostess's plum upside-down cake. When she got home that night she felt she had done it again—fallen off the wagon before the trip had barely begun. To console herself, she smeared peanut butter and jelly on half of a loaf of bread as a midnight snack, even though she almost had to force herself to eat because she was so full.

Trudy might have told herself that she had made a mistake and would have to be more careful in the future. She could have consoled herself by thinking of how well she had done all day long—might even have realized that she had eaten just one and not two slices of plum cake. Rather than magnifying her error and forgetting her achievements, she could have kept her error in perspective.

The Fourth Mistake: Terminal Thinking

The fourth mistake, like the second and third, can point the dieter toward disaster. When Trudy arrived home after the plum cake caper, she wondered *why* she had made a bad mistake. In answering, she told herself that she was "weak," that she had "no willpower," and that she was "born to be fat." Just as night follows day, she concluded that "weak," "willpowerless," and "born to be fat" people have no chance for self-control. The *dead-end language* that she used— "weak," "no willpower," and "born to be fat"—left her paralyzed by terminal thinking with no possible way to overcome the obstacle that she faced.

Instead of thinking about *why* she had gotten into difficulty, Trudy could have pondered *how* she could have handled herself differently. Answers to "why" questions, if they can ever be found, do little more than justify failure and direct attention away from remedies. On the other hand, answers to "how" questions point toward the *process of problem solving*.

The Fifth Mistake: Reversed Thinking

Trudy would like to work on weight control. But she feels down in the dumps and for the past several months has told herself: "When I feel better about myself, then I'll start to do something for me. For now, I'd better not rock the boat." This is a perfect illustration of reversed thinking.

Trudy believes that her mood should change *before* she

changes her behavior. But her moods are a *result* of her actions. When she acts positively, she and others react positively. When she acts negatively, she and others react negatively. *Until she changes her behavior, nothing can change her mood.* In her thinking she has reversed the natural sequence of events in the thought–feeling–action–reaction chain, and constructive action is hardly possible.

In reversed thinking, goals are considered in place of the steps that are necessary to reach the goals. It is like trying to complete the roof of a building without having built the walls: there is no chance for success. To unscramble reversed thoughts, it is necessary to think in terms of first things first, or cause and effect. To feel better, you must change what you do. To change what you do, you must change the way you think. To lose weight, you must change what you eat. To change your use of food, you must manage your urge to eat. With reversed thinking, you back yourself into a box with no way out: straight thinking is the only way for you to plan to reach your goal.

The Sixth and Probably the Worst Mistake: Fatalism

Dr. Albert Ellis founded what has come to be called the Rational–Emotive Approach to therapy. He observed that many people share the same general kinds of fatalistic, irrational ideas and that so long as these ideas persist, failure is a foregone conclusion.

Researchers, stimulated by Dr. Ellis's work, conducted a survey among several hundred people who had embarked on a weight-reduction program. As predicted, several beliefs about the inevitability of personal failure were widely held. As you read through the statements listed in Figure 3.1, see how many of them have crept into your thinking.

FIGURE 3.1

Some Common Fatalistic Ideas

Doesn't Fit	Fits Me	
1	2	1. Unless people consistently like and show respect for me, there is something wrong with me.
1	2	2. Because I had eating problems as a child, teenager, or young adult, I can't learn new self-management skills now.
1	2	3. It's my fault when things don't turn out the way that I would like them to be.
1	2	4. It's perfectly natural to turn to food in response to all emotions, from happiness to despair.
1	2	5. Things just happen to me: I can't do anything to improve matters for myself.
1	2	6. It is not fair for anyone to expect me to control my actions whenever I feel upset.
1	2	7. Because I don't expect to succeed at developing better self-control, I don't really expect to do so.
1	2	8. I seem to be jinxed: I'm always the one who has bad luck, who misses out when good things happen.

If you checked "Fits Me" for even one of these statements, you have a tendency to create unnecessary problems for yourself. Among the would-be reducers who were tested at the time that they began their weight-loss efforts, those who ultimately succeeded chose an average of 2.3 of these statements; among those who failed the choice was 4.4. Therefore, fatalistic ideas that you accept at the start of your weight-control efforts can be expected to influence your level of success when your efforts are under way.

Cleaning Up Your Troublesome Ideas

To the extent that you make any of these six mistakes (and we all make some of them some of the time) you will be hindered in your effort to reach your goals, no matter what they might be.

Knowing the more common errors that you might make, you can be alert to their occurrence. When you find yourself slipping into any of these errors, hold an internal dialogue to set your thinking straight. Pretend that you are a member of an international debating team. The other team has just made a case for your negative thought. For example, they have just defended the position that "Every time you feel that you are socially rejected you must resort to food to keep your sanity." Your job is to prove them wrong. You might argue that no one is accepted by everyone and that some rejection is an everyday occurrence. You could also contend that just because someone does not respond positively to you in one encounter they are not necessarily rejecting you. And you could go on to say that they obviously did respond to you with some genuine positive regard even if they were not as overwhelmed by you as you might have hoped. You did handle many aspects of the encounter very nicely and you are learning, now, how to come out farther ahead in the future.

Irrational ideas by definition defy logic. Therefore, one way to get the better of them is to challenge them head-on by attempting to prove them false rather than simply acquiescing in their coercive control of your behavior.

Once you have weakened the strength of the negative statements by refuting them in your own words, the next step is the development of your own positive, alternative messages. To the extent that you confidently expect positive results, you will act in a positive way. To the extent that you act positively, you will enjoy positive outcomes. But merely thinking about positives in general terms is not enough.

Dr. Donald Meichenbaum of the University of Waterloo, who has pioneered in this technology of thought reengineering, found that self-directed statements do little good if they are hollow, overly general sweetness-and-light pronouncements.[3] For example, "Day by Day, in every way, I'm getting better and better" is a statement that does little good. While positive, it does not point the way to any new action. Only when thoughts lead to actions and actions to results can one begin to feel more positively about oneself. Therefore, *the phrases that you use to cue your positive thinking must suggest new things to do.* The following examples illustrate this point:

I. *Irrational thought:* I would like my husband to have dinner alone with me one night each week so that we can have time together without the children. But I'm afraid that he is bored with me and so I'd better not make any new requests of him. *Constructive thought:* My husband probably feels as I do that we are not as close as we used to be. He, too, will like the chance to be alone together one night each week, so I'll suggest that we have dinner after the children have eaten on Friday night.

2. *Irrational thought:* I am not as capable as most of the people I meet so I'd better avoid joining any social groups so that I do not embarrass myself and waste other people's time.

   Constructive thought: All people have different talents. I can do some things better than others and I can gain from being with people who have abilities which I lack. Therefore I'll join the library discussion group, the fund drive for the hospital, or I'll volunteer to work with the Parent–Teacher Association.

3. *Irrational thought:* I cannot control my eating at parties. Everyone sees me make a pig of myself and they think that I'm awful. So the best thing for me to do is to refuse invitations so that I can avoid embarrassment.

   Constructive thought: I can manage my eating at parties by having a snack before I leave home and by drinking only club soda with a twist of lemon while I am there. Even if I do eat something which is not on my food program, people will not notice because they will be interested in the conversation and other things which are happening. Moreover, I will enjoy being among friends and will really feel little urge to eat what I am supposed to avoid because I will feel satisfied by the social contact.

Can you see the irrationality in each of the first thoughts? Can you see how the constructive thought creates the condition for positive action? You should now be ready to purge your thinking of mistaken ideas whenever they occur, first by refuting them and then by formulating constructive alternative plans for your own new actions.

Making Effective Plans

Effective planning is much easier when the ideas that guide you are sound. To plan effectively you must:

1. Start with facts, not fables;
2. Think in terms of partial success, not total victory or defeat;
3. Take a balanced view of yourself, giving your assets their full credit while recognizing your liabilities;
4. Think in precise terms about how to take advantage of the opportunities posed by challenges rather than pondering why obstacles have made you powerless; and
5. Plan a course leading from cause to outcome rather than expecting results before action.

Many of these errors may have insinuated themselves into the basic logic of your thoughts. They can be as subtle as they can be destructive. You can begin to identify them by jotting down a few key words as you think about the challenges you face at critical times. Just relax and use an uncensored free hand. What are the things that you "know" about the situation? Are they facts or beliefs? Are they true or false? What are the words that you use to describe yourself and the situation? Are they absolute or relative words? As you ponder your relationship to the situation, do you include an accounting of your assets or do you focus entirely on your liabilities? Do you wonder why you got into the mess or do you concentrate instead on how to meet the challenge? Is the horse where it belongs, before the cart? Have you thought in terms of causes leading to desired effects? And have you purged yourself of fatalistic ideas? Self-analysis of this sort can help you clean up faulty thinking that can lead you into one blind alley after another.

A Plan of Action

Planning action requires straight thinking. To think straight you must know:

1. Exactly what you hope to accomplish;
2. Exactly where you stand at the beginning;
3. And what steps you can take to move from where you are to where you want to be.

The goal must be specific. The knowledge of where you are beginning must be precise. And the steps that you plan to take must be small, positive, and all in the right direction. Frank's story shows how it can be done.

Frank knows that he has a problem in managing his eating on weekends. A survey taken among members of Weight Watchers classes revealed that people were more than twice as likely to have trouble managing their eating on weekends as compared with weekdays, and, also, more had difficulty in managing weekend crises than those that cropped up between Monday and Friday. Frank is not alone.

His goal was to follow his food plan all week long, but from 6 P.M. Friday till bedtime Sunday night his motivation was put to the test. He knew exactly what to eat. His self-recording chart told him that middays were his downfall. He analyzed his actions at these times and realized that on weekends he tried to catch up on paperwork from the office and generally worked at the kitchen table. Since he was unhappy that he had to work when he could have been playing, and was surrounded by cues to eat, it is little wonder that he gave in.

Frank sized things up in the following way: "I do well in the evenings and all week long. I have trouble when I work on weekends, and trouble with where I work. Another problem is that when I sit down to work, I never know how much I should accomplish and therefore no matter how much I do, I never feel finished. I also have difficulty in not eating food that I can see and reach. So I had better do two things: I'll decide ahead of time exactly how much work I'll get done, and I'll work in the living room where food is out of sight. If I still have trouble, I'll try to set smaller goals to avoid feeling overwhelmed, and I'll try working in the public library or another place away from home."

Note that Frank didn't try to convince himself that a little extra food wouldn't hurt. He didn't think he was a total failure all week long because weekends were a challenge. He didn't forget his strengths and dwell on his weaknesses. He didn't wonder why it had to be him, and he didn't try to convince himself that he would take constructive action *after* he began to feel more in control. He did chose a goal, learn where he was at the start, and plan small and positive steps, and so he quickly reached his goal.

In A Nutshell

Your ideas are an important starting point for your actions. Positive ideas engender constructive actions; negative ideas lead to self-defeating actions. Your thinking is troubled if what you take for facts are fallacies, if you think in either/or terms that give negatives more weight than positives, and if you stress obstacles instead of opportunities. You're also off the track if you expect results before actions and if you do not move from a knowledge of where you are to where you want to be in a series of small and positive steps.

Jot down the key words that you use when you think about your life at times of stress and try to find positive substitutes for fruitless words and ideas. Also, decide upon specific means for meeting focal challenges so that you always know where you are en route from where you were to where you want to be.

4/ Making Ideas About Yourself Work For You, Not Against You

We all have our own ideas about what we look like and how we behave. The picture of our appearance that we carry about in our mind's eye is our "body image." The notion that we have of the way we act is our "self-concept." Sometimes these pictures are accurate, sometimes less so. Accurate or not, they can give us pleasure or cause us pain. Right or wrong, pleasing or troubling, these ideas about our bodies and ourselves always have a profound impact upon the way that we behave.[1]

Body Image

If we view ourselves as tall, we act as we think tall people should. If we think of ourselves as short, we take on what we believe the manner of short folk to be. If we like our height, we think happily about at least one aspect of ourselves, but if we feel too tall or too short, we constantly stoop to look shorter or stretch to gain an inch or so.

Unfortunately, as a nation, we seem doomed to think that we should be something we're not. In an appearance-conscious culture in which "slim is in" and "fat is ugly," the overweight suffer sorely. Almost as soon as they can talk, children are taught to accept or reject themselves because of the way that they appear. Whether smart or dumb, rich or poor, every child learns that he or she will be accepted if he looks like others and he will be rejected if he looks different. Weight is a very visible difference and one that many a layperson believes to be wholly self-induced. Therefore, many a sad plump child is forced to spend years on the outside looking in.[2] Nor is self-consciousness about weight shed in later years. Few adults avoid the urge to suck in their stomachs or conceal their bulges from the public eye.

If you do not accept your body, there is little chance that you will accept yourself. It is difficult to measure body acceptance objectively, but two researchers did produce a scale that will give you some idea of how you view yourself.[3] A modification of this scale can be found in Figure 4.1.

Along the left side of the figure is a list of personal features. Along the top you will find a list of reactions to these physical characteristics. On the scale of from 1 (strong to moderate desire to change) to 5 (feel fortunate to have it like it is), rate your reaction to each of the aspects of your own body, and then add to find your total score.

A score of 50 indicates perfect body acceptance on this scale, a feat not achieved by anyone in a group of weight losers who were tested. A score of 10 signifies complete rejection of one's sex, age, and body composition. It, too, was not approached in the sample studied. A score above 34 indicates a trend toward body acceptance, with higher scores naturally indicating greater acceptance, while a score of 26 or less indicates a trend toward body rejection. Between 33 and 27, you're indecisive.

While weight is only one dimension of this scale, it has been found that people who lose weight are likely to improve

FIGURE 4.1

Body Acceptance Scale

Rate each feature of your body by circling the appropriate number that shows the extent to which you would like to change it or are completely satisfied with the feature as it is.

	Strong to moderate desire to change it	Willing to put up with it	No particular feelings about it	Satisfied with it	Feel fortunate to have it
Your sex (male or female)	1	2	3	4	5
Your age	1	2	3	4	5
Facial features	1	2	3	4	5
Complexion	1	2	3	4	5
General shape	1	2	3	4	5
Muscle tone and bone structure	1	2	3	4	5
Weight	1	2	3	4	5
Height	1	2	3	4	5
Age	1	2	3	4	5
Sexual characteristics (body hair, breasts, genitals)	1	2	3	4	5

their self-ratings not only on this feature but on others as well. Weight is thus a pivotal dimension in our current images of how we think we ought to look. For example, a group of overweight adults completed this scale upon joining a weight-control program for the first time. They rated themselves as they saw themselves on Day 1 and at the same time indicated the kinds of ratings which they thought they would select when they reached goal weight. Their projected ratings were an average of 14.5 points better, with satisfaction with sex, age, muscle tone and body structure, and sexual characteristics all showing improvement. Moreover, when they lost an average of only 12 pounds, their average body image score increased 5 points for every 1-point increase in their satisfaction with their weight. In the end, those whose initial scores ranged between 15 and 20 points evaluated themselves at the 30+ level once their weight loss began to improve.

It is important for people to go beyond body-image change into behavioral change as well. As reducers become more satisfied with their body images, they must change their behavior to conform to these images. Some who lose weight maintain a "phantom body size" by continuing to imagine that they still carry about with them the fat they worked so hard to shed. They have been called "thin, fat people"; they are no longer obese, but they remain preoccupied with body size, dwell constantly upon thoughts of food, and even draw pictures of themselves as much heavier than they actually are.[4]

There are many outward behavioral indications of the tendency to preserve the old body image despite a new physical reality. For example, some people continue to go automatically to the size 20-and-over dress racks or to the section of the men's shop offering "portly" sizes, even after they've lost weight. They may continue to walk by shuffling from side to side rather than by thrusting their weight forward by pivoting over the leading leg. (By shuffling from side to side, heavy people can keep their weight distributed on both hips for a greater proportion of their walk time than would be true for a forward-thrust gait. While bone and joint strain is saved, a price is paid in walking speed.) People who fail to adjust their body images to their true proportions also continue to turn slightly rather than walk through doorways in the normal full-front position. They may also hesitate before sitting down as they search for the sturdiest chair in the room. They are likely to decline invitations for social activities, particularly those that require them to wear sports clothes, and when pressed into accepting, they assume the least obtrusive positions in order to avoid calling attention to themselves.

All of these "fat behaviors" are throwbacks to their overweight days. As long as they act as though they were fat in these small ways, the likelihood is great that they will act as fat people do in eating ways as well. Fat behaviors continue as long as fatness is part of one's body image. Therefore it is imperative for all reducers to start early in their efforts to bring body image into line.

There is no vanishing cream that can make a fat body image disappear, just as there is no magic that can hide unsightly flab. You can, however, begin to study your own self-judgments and your own behavior. Do you tend to think of yourself as fat? Do you begin to size up your appearance by checking first to see whether you are thin and trim? Do you think about others first in terms of weight and then in terms of other characteristics?

Any time that you become aware of these telltale signs of fatness in your body image, repeat the thought but replace "fat" with "thin." If you think of yourself as fat, repeat the thought with you as "thinning." Choose other aspects of your appearance for special note as you dress or prepare to leave the house. And when you think of others, concentrate on how they behave instead of on their good looks. Anything that you can do to train yourself to shift your attention away from a preoccupation with excess weight can work to your advantage in giving you a better balanced, thinner body image.

Self-Control

Your behavior is the key to the way others know you and the way that you understand yourself. As far as other people are concerned, *you are what you do.* After an initial meeting, when your appearance can play a role, others will evaluate you mostly in terms of the way that you act. Act in a way that others consider positive and you will be seen in a positive light; act negatively and the evaluation will change.

Your assessment of yourself is very much more complicated, however. While others may know you in only one situation, you know yourself in many. While others see only what you do, you know what you intended to do and the alternatives that you rejected in selecting a course of action. Others have a relatively simple task in deciding who you are and what can be expected from you. For you, the job is huge if only because you have so many of the pieces of that very complex puzzle that makes you what you are.

We work hard at developing a concept of ourselves and we know that this concept will be ever-changing. Most of us have a tendency to be a little kinder in our judgments about ourselves than others might tend to be, but at times we can be harsher. Right or wrong, kind or cruel, our concepts of ourselves strongly influence everything we do.

Norman knows that he "can't" resist chocolate and Susan

knows that she has "never" controlled her eating at parties. What Norman "can't" do and Susan "never" did become the ground plans for the future because words like "can't" and "never" are almost sure to become self-fulfilling prophesies.

Fortunately, we can weaken this link in the chain of self-destructive behavior: we can change the messages that we give ourselves and thereby help to change the course of our future behavior. To do this, we must change what we think *and* what we do. We must begin to give ourselves positive messages, but these messages will ring true only if we change our behavior as well.

Take the case of a woman whom we will call Jane. She was a bridge player and snacking was part of her game. She knew that she "always had to eat to keep her tension down." One night she decided that she could change that old familiar tune. Instead of telling herself that she *couldn't* manage her eating while sitting South, she told herself that she *could and would.* To back this up, she had a small snack before she went off to the game and asked that the pretzels and nuts be placed within North's reach and out of hers. She had a nut or two that first night but much less than ever before, and at the next bridge game she was even better.

When Jane began to think back over her old "I can't" statements, she realized that she was really saying "I won't." Then she realized that "I won't" could become "I will." When she turned this corner, she began her first real change toward better self-control by changing the person she thought she was.

It is helpful for you to start your weight control efforts with a knowledge of how you truly size up your self-control potential. Are you in the "I have never had and never can have power to manage my own behavior" camp? Or do you realize that you do have the power to control your own fate?

The Self-Control Potential Scale in Figure 4.2 will help you to learn about this very important dimension of your self-concept.

The items in this scale are developed from the original work of one American and two Canadian psychologists.[5] The scale has proven useful in predicting who will and who will not maintain their goal weights once extra pounds are lost. If you know that you tend to take an "I can't" point of view at the start of your program, you can concentrate on developing your "I will" potential; in that way you can increase the chances that you will both lose weight *and* maintain the loss once it has been achieved.

Please read the instructions on the scale and choose one of each pair of alternatives. In scoring the scale, "A" and "B" items have different values. Each "A" item counts 1 point and each "B" item is valued at 2 points. When you have added up your score, you will find that the possible range is from 12 to 24 points. A score of 12 indicates a complete lack of faith in your ability to manage your own behavior because you see your impulses, fate, and other people all pulling the strings that control your movements. On the other hand, a score of 24 indicates that you view yourself as fully in control of your own actions at all time.

The Self-Control Potential Scale consists of three sets of items. Items numbered 2, 4, 7, 9, 11, and 12 refer to the extent to which you feel that you are in control of your own thoughts, feelings, impulses, and actions. Low scores on these items suggest that you feel relatively powerless to manage forces within yourself while high scores indicate a feeling of self-mastery. Items 1, 5, and 8 measure the extent to which you feel that your behavior is under the control of other people, while Items 3, 6, and 10 assess the extent to which you consider yourself to be in the hands of fate.

FIGURE 4.2

Self-Control Potential Scale

Each of the following twelve items has two alternatives. Please read both alternatives carefully and circle the letter of the item which best characterizes the way in which you have felt during the past two weeks. Please be sure to circle one of the alternatives in every item.

---

1. A   My behavior is frequently determined by other influential people.

   B   I always feel in control of what I am doing.

---

2. A   There are moments when I cannot constrain my emotions and keep them in check.

   B   When I put my mind to it I can constrain my emotions.

---

3. A   Many times I feel that I might just as well decide what to do by flipping a coin.

   B   In most cases I do not depend on luck when I decide to do something.

---

4. A   People cannot always hold back their personal desires: they will behave out of impulse.

   B   If they want to, people can always control their immediate wishes, and not let these motives determine their total behavior.

---

5. A   In this world I am affected by social forces which I neither control nor understand.

   B   It is easy for me to avoid and function independently of any social forces that may attempt to have control over me.

---

6. A   Most of my present behavior is determined by genetics and by my experience when a very young infant.

   B   I have the power to work hard enough to be able to achieve my major objectives in life.

7.	A	I frequently find that when certain things happen to me I cannot restrain my reaction.
	B	Self-regulation of one's behavior is always possible.
8.	A	I feel that I must yield to social pressure because I am very uncomfortable when I go against the wishes of others.
	B	I generally feel that it is more important to act on my own good judgment than to do what others advise me to do.
9.	A	Even if I try not to submit, I often find I cannot control myself from some of the enticements in life such as overeating or drinking.
	B	When I make my mind up, I cannot always resist temptation and keep control of my behavior.
10.	A	I often realize that despite my best efforts some outcomes seem to happen as if fate planned it that way.
	B	The misfortunes and successes I have had were the direct result of my behavior.
11.	A	Something I cannot do is have complete mastery over all my behavioral tendencies.
	B	Although sometimes it is difficult, I can always willfully restrain my immediate behavior.
12.	A	I have no control over the way that I feel, the things that I think, or the way that I act upon my feelings and thoughts.
	B	I can control my thoughts and behavior and therefore I can control the way that I feel most of the time.

If you have chosen items in the first series that indicate that you feel you are in control, you are likely to choose few items in the final two series attributing control of your behavior to outside forces. If you checked low-self-control items, you might or might not have checked items that put your behavior in the hands of others or of fate because you might feel that your actions are under the influence of the deeper recesses of your own being.

To the extent that you accept responsibility for your own actions, you will take steps to improve your self-management behavior. However, if you feel that you do not have control, you will be much less likely to do what you should do in order to accomplish your goals. If you have recorded a low score on these items, take special precautions to overcome your initial doubts about your abilities as you approach the recommendations in this book. Furthermore, be sure to interpret every success, no matter how small, as proof that an "I can't" statement can become an "I can, I will, I did!" statement.

Some Steps to Take

There is no guarantee either that weight will be lost or the loss maintained when self-concept is changed. But the probability is great that the process will neither be started nor sustained unless positive changes in self-regard are accomplished. This means that you must change the persistent wallpaper of your consciousness—the kinds of things that you tell yourself about yourself from morning to night every day of your life. You have had many years of practice for your negative thoughts so you must expect to work very consistently to change these crucial ideas about yourself. The success of your efforts depends upon the *seriousness* with which you approach the task and your *consistency* in following through.

First, you have to think about the most negative things you tell yourself. Norman told himself that he was a "chocolate freak, who could never say no to a piece of candy." Susan told herself that she "couldn't resist canapés and cakes at parties." Jane told herself that "for me, bridge decks and peanuts go hand in hand." Toby knew that he was "born to be fat," Natalie that she was "still a fat mind in a slimming body," and Marilyn that her "appetite was in the driver's seat." What are the two or three *negative* self-statements that you make to yourself time and time again every single day? Write them in the spaces below:

1. _____
2. _____
3. _____

Now go back over these negative messages and change them into positive self-statements. Norman can tell himself: "I can control my eating candy as well as anyone else." Susan can say: "By having a snack before the party, I can keep from eating anything while I am there." Jane can tell herself that her "interest is card play and not junk foods," Toby that "thin is a set of behaviors that he has already begun to develop," Natalie that she has a "new thin sense of self," and Marilyn that she has "her urges to eat on the run." In each instance, the message is simple, easy to remember, and to the point. Above all, each one is concerned with what can and will happen, and weakens old ideas about what can't or won't.

Looking back over your original negatives, rewrite them now as positive self-statements.

I. _____

2. _____

3. _____

There are two different sets of times that you should select to begin making these statements to yourself.[6]

First, every time that you catch yourself making a negative statement in that inner dialogue we always carry on within ourselves, silently order yourself to "Stop that nonsense!" and then repeat the positive message.

Second, plan to repeat these important positive messages to yourself at regular times every single day. For example, if you drive to work, make a positive self-statement every time that you stop for a red light. If you do something several times each day like washing dishes or straightening your desk, repeat the positive message before you do the chore. Or if you look at your wristwatch several times each day, try to train yourself to repeat a positive self-statement every time you do. List below the times and situations when you will choose to cue your new self-statements every single day:

In the morning: _____

In the afternoon: _____

In the evening:_____

Only by interrupting the thought chains that begin with self-criticism and by developing high-strength habits of positive self-statement can you begin to be successful in changing your self-concept in a way that keeps pace with your slimming self.

Any task worth doing is worth counting. As a way to help you to remember to think kindly about yourself, and as a way of helping you to assess the consistency with which you have applied yourself to this vital self-redevelopment task, use the left-hand segment of the fourth column of the Self-Monitoring Chart on page 27 to keep track of the times that you do remember to reprogram your concept of you. If you change bad messages into good and restate the positive messages inwardly ten or twelve times each day, you will be well on the way toward bringing your self-fulfilling prophesies into line with your personal goals for change.

In A Nutshell

We all have inner ideas about our bodies and about our behavior. Whether these ideas are right or wrong, pleasing or painful, they do influence our behavior. If we think of our bodies as fat and ourselves as weak, we are very likely to perpetuate self-defeating behaviors. On the other hand, if we can change fat body images to thin ones at the proper time, and replace doubts about our abililty to exercise self-control with confidence in our abilities as our strength in self-control grows, we have a much stronger chance of accomplishing our behavior change objectives. In this chapter you have had an opportunity to size up your body image and your belief in your potential for self-control. You have been offered ways in which you can improve your scores on both important dimensions; as your body begins to shed its weight, your body image will be slimming, too. Even before your shape begins to make visible change, start to rethink your ideas about your own behavior so that you think of yourself as "thin behaving" and stop cueing yourself to act as though you were doomed to everlasting fatness.

5/ Getting the Goods on Your Pantry Shelves

The diet of the average American is changing—and changing fast. Since 1935, the typical adult in this country has increased his or her consumption of red meat by some 50 percent, to 187 pounds annually. We have more than tripled our poultry consumption to 50 pounds per year. We eat more than twice as much cheese as we did forty years ago (some 15 pounds per person per year). We eat about the same number of eggs per year (285), put away about the same amount of sugar (100 pounds), and wash it all down with about the same amount of coffee (14 pounds). At the same time, our intake of fresh vegetables has declined by close to 15 percent, we drink about a third less milk than was consumed in the past, and we eat over 40 percent less fruit.[1] In place of reaching for a carrot, a glass of milk, or an apple, our hands fall instead on pastries (up 70 percent), soft drinks (up 80 percent), and "munchie" foods like potato chips (up over 85 percent).[2] While we talk more and more about healthful eating, we are turning away from fresh nutritious food to processed foods with empty calories. So great is the impact of this change that the U.S. Department of Agriculture has found that over half of all Americans now have inadequate diets, up 10 percent in a single decade.

If our incomes are small, about thirty cents out of every

dollar spent goes to pay for food. If we are more fortunate and find ourselves with more generous incomes, we spend about twenty-one cents of each dollar earned for food. It seems as though with each increase in food prices, we become less concerned with the declining nutritional value of the foods that we eat. What has helped to blind our vision so?

Technology on the March

Prior to World War II, foods were processed primarily to improve their shelf life and food advertising was limited basically to print ads advising consumers about the price and availability of foods. During the war, technologists were called upon to produce new methods and materials at an unprecedented rate. Transportation, munitions, human engineering, and communication technologies produced innovations with unprecedented speed and dependability. One of the challenges posed by the war was the need to bring preserved foods to servicemen in the field in easily consumed individual portions. Rising to the challenge, the food industry developed the infamous "C" and "K" rations which both assured the survival of hundreds of thousands of GIs and dulled their palates for years to come.

After the war, we had surpluses of manpower and technology. It did not take long to find ways of putting both into action again. The workers and the machines that brought hardtack and beef jerky to the servicemen were employed to bring convenience foods into the homes, offices, and factories of America. Technology was used to devise new forms for food that would have staggered the imagination of the chief cook and bottle washer on Buck Rogers's interplanetary space rocket.

Where Has All This Gotten Us?

We eat about the same number of calories today as we did in 1940 but the nutritional value of this food has suffered a steady decline since the end of the World War II.[3]

Several technologies have played crucial roles in this change. The technology of food processing has developed an unprecedented array of new foods and new forms of familiar foods. The technology of advertising has had a large impact upon changing public attitudes toward these foods. And the technology of marketing has worked to lower buyer resistance in the actual marketplace. Consumers ultimately pass judgment on the success of these technologies and their vote must be seen as one of resounding approval as they buy increasing quantities of the new foods and shrinking quantities of the old. "Synthetic" seems more valued than "natural," and "convenience" has come to dominate "economical" as values among the food buying public.

Unfortunately, many of these new foods are made palatable by the addition of unprecedented amounts of sugars and fats, and the packagers, advertisers, and marketers have become so skilled at their trade that the food-buying public is bombarded to buy more than they need—and more than they should have. Food on the shelf cries out to be eaten and, therefore, it is important for weight-conscious people to develop the skill necessary to buy what they need and only what they need.

TV and the Urge to Act

Which tablets absorb over forty-seven times their weight in acid? Which bread builds bodies twelve ways? Which mouthwash tastes bitter but fights bacteria? Nearly everyone over the age of twelve can answer these and dozens of questions like them. We know more about the absorptive capacity of some antacids than about the caloric value of fat. We know more about the supposed virtues of some breads than about the importance of fruits and vegetables. And we know more about how to keep our breath smelling sweet than about how to choose foods wisely.

All of us have learned these tidbits in the privacy and comfort of our own living rooms while watching one of the some 122,000,000 television sets that carry their message into 90 percent of the homes in America.[4]

It has been estimated that children view between 8,580 and 13,260 televised commercials per year, or an average of over 100 running hours of commercial messages. During what is believed to be "kiddie prime time," advertising is limited to 9.5 minutes per hour on Saturday and Sunday mornings and to 12 minutes per hour on weekday mornings. Also, during these hours, advertisements urging children to ask their parents to buy certain products are prohibited and stations are prevented from running ads in which the cartoon heros of adjacent programs are used to hawk a product. But children watch many hours of television during the afternoon and early evening hours and no such protections are afforded during these important times. Children are thus unprotected during all but about 10 percent of their TV-viewing time.

Repeated time and time again, and presented in picture and sound that often competes successfully with the program itself, televised commercials have a great capacity to influence. They can help to disseminate an understanding of nutritional principles and to market healthful and nutritious foods. Or they can promote the consumption of foods which are as destructive in their effects as they are costly in price. Unfortunately, it is clear which end comes out on top in the choice between education and commercialism.

A look at the list of products that are offered to children by the clowns and cartoon figures who prance across the Sunday morning TV screen is frightening indeed. Consumer activist Robert Choate took notes one Sunday morning in his hometown, finding that on children's programs all of the products advertised between 10 A.M. and noon were empty-calorie, highly sweetened junk foods.[5] The child who fell victim to all of these ads would spend his adolescence in the dentist's chair if he were not too fat to make the trip to the dentist's office. Clearly, the foods sold to children by TV stations in Choate's hometown rank high on the list of nutritional bombshells.

According to the *Broadcast Advertisers Report,* during the first nine months of 1975, and on the three commercial networks only, there were:

  8,166 cereal commercials
  4,083 ads for candy and chewing gum
  3,208 ads touting shortening and cooking oils
  3,024 soft drink commercials and
  2,129 cookie and cracker ads

During the same time, you could count on one hand the number of national ads for fruits other than oranges and vegetables of any description.

Many of the ads which are aired on TV are aimed primarily to child viewers. A review of which ads are slotted during children's viewing times and which during adult hours is informative. The following figures were also adapted from the *Broadcast Advertisers Report:*

Product	Percent Sucrose	Number Weekend Broadcast	Number Total Broadcast	Percent Weekend Broadcast
Cereal A	55.1	279	334	83.53
Cereal B	50.0	141	143	98.60
Cereal C	48.8	279	288	96.88
Cereal D	46.6	121	122	99.18
Cereal E	45.9	187	201	93.03
Cereal F	10.6	37	259	14.29
Cereal G	8.1	0	219	0
Cereal H	4.4	0	260	0
Cereal I	4.1	0	278	0

Notice that the cereals with the highest level of sucrose (refined sugar) are those with an overwhelming percentage of their ads scheduled during prime time for the kiddies, while the cereals with modest sugar content are virtually hidden from childrens' view. What does this tell children about which foods are good to eat? What will they ask their mothers to buy? And what impact will eating presweetened cereals, candy, and soft drinks have upon their waistlines and their health forty, fifty, or sixty years later?

Children are not alone as targets of the food advertisers. According to a summary in *Advertising Age,* during 1973, large food manufacturers spent as much as $180 million on advertising. Close to 90 percent of these expenditures were allocated to television by these major advertisers and by others who help to push food advertising past $1.5 billion per year.

Some of this money is used to fund ads that present simple facts about foods that are offered for sale. But some of the money goes into ballyhoo ads that by inference and innuendo try to represent a product as something which it is not. The goal of most of these ads is at best to inform consumers about the availability of services and goods that might not other-wise come to their attention. At their worst, however, un-scrupulous advertisers urge consumers to make purchases that otherwise knowledgeable buyers would fail to make.[6]

The common threads in these legal, yet deceptive, ads are juxtaposition and inference that lead consumers to false ideas. The following is a listing of several different types of deception:

1. *Virtue by Association Ads.* The background for these com-mercials is the information that consumers tend to associate certain virtues with certain product characteristics. For ex-ample, if it is known that consumers believe that athletes gain their strength by eating certain foods, the suggestion that athletes eat a particular product activates an expectation that eating that product will lead to athletic prowess.

2. *Incomplete Statements.* How often have TV announcers pro-claimed that "three out of five doctors recommend brand X diet supplement pills?" We, naturally, assume that a majority of physicians endorses the supplement in question. But are the doctors physicians? biochemists? doctors of divinity? or doctors of veterinary medicine? Under what conditions do they recommend the pill? For what disorders? Against which alternative? And did literally three out of five make the recommendation or was it 30 out of 50 or 3,000 out of 5,000? Clearly the "three out of five" statement is intended to reach far beyond the simple meaning of the words.

3. *Incomplete Remedy Ads.* "Buy XYZ formula and lose pounds in hours, inches in days!" What's implied? That XYZ formula alone will produce dramatic weight-loss results. But read the fine print on the package liner when the magic elixir arrives: it also requires a 600-calorie-per-day diet and two hours of hearty exercise every day. Then ponder the situa-tion: the diet and the exercise alone can produce the weight loss—Dr. X's magic potion is harmless (we hope) and useless

(we know) icing on the cake. The same kind of logic is found in ads that promise 50 percent of the minimum daily requirements of certain nutrients when one cup of "Breakfast Delight" is included with four ounces of orange juice and a glass of milk every morning. Check the tables and what do you learn: the nutrients are in the orange juice and milk!

4. *Fool's Gold Ads.* These are the ads urging consumers to buy a product in order to take advantage of its fundamental element. "Buy Wonder Vitamins and give your vision a boost with retinol!" Retinol does help to improve vision but it is another name for vitamin A_1 and it is found in virtually every multi-vitamin capsule sold over the counter.

5. *Food Is Love Ads.* This ad preys upon human frailty. We all want to be loved. If we are parents, we want the affection and respect of our children. If we are spouses, we want our husbands and wives to know that we care. If we are friends and relatives, we want them to know that we are wise and gracious. Therefore, many, many foods are sold with the following senario:

> Junior rushes into the house after a long day at school: "Hey Mom," he shouts, "I'm home. What ya got to eat?"
>
> Mom reaches into the cupboard and comes out with an instant treat.
>
> "*Wow!*" says Junior. "At Billy's we never get things as good as this!"
>
> Moral of the story: If you want to outdo Billy's Mom and score high on your child's hit parade, buy a treat which he should probably never eat.

The key to these ads is thus the inference that some positive social feelings are tied to serving a particular foodstuff, an inference which is as absurd as it is destructive.

All of us, old and young, white and black, male and female, rich and poor, fat and skinny—yes, all of us—are vulnerable to the ads. Unfortunately, some of us are more vulnerable than othes, especially the young, the less educated, and, where food ads are concerned, the overweight as well.[7]

The overweight were shown to be vulnerable to the lure of ads in a simple experiment. Researchers at the University of California at Davis showed some food slides to groups of heavy and normal-weight subjects and slides of pretty scenery to other subjects of varying weight. All subjects were then asked to rate the taste of crackers and to indicate whether or not they would purchase packages of the crackers which they were tasting. You guessed it: while normal-weight subjects did not seem to be influenced by the slide show, overweight subjects seemed willing to buy more types of crackers after having been shown food slides than after having been shown scenery slides.[8]

The Plot Thickens

Food packaging is big business. In 1971, the average American made use of 591 pounds of food-packaging material. Forty-seven percent of all paper products, 14 percent of the national aluminum production, 75 percent of our glass output, and 29 percent of the plastics go into materials used to package food. All of this is quickly processed by the family and becomes one-third of all household refuse, the largest single component of municipal waste-handling systems.[9]

Packaging, of course, does help to preserve food and to protect it from damage. But it has two other very important functions. It facilitates handling of foodstuffs by market managers who can cut labor costs when cream cheese comes foil-wrapped and placed in cardboard boxes (rather than in one solid brick needing cutting) or when tomatoes come nestled in cellophane-wrapped plastic trays (rather than being displayed loose on large counters). While serving these utilitarian functions, the packaging in which food is marketed is also a form of *point of sale advertising*. Its purpose is to attract attention.

Food packagers spend large sums of money in order to determine the best way to present their wares. Some cookies have been found to have great eye appeal and are resistant to breakage and easily stacked; they are sold in see-through packages. Other cookies would look attractive if they were not so fragile and if they held their positions in columns; their pictures are printed on wrappers. And still others are not very interesting to look at; they are decked out in packages with fancy lettering but no likeness.

The colors of the wrappers are scientifically chosen and the choice of the brand name and the wording of the package label are both as carefully test-marketed as is the food itself.

All decked out in attractive garb, the product is then passed along to the market manager who has some very important decisions to make. Products that are displayed between waist and eye level naturally attract more buyer interest than do those that are on low or high shelves. Staples, the items that customers will seek out, can be placed where they are more difficult to see, with the most visible display area assigned to those products for which the store manager would like to attract buyer interest. Other foods are more easily seen in open display cases, so considerable energy is consumed by keeping frozen foods frozen and chilled foods chilly in refrigeration units, the doors of which are constantly open—a feat that astounds utility-bill-paying homeowners.

Some surplus and hard-to-market items are placed in sale

bins at the ends of aisles so that customers are certain to see them as they round the bend en route from fruit juices to breakfast cereals. Other items are placed in racks adjacent to the lines in which customers must stand while waiting to pay for their purchases. These are often items with appeal to children, who nag their parents to make an unnecessary purchase under threat of a row that will bring disgrace to one and all. At other times, items which shoppers would normally pass up, but which they might drop into their carts when given several minutes of boredom and inactivity, are put on display before customers in checkout lines.

Such, then, is the industry that has developed to manufacture need. Advertising seeks to condition favorable responses to products, from techniques as simply as merely repeating brand names so that they are recognized in stores, through the communication of information which can aid intelligent selection of the product, to ads which intentionally mislead through implication or outright lie. Some advertising also seeks to build demand by programming children to ask for products which they do not need and would often be better off not having. Meanwhile, the food packagers and store managers are making ready to close the sale by decking foodstuffs out in fancy wrappers and by arranging displays which all but guide the hand to discretionary (read *unnecessary*) merchandise.

How to Evade the Shopping Traps

The unwary consumer who watches his or her television set in earnest and who goes unprepared into the marketplace is a "sitting duck." Armed with the clichés of the ad men, still hearing junior's request for What-Not Honey Flakes, and scanning the shelves for "good" buys, the unprepared shopper is very likely to shell out dollar upon dollar for unnecessary food, leading to pound upon pound of extra fat. On the other hand, the wary shopper who analyzes the commercial messages and who prepares for the foray into the marketplace has a much better chance of arriving home with only the items which are needed.

The key to successful shopping is to apply the cardinal principle that has been used throughout this book: *break the chain at the earliest possible point, and be ready with an escape plan if avoidance fails.*

- The buying chain starts with the manufacture of demand by advertising: try to resist the entrapment of ads.
- The chain continues when demand for items is voiced by other family members: try to resist acceding to requests which you consider unwise.
- The chain is lengthened when the decision is made to go forth to the market: make certain that this decision is made at the best moment for you.
- The chain ends in the store as you make your purchases: arm yourself so that you steer clear of the snares set by the packagers and market managers.

Here, as elsewhere, the chain is strong and it can be broken only with careful advance planning. Let's explore ways to break the chain at each of its critical points.

1. Build your Resistance to Promotions of Food on TV

As in love and war, the best defense against the onslaught of TV is a good offense. It is also essential to have a good defense in reserve.

As an offense, *cut down the number of food commercials*

to which you and your family are exposed every week. This can be done by a range of different stratagems which vary in strength.

A. For starts, try to reduce your TV viewing time. Watching television is about as passive a pastime as humankind has conceived. It requires no activity and little if any imagination and/or intellectual ability. Long hours of televiewing can fatten the body and dull the senses. Therefore, finding activities that provide more stimulation can both help to flatten the belly and sharpen the mind.

B. If TV's your affliction, try to vary the programs you watch by turning in to at least some noncommercial broadcasts. Many cities now have educational television stations where some of the best broadcast fare can be found.

C. When commercial television is your choice, plan in advance activities which you will pursue during the typically two-minute program interruptions. You could, for example, turn the TV volume down and

  (1) Converse with friends and family members—you'd be surprised how much family business can be discussed in nine to fifteen minutes of every TV hour;

  (2) Begin a solitary pastime such as crossword puzzles, a craft project, or a jigsaw puzzle, or start a family game in which each member of the family takes one to two turns during each break;

  (3) Use the commercial time to get a little exercise by climbing up and down a flight of stairs once or twice or strolling around the house. The activity can help to pep you up while shielding you from the commercial.

D. When you do watch commercials, try to psych them out. For example, on a typical evening you might see ads for many of the following items:

A presweetened cereal _____

A snack food _____

A soft drink_____

A cleaning compound _____

A toiletry_____

An automobile or _____

An appliance. _____

Watch the ads with a critical eye and, with pencil in hand, try to decide whether the ad (1) gives straight information or whether it (2) is a virtue by association ad, (3) uses incomplete sentences, (4) offers an incomplete remedy, (5) is a fool's gold ad, or (6) tells you that food is love. Write the number of the ploy after each product type and see how often you are exposed to each.

Only by training yourself to interpret the advertisers' messages can you begin to make yourself immune to their effects.

When you work on cracking the advertisers' code, you are working on your own reeducation. It is a good idea to enlist the cooperation of your family. If you are the family food buyer, you can reeducate others so that they do not pressure you to bring into your home those troublesome excess foods. Even your preschool-age children can understand simple concepts like "good to eat" and "not good to eat" and they can begin to learn which messages tell less than the whole truth. Older children and spouses can join the game of "find the villain" as you all build your skills in wise consumerism.

2. Plan Your Attack

Frequency of exposure brings greater hazards of risk. The more frequently you enter the supermarket, the greater the possibility that you will make an unwise purchase. This is particularly true when you go into the market to buy only one or two items. You feel that you want to make the most of your trip or that you "should" buy several items, and therefore you pick up unnecessary items just to round out your purchases. Therefore, it is wise to *plan your shopping well in advance. Make as few shopping trips as possible, trying to go once each week or less.* If you have a tendency to run out of certain items, build up a supply. For example, if yours is a family which puts away two gallons of milk one week and three quarts the next, keep on hand a supply of powdered nonfat milk to draw upon in emergencies. If you have unexpected children staying for lunch and extra bread for sandwiches is needed, keep several loaves in the freezer so that you can avoid a shopping trip just to pick up a loaf of bread.

Prepare a list before you enter the store. It is a good idea to take advantage of weekly food specials. If you have the choice, shop at the market that has advertised specials on items which you need that week and try to buy only those things on your list. The three-for-a-dollar cookie specials and the day-old bakery items are problem merchandise for the market manager: let them be his problems and not yours— leave them alone! In order to plan your shopping in advance, *plan your menus at least a week in advance,* making certain that you estimate leftovers that will be available for lunches. If you go into the store without a list and look over everything on the shelves, there is a good chance that you will be hooked by the marketing and packaging specialist.

Shop only after you have eaten a satisfying meal and then only when you are feeling comfortable and rested. If you go into the store hungry, many food items will look good to you. If you feel hassled and harried, you will face the natural human inclination to buy a few treats as "pick-me-ups." Before you cross the threshold of the market, be sure your stomach is comfortably full and your spirits high.

3. On the Field of Battle

Store managers have become increasingly sophisticated. Music is now piped into climate-controlled emporiums. Display techniques have been developed in a way that offers products maximum eye appeal. Some larger markets even have snackbars. All of these creature comforts are designed to keep you in the store as long as possible because the longer you are "in house," the greater the possibility that you will snap up the bait. Therefore when you go into the store, *walk quickly, not slowly,* so that you minimize exposure to problem foods. *Walk only through the aisles that display foods that are on your list.* Again, the goal is to minimize your contact with problem foods. If possible, *shop with a friend* because this will help to sharpen your awareness of the products which you select. Take turns cross-examining each other: "Is this product really necessary?"

Remembering that the store manager displays products in a way that intensifies the likelihood of discretionary purchases, you can take the offensive and ask that staples be given prime shelf space. Ask that food bins near the checkout counter be replaced with magazine racks: you may as well thumb through the latest weeklies while you wait instead of trying to stiffle your urge to buy things that you don't need. When you make progress with a store manager, tell your friends: help that manager make up in volume what might be lost through less impulse purchasing of unnecessaries.

IN A NUTSHELL

It is important for you to have in the house only those foods that you should eat. To help you restructure your buying to these and only these things, a multi-stage program has been suggested:

1. Build your resistance to commercials by watching as few as possible and by carefully analyzing the overt and covert messages of those that you do watch.
2. Cue other family members in so that they cut down their pressure on you to make unnecessary purchases.
3. Plan your shopping in advance, shop as seldom as possible, prepare your menus in advance and then develop a shopping list, and go into the store only when your resistance is high —when you're full and happy.
4. Finally, treat shopping like work instead of play: shop briskly, avoid contact with any foods that are not on your list, and try to shop with a friend with whom you can discuss the merits of problem purchases.

This program can go far toward helping you break the chain of problem eating at an early link by keeping problem foods where they belong: on the grocer's shelves instead of in your kitchen.

6/ Out of Sight, Out of Mind

Some people seem to eat too much too often. Others seem to eat just the right amount most of the time. How can we explain the difference? We could say that the people are different. However it would be closer to the truth to say that the people may be *slightly* different, but their major differences are to be found in their *eating environments*.

A number of factors help to clarify the picture of eating-urge control. The first is how hard one must work to find the food one eats. In one early study, newborn babies were given normal nipples on the first and third days of their lives and nipples with slightly smaller holes on their second day among us. Normal-weight babies worked a little harder and drew the same amount of milk on the second day as they did on the first and third. Overweight babies, however, drank 20 percent *less* on Day 2 than they did on Days 1 and 3.[1] Therefore, it should come as no surprise that overweight adults were later found to eat fewer nuts that required shelling and fewer chocolates that required unwrapping while ease of access had little or no effect upon the treats that the lean would eat.[2] Ease of access is therefore one important consideration.

The simple visibility of food is a second factor. When food

is out of sight, the overweight are less likely to think about it than are the lean. When food is plainly in view, on the other hand, the overweight will eat—mealtime or not—and they will clean their plates of every morsel. The lean are more likely to say "no thank you" or leave a scrap or two.[3]

A third factor makes the picture even clearer. Research at Yale University has shown that the overweight outperform the lean on tasks that require great attention to detail —as long as there are no distractions. Add a stimulus that can divert their attention, however, and the performance of the overweight falls far below that of the lean.[4] That tells us that the overweight attend more closely to detail than do the lean, but perhaps because of this their attention can be more easily distracted than can that of their normal-weight peers.

Using just these three factors, we can construct an environment that would make problem eating more likely for the overweight although perhaps not for the lean: make food easy to eat; put it in plain view; and provide activities that are not totally absorbing so that the heavy person's attention can be drawn to food.

We can also arrange an environment in which problem eating is *less* likely to occur, by providing foods that take some effort to eat, by keeping these foods out of view, and by providing strong non-food-related stimulation.

A Plan of Action

These important studies have given us the foundation for a plan of action that can help to reduce the number of times that eating is stimulated by carelessly managed cues. If first you take the time to clean up your living environment, you will help yourself to *avoid* the temptations posed by food within easy reach. You will break the chain of eating urges early and preserve your second-strike capability. If, on the other hand, you leave your life space as it is, your only recourse will be to attempt to *escape* from temptation once it has arisen. The urge to eat will not only be stronger, but you will have no second chance. Therefore, great dividends can be gained through your willingness to act now to reduce the occurrence of eating crises.

Strategy 1. Clean House

Many temptations exist in every home and office. Any food that is on display or open for easy access is a trap. When your favorite bread is in a glass container, it is a temptation. The temptation is less when the container is opaque, and still less when the container is in a closed cupboard. Of course, buying breads that are not your favorites is an even better solution. If we reverse this sequence, we can list ways of managing the external environment so that problem eating is less likely to occur:

Don't buy foods that you have trouble resisting.

If you do buy these foods for others, keep them out of sight and reach.

Those foods which you can reach should be covered so that they offer as little temptation as possible.

Chapter 5 suggested ways to build control over the things that you buy. Now you can take steps to keep these foods out of reach and out of sight at home, at your office, and even when you go out to eat.

At home in your kitchen:

1. Put all foods in covered containers, whether they are on the counter, in the cupboard, or in the refrigerator;
2. Put favorite foods in the *least* obvious and most difficult-to-reach places;
3. Keep on the fronts of shelves only those foods whose temptation quotient is low.

At your *place of work,* have *no* food in your immediate work area. Develop ways to handle food cues in the place that you eat your lunch. If the danger area is a cafeteria where you must pass a variety of tempting foods, plan to bring your lunch. If that is not practical, see if you can find someone who will buy your food for you so that you can skip the line entirely. And if that is not possible, try to find someone who will choose food for your tray while you choose food for his or hers.

In *restaurants,* you have the same goal: keep your contact with tempting foods to a minimum. You can do this by following the same food-cue hierarchy:

1. Select restaurants that serve the foods that you can and should eat;
2. Do not open the menu—order only what you know you should have;
3. Be the first to order, so that the foods chosen by others do not tempt you;
4. Request that condiments and rolls be moved to the far side of the table or be removed entirely, after others have had their fill.

Exotic restaurants may not serve the foods that you need: avoid these restaurants. Menus are written *in order to tempt you:* avoid reading them. If you must open a menu, look only at the salad and entrée section and avoid discovering that your passion foods are on the bill of fare. Even if the foods that you order are *not* on the menu, restaurants can often accommodate your wishes, so do not hesitate to ask. If you order your own food first, the choices of others will not tempt you. Finally, the removal of foods that are not part of your planned eating will help to curb your urge to eat them.

List the steps that you will follow in reducing contact with food cues in each of these environments:

1. _____
2. _____
3. _____

Strategy 2. Keep Busy

No matter how careful you are in eliminating eating cues from your environment, you must have food in the house. To keep from being drawn into the trap of eating the food that is unnecessary and unwanted, make sure that your attention is always occupied as constructively and enjoyably as possible. Food cues can distract you from your task, but a task that is interesting and challenging can also distract you from food!

Keep your mind busy with a range of absorbing activities. Crafts work well, and so do hobbies. If possible, have the supplies at hand and the work area already set up, so that you can pursue your activity at a moment's notice.

Often new books can be experienced as strangers. It takes effort to develop a "feel" for a new book so reading the first chapter can seem more like work than relaxation. Also, books have their own character and different books suit your needs when you experience different moods. At times when you feel bored or lonely—the kinds of times that usually trigger your urge to eat—it is useful to have at hand several books, the first chapters of which you have already read. That makes it easier to turn to reading as a source of stimulation. Having several books on hand will also make it more likely that you will have a novel, a book on current events, a humorous book, or any other kind of book that will meet your need when your urge to eat arises.

Phoning friends, doing chores—which could be anything from washing floors to balancing the checkbook—and listening to music or working on a craft project are other useful ways of attaining the goal of eating-urge control.

All of these strategies keep you in the situation in which the urge arises. If your eating urges occur at home, you might think of things to do outside the home during troublesome times. A visit to friends, a trip to the library, a full- or part-time job, or volunteer work can all help to divert you from the urge for food.

In the spaces below, list activities that you *now* enjoy that could be helpful in avoiding the urge to eat:

1. _____
2. _____
3. _____
4. _____

Now think of things that you do enjoy but have not done in some time, and other things that you would like to begin to do. List them in the following spaces:

1. _____
2. _____
3. _____
4. _____
5. _____

Look back over your lists and see which items you can do now with little or no preparation; star these. See which can be done with a small amount of preparation and put a plus by these. Next, make arrangements to get the activities under way. Start with those you have starred, move on to those that require a little more preparation, and finish with those for which the most preparation is necessary.

Specifically, your job here is:

PLAN TO USE AT LEAST ONE ACTIVITY
(WITH *TWO* OTHERS AS FALL-BACK PLANS)
DURING THE TIMES YOU NORMALLY FEEL
STRONG, TROUBLESOME URGES TO EAT.

To determine these times, look at the ratings that you gave your urge to eat in column 2 of the Self-Monitoring Chart on page 27.

What were the days when you were most likely to report more frequent non-hunger-related urges to eat?

At what hours did these urges arise?

What do you know about these particular days and these particular times that would allow you to plan activities that could subdue your urge to eat?

For example, Elaine found that her appetite was powerful in the late afternoon. Part of the problem was that she prepared dinner at this time and she tended to feel lonely by the end of the day. She decided to work on dinner right after lunch and use the time from 3:30 to 5:00 P.M. to do her gardening in good weather and her sewing when the weather was bad.

Bill found that he tended to start eating at dinner and to eat right through the evening. He realized that if he could break the grip of this habit of "needing" food, he would be home free all evening. He worked out an arrangement with his son Dan so that the two would work on their stamp collections together immediately after dinner. In short order,

Bill's evening eating was brought under control and the D & B Stamp Plan Company was underway. These are the kinds of activities that you should arrange to help you cope with your high-stress times.

IN A NUTSHELL

Researchers are gradually arriving at a description of those events in the environment that cue problem eating by the overweight. Easy access to food, food in full view, and vulnerability to distraction by food cues—all contribute to a buildup of eating urges. You can avoid giving in to temptation by following a two-stage plan of action. First, arrange your living environment so as to limit your access to problem foods. Second, build up your resistance to the food that must exist by providing for yourself a rich array of interesting activities that will draw your attention away from food.

7/ Making Eating a Pure Experience

Cynthia has been divorced for several years and she lives alone in a small apartment. She works hard at the office all day and comes home tired every evening. Because she puts out so much effort on the job, she likes to take it easy at home so dinner is usually broiled food eaten before the early-evening movie. When the film is over she clicks the TV off, does the dishes and a little straightening up, and spends an hour or two on work that she has brought home from the office. Then it is her custom to turn the TV back on to catch an interesting guest on a talk show or watch part of a late-night movie. Her problem is that she has grown from a size 10 to a size 16 in the past few years because her late-night televiewing is almost always coupled with an apple, then a slice of bread with a dab of peanut butter, and, when these have not hit the spot, a dish of ice cream with a handful of cookies.

What's happened to Cynthia? She has *trained* herself to turn to food whenever the TV tube comes to life. In this conditioned behavior she is not alone; millions of others put themselves to this same test every day. Let's look at just one of her fellow sufferers.

Ray is a member of a weight-conscious family. Everyone

has a good breakfast and a well-planned, healthful dinner. There is no eating after dessert in the evening and everyone except Ray is trim and fit. What's Ray's problem? Well, he leads a very pressured day at work. He has a mountain of paperwork on all of his accounts and so he takes his coffee breaks at his desk and eats lunch there as well unless he has an appointment with a client (which almost always involves either lunch or coffee and a sweet roll). Over the months, Ray has learned that eating and working go together. As a result, he feels that his wits are dull and his concentration wanders unless he has a bite to eat. For his efforts, Ray has a full belly from nine to five, a paunch that makes him the black sheep of the family, and suits that come from the "Portly Shop" of the downtown department store.

Cynthia and Ray have learned to turn to food automatically when they do some of the important things in their lives. They are probably unaware of this self-programming, but they are painfully aware of its consequences. By being careless in allowing themselves to associate unnecessary eating with watching television and working, they have programmed into their lives habits that will be difficult to break.

We "program" ourselves to act in certain ways when we repeat several behaviors in the same sequence a few times over. This builds the habit strength of a chain of behaviors and in the future the occurrence of one response in the chain will make the next one very likely to occur. For example, Cynthia programmed herself to come home from work, put the groceries away, read the mail, put something in the broiler before hanging up her coat, splash some water on her face, and then wash the salad greens while the broiler does its work.

Ray arrives at his office at 9 and his first stop is at the coffee machine. He glances at the headlines of the newspaper as he sips his coffee and eats a Danish pastry as he opens his business mail and gets down to work. Like clockwork, one action follows upon the other and any step that is missed leads to an uncomfortable disruption of the routine.

As we move through our self-programmed paces, we also learn to associate certain stimuli with each action. Cynthia listens to the 6 o'clock radio news while she reads the mail: the news and mail go hand in glove for her. Ray opens the mail and eats his pastry: papers and pastries are a strong combination for him. After several weeks of these pairings, Cynthia's interest and comfort in reading the mail is "conditioned" to her hearing the newscast, and Ray's correspondence creates an urge to eat. This is the same conditioning that Pavlov discovered as a means of training his laboratory dogs to salivate when a bell was rung, after previously giving them food powder at the sounding of the bell. The only difference is that while Pavlov worked hard to condition his dogs, Cynthia and Ray simply *relaxed into their natural behavior chains to condition themselves in unintended ways.*

Why Should You Decondition Your Reactions?

Some conditioning is inevitable in everything we do. We cannot help but grow habituated to our routines and when we repeat behaviors in the same contexts, the contexts become cues to act. Much of this programming is harmless. For example, we dress ourselves in a fairly individual sequence —so what? We follow a common route in our drive or walk to work—that's okay too. We follow a routine when we settle down to relax in the evening and any change from that routine can interfere with our relaxation. That, too, is no problem. There is a problem, however, when the routines that we establish lead to an association between urges to eat and to activities that can and should be entirely free of food. When we are careless and allow diverse activities to stimulate our appetite, we create for ourselves a continual pressure to suppress our appetite. It is easier to develop a negative reaction of this type than it is to bring it under control, but through effort we can learn to suppress the reaction entirely.

One advantage of *de*conditioning ourselves in this way is the freedom from an abiding preoccupation with food when we engage in diverse activities. Another advantage is that we can learn to perform these acts better and with more enjoyment if we can disasociate them from food. It has been pointed out that the overweight tend to be more distractable than those of normal weight. When appetite competes with another activity, the overweight experience difficulty in focusing their concentration. Therefore, eliminating food from other activities frees the individual to become involved in these tasks with total energy.

Separating eating from other activities can also help the reducer achieve a more accurate awareness of how much or how little he or she eats. Dr. Susan Wooley of the University of Cincinnati asked normal-weight and overweight subjects to recall the amount of food that they ate during an experimental meal. No group overestimated what they ate. Normal men underestimated by an average of 26 percent while overweight men underestimated by a full *44 percent*. Women did considerably better, with the normal-weight group testing out at an average of 7 percent off the mark as contrasted with 19 percent for the overweight group.[1] What this tells us is that under stimulus-controlled laboratory conditions, the overweight have a tendency to underestimate what they eat. When they are distracted from concentration on their food, it is reasonable to expect their accuracy to deteriorate even more.

Finally, when the overweight eat they experience what has been termed the "warm glow" syndrome. Their receptivity to many different stimuli is heightened and they predispose themselves to accept ideas that they might otherwise reject. For example, watching television commercials while eating increases the likelihood that the overweight will believe what they hear, while watching the same commercials with no food at hand denies the sponsor this unearned advantage.[2]

In summary, there are at least four advantages to be gained from a serious effort at dissociating appetite reactions from nonfood events. You can earn freedom from a preoccupation with food at certain times, you can gain more from the activities because you will not be distracted by food, you can increase the likelihood that you will be aware of what you eat, and you can strengthen your critical faculties as you receive messages aimed at influencing the way you think and feel.

Your Personal Deconditioning Program

To start your deconditioning program you must know which situations are associated with your unguarded eating. Typical cues are:

- Places,
- Activities, and/or
- People.

By looking at the times when you recorded a "—" in columns 3 or 4 of your Urge to Eat Self-Monitoring Chart (page 27), you can learn when you ate the wrong foods or too much of the proper foods. Working backward, you can then determine which places, activities, and/or people tended to be present when these eating problems arose.

Places

It is quite natural to think of food when you are in the kitchen or dining room. If you have been careless about the way in which you program your eating urges, you must also have the urge to eat when you are in other rooms of the house or other places in your life space. For example, if you keep a candy dish in the living room, walking into the living room can trigger the urge to eat a piece of candy. If you keep a dish of popcorn and nuts in the den, then merely stepping into the den can turn your attention to some nibbles. Therefore, you will have to make certain that you *keep food in the kitchen only* and that you *eat only in the kitchen or dining room.* This may mean removing the candy bars from the glove compartment of your car or the half-eaten packages of cookies that lie in wait in your lower right-hand desk drawer, in addition to purging the living room and den of their booby traps of treats.

Activities

Reading and watching television are the two most common activities which are associated with unguarded eating. Something as innocent as reading the morning newspaper while having breakfast can lead to the urge to eat when you read later in the day. Watching television while having dinner can program you to have that "empty" feeling when the television is turned on later in the evening. Some people eat when they work on craft projects, others when they engage in certain social activities like card playing and bowling. Whatever the activity, it is playing with fire for overeaters to condition themselves to feel the urge to eat at times of the day when by rights they should be urge-free.

People

Sometimes people are the cue for problem eating. Jane's sister used to bring homemade cakes and pies with every visit. Jane and Ellen could linger for hours over "coffee and . . ." When Ellen saw that Jane was putting on weight, she stopped bringing goodies. But Jane made certain that the table was spread, and in keeping up the tradition her bottom spread as well. For Jane, Ellen became a conditioned cue for the urge to eat. To keep the cost of sisterly love within bounds, Jane would have to work hard to reprogram her contacts with Ellen for both their sakes.

A Plan of Action

Working from these data you are now ready to get down to business. Make a pact with yourself to do three things:

1. Go through your home, car, and place of work on a shake-down search for any food. Remove all food to the kitchen.
2. Make a commitment to do all of your eating only in specified places—
   a. In the kitchen, eat only when seated at your own place and then only when you use your own special placemat;
   b. In the dining room, also confine yourself to one chair and try to use a distinctive placemat;
   c. At work, eat only in the areas set aside for all workers to eat, or leave the building.
3. When you eat, make certain that eating is a pure experience by dissociating any and all activities other than socializing with family or friends.

Restricting all food to the kitchen will help you to overcome absentminded eating elsewhere. Eating at only one place in the kitchen or dining room will help you limit your eating urges to only these places.

Using a distinctive placemat will help you to gain even better stimulus control over the cues for eating urges because, when you have learned to allow *only the placemat* to trigger eating urges, you will be able to use your place at the table for other things as well. Finally, breaking the association between eating and other activities will allow you to enjoy both eating and the activities as uncontaminated, pure experiences.

In mounting this plan of attack you can anticipate two important difficulties. First, you must work toward *perfect consistency.* One or two slips will trigger the old expectancy mechanism all over again and you may spend weeks trying to regain your self-management controls. Therefore, once you make the decision to gain mastery over your urges to eat in this way, you must guard against a single error. With every slip you run the risk of telling your memory bank that the old rules are back in effect.

The other problem is faced by people who eat some or all of their meals alone. Singles or people whose spouses and families live and work on schedules different from theirs may find themselves in the habit of reading or watching television while eating. However strong the justification for pairing activities and eating, the effects are always the same: a constant need to fight a personal holding action to squelch the urge to eat. After trying to concentrate exclusively on eating for a week or two (once or twice is not enough!), try to choose as an eating activity something which you will do *at no other time of the day.* For example, if you tend not to read the newspaper you might pair it with eating. If you tend not to read magazines or books, they might be your mealtime company. If you generally ignore the radio, listening to local newscasts or to music might break the mealtime silence for you. It is best that you do nothing, but if you must do something try to make absolutely certain that it is not an activity which will cause eating-urge difficulties for you at other times of the day or night.

The simple steps suggested in this chapter can buy precious freedom for you—freedom from place-, activity-, and people-triggered urges to eat. By overcoming faulty conditioning in this way you can have the same degree of enjoyment of your life space that others have without feeling the need constantly to inhibit the desire to reach out for something to eat.

Use your Self-Monitoring Chart to keep track of your progress. In one of the unused sections of column 4, draw a circle opposite the hours when you plan to take particular care to work on your deconditioning program. Look over the chart at the start of each day to remind yourself when special effort will be needed. Then, as you go through the day, use these circled hours to record a "+" if you have accomplished your objective and a "−" if greater effort is needed. Remember that in this task *a perfect result is your goal.*

IN A NUTSHELL

In this chapter you have learned that there are routines in your behavior of which you may have been unaware, and that many elements in this chain of behaviors are associated with stimuli in your immediate environment. You may have allowed certain places, activities, or people to stimulate your urge to eat, and merely going to certain spots, doing certain things, or being with certain people can bring your appetite to the fore. These are conditioned associations between non-food stimuli and the urge to eat. To free yourself from these unnecessary urges, you must work on deconditioning your-self. You do this by making eating a pure experience, one that is not associated with any other event. Make sure that all food is kept in your kitchen, that you eat only in designated places, and that you engage in no activity other than socializing with family, friends, or business associates while you eat. Use your Self-Monitoring Chart to identify your danger signals and keep track of your success.

8 / Eating Speed and Satisfaction

When you are hungry, you will take frequent bites of your food and you will chew your food less thoroughly before you swallow. When you like the food, you will also take more frequent bites and chew less. When you are hungry, then, you are likely to eat as though you like the food you eat even though it might have little appeal at other times.[1] If you are overweight, you are also likely to take more bites, chew your food less, and take more food into your mouth per bite.[2]

The lean fill the between-bite time with many "thin eating behaviors." They put down their utensils between bites, they "toy" with their food, they wipe their mouths with their napkins, they leave scraps on their plates, and they rise from the table as soon as the meal has been eaten. The overweight, on the other hand, are all business. They eat quickly and efficiently, clean their plates completely, and yet linger at the table after the last morsel is gone as if hesitating to part from a beloved.[3]

The disadvantages of the rapid eating of the obese are obvious: they eat more than the lean per mealtime minute, they chew their food improperly so that it is less readily digested and absorbed, and in their haste they enjoy it less.

When obese and normal-weight volunteers were given exactly the same amounts of food and some were asked to eat quickly and others slowly, it was found that an hour later those who had eaten slowly were less hungry than those who had eaten at a more casual pace.[4]

Studies have shown that approximately twenty minutes are needed for the food that reaches the stomach lining to be broken down so that it can be absorbed into the bloodstream, for the absorption to take place, and for the blood to carry the message that nourishment has reached the stomach to the hunger centers in the brain. A surprisingly small amount of food is sufficient to trigger this "I've had my fill" signal, but a great deal of food can go down the hatch within that twenty minutes if the eating pace is fast.

Several explanations have been offered for this slow-eating/less-hunger relationship. When eating is slower, more chewing takes place and food is kept in the mouth longer. This means that the sensitive taste buds are stimulated longer and that the muscles in the jaw and tongue are more fully utilized. Both of these sensations can contribute to the feeling of satisfaction. (Children seem to know this. Given one cookie for dessert, most children learn to suck it slowly both to make it last longer and to increase satisfaction with the treat.) Chewing the food longer and extending the length of time that it is kept in the mouth can also help to increase its digestability.

Chewing grinds food into smaller pieces which are better exposed to the digestive chemicals in the stomach and small intestine. Also, chemicals in the saliva help to start digestion before some foods reach the stomach and small intestine where digestion will be completed. Therefore, the chemical transformation of food from its solid state to a state in which it can pass into the blood system is expedited by slower chewing. The more efficient the digestion process becomes, the more quickly do chemical messages reach the brain to signal a stop to eating. Eating slowly, therefore, has the triple advantage of: (1) cutting down the amount which is eaten; (2) making the food that is consumed more digestible; and (3) increasing the feeling of satisfaction that follows the consumption of moderate amounts of food.

What Can Be Done?

Are you likely to be the first to finish a meal? Does the serving of food cause you to stop talking and start eating while others continue to participate in conversation? Do you tend to hold onto your fork or spoon from the first bite until the last bite of food has been eaten? Do you tend to put more food into your mouth before you have swallowed the food which was already there?

Whether or not you think about eating all day long, are you relatively unaware of the taste, smell, and texture of the food that you eat while you are eating it? Can you recall whether you can feel the seeds in tomatoes with your tongue? Whether eggs have a distinctive aroma? Or whether roast beef is sweeter or saltier than steak? And do you find yourself still thinking about food when you have finished what you know to be an adequate meal? These are the signs of *someone who must learn again how to eat*—strange as that may seem.

What you must learn to do is to s–l–o–w d–o–w–n the rate at which you eat. To do this, you will have to select one or more of the following steps to follow *at your main meal:*

1. When you sit down at the table with others, keep your utensils on the table for the first two minutes of the meal as you

think quietly to yourself about how you will work on slowing down the rate of your eating.

2. Before you start to eat, cut the food on your plate into small bite-sized portions.

3. Pick up your fork and put one portion in your mouth, putting the fork down as soon as it is empty.

4. Chew the food carefully and thoughtfully. Feel the texture of the food with your tongue as it is ground into smaller morsels by your teeth. Try to sense its saltiness or sweetness, its bitterness or its sourness. Concentrate on smelling its aroma. Focus your attention upon the experience of eating so that you can capture its full enjoyment.

5. When the food has been swallowed, join in the conversation before picking up your fork for another bite which will again become the focus of your attention.

6. Finally, make certain that you are the last person to start to eat each new course as it is served. You will do this in order to extend to the maximum possible the time which you spend eating your meal.

Steps one, five, and six will help to extend the length of time that you spend eating. Step one is particularly important because it has been observed that eating rate during the first five minutes of the meal sets the rate of eating throughout the meal.[5]

Steps two and three will help you to take smaller bites and to keep only a moderate amount of food in your mouth at any one time.

Step four will help you savor the food that you are eating, and this will ultimately help you to enjoy your eating more. Strange as it may seem, while many overweight people spend their lives thinking about food, they often eat it so fast that they hardly ever fully experience it.

Which of the steps will you choose to follow? As with all

Self-Monitoring Chart for Rate of Eating

	How many minutes did you spend eating your main meal?			Did you take these steps?				After eating your normal meal, how did you feel?	
	Time start?	Time stop?	Total time?	2-min. wait?	Cut food?	Put fork down?	Sense taste, texture, smell?	Less satisfied than normal?	More satisfied than normal?
Monday									
Tuesday									
Wednesday									
Thursday									
Friday									
Saturday									
Sunday									

of the other recommendations in this book, it is important to be able to keep track of your progress. A special self-monitoring chart (see Figure 8.1) should be used for following your progress with this particular series of steps.

Bring this chart to the table with you for your main meal for seven consecutive days. Check your start and stop times. Become aware of your effort to develop the "thin eating behaviors": pause before starting, cut food carefully, set your utensils down between mouthfuls, and concentrate on the taste, texture, and smell of the food that you are chewing slowly. Then, when the meal is done, rate your satisfaction with your new eating style. You should find that satisfaction mounts as your eating rate declines.

IN A NUTSHELL

The obese and lean eat at very different rates. The obese eat normally in the same way that the lean eat when they are very hungry and are eating a favorite food—that is, with little time between bites, larger bites, and little time to chew. This "fat" eating pattern leads to consumption of a large amount of food before satiety is experienced, to swalloing food in relatively undigestible form, and to a diminished sense of satisfaction after the meal has ended. The result is that the obese are ready to eat sooner after a meal than the lean. To correct this situation, it is recommended that the overweight adopt a program of six steps toward the development of a "lean eating pattern." Included among these steps are recommendations that you wait two minutes before eating while you plan your slower eating pace, that you place your utensils on the table between mouthfuls, and that you chew your food very slowly, concentrating on its taste, smell, and texture.

9/ Timing Your Urge to Eat

Invisible rhythms underlie most of what we assume to be constant in ourselves and the world around us. Life is in continual flux, but the change is not chaotic. The rhythmic nature of earth life is, perhaps, its most usual yet overlooked property. Though we can neither see nor feel them, we are nevertheless surrounded by rhythms.[1]

Do you like to eat a hearty breakfast or does food taste like sawdust in your mouth before midday? If you have a "taste for food" one morning, you are almost sure to have it the next; and if you escape breakfast one day, food will taste no better at dawn the next. This is because your taste sensation follows a circadian or 24-hour cycle along with nearly all of your important bodily functions.[2] Indeed, in you and in all life around you, rhythms measure and control the pace of life.

Rhythm implies time and time is a crucial dimension in eating control. You may not be able to change the diurnal nature of your taste sensation, but you can alter the time each day that it is strong or weak. People who have been closed off from all cues of natural day or night nevertheless follow almost perfect sleep–wake cycles in a 24-hour pattern. Others whose fluid intake varies greatly from one day to the next produce urine with remarkable regularity. Just as you could, with difficulty, shift the time of your taste for food by training yourself to start your circadian rhythm in motion at different times of day, so, too, can you train yourself to experience the urge to eat at different times of day.

Research done at Columbia University in the mid-1960s

103

first alerted weight-control experts to a very important fact: overweight people tend to feel the urge to eat when *they think* their mealtimes have arrived.[3] Student volunteers were seen in an experimental room in which the time shown on the clock was artificially manipulated. For some subjects the clock time was regulated to pass much more slowly than real time, while for others the time shown on the clock was speeded up considerably. During the experiment, subjects were given the opportunity to eat crackers, and the number eaten was carefully observed by the research team. It was found that normal-weight people were not influenced by manipulated time: they ate the same number of crackers whether the time was apparently passing quickly or slowly. Overweight people, on the other hand, seemed to be very much influenced by apparent time. They ate significantly *fewer* crackers when they thought that their normal dinner hour had *not yet arrived* and they ate significantly *more* crackers when they believed that their dinner hour had *already passed.* Overweight people, unlike those of normal weight, appeared to be more influenced by the clock than the natural time of day.

Elsewhere it has been shown that when overweight people were denied access to any external cues about time, they were much more varied in their estimates of lapsed time than were normal-weight subjects who seemed to be less dependent upon external time cues.[4]

On the basis of the above facts, there is good reason to believe that *scheduled* eating can have an important *positive impact* upon the urge to eat experienced by overweight people.

Patterns of Eating

People eat on some very different schedules.[5] In general, three different patterns have been demonstrated. In one, certain quantities of food are eaten at certain times every day. When this plan is followed for several weeks, thoughts of eating are confined to the scheduled times. If the eating times coincide with the best conditions for controlling the amount and selection of food for that individual, this kind of eating pattern is constructive and well adapted to the individual's needs.

A second pattern is found among those who decide to "diet" every day. This decision usually means delaying any eating as long as possible, sometimes throughout the entire day, and eating at will during the evening. Hunger is rarely experienced during the daylight hours but it is a constant companion during the evening.

A third pattern is one in which eating is scheduled but the times selected are not those designed to produce the best self-control. Breakfast is likely to be skipped, as is lunch. Dinner is generally a full meal with snacks planned for several times during the evening. Eating during the evening is often a problem because most people are less occupied then as opposed to during the day and therefore they have fewer opportunities to distract themselves from food thoughts once the thoughts have begun. The problem with this third eating schedule is that food is not available when eating is most controllable and is available when eating is most likely to resist control.

A Plan of Action

In order to achieve freedom from obsessive preoccupation with food, you must set up a systematic program whereby you eat at only specified hours. This will condition your body to expect food at certain times and not at others. Our bodies are dominated by patterns of consistency, despite their vast complexity. Therefore, the achievement of urge-free times during the day requires a highly consistent retraining effort. Two things are necessary:

> FIRST YOU MUST DECIDE WHEN
> YOU WOULD LIKE TO EAT EVERY DAY.
> THEN YOU MUST FOLLOW THIS SCHEDULE
> FOR SEVERAL CONSECUTIVE WEEKS.

How often should you eat? This is a question that has interested health professionals for many years. No one knows what our natural eating rhythm might be because throughout human history we have sacrificed our natural tendencies to cultural conventions.[6] Meat-eating animals tend to gorge themselves when they make a kill while grass-eating animals tend to take in small amounts of food constantly. Because man is both meat and vegetable eating, our natural pattern would probably be a cross between the gorging of the meat eaters and the nibbling of the grass eaters.

Different eating patterns can have some impact upon health. Research has shown that people who have fewer than three meals each day tend to have slightly higher cholesterol and triglyceride levels and lower glucose tolerance levels.[7] Both of these are problems for the overweight. Other studies have shown that those who eat fewer than three meals per day also have a slightly greater chance of experiencing certain kinds of heart disease.[8] Eating three meals per day and avoiding the urge to skip breakfast and lunch can therefore bring with it some important health advantages. Although other studies have shown that it may not have a *necessary* impact upon the management of weight,[9] eating three meals per day can also help to reduce that "psychological caloric deficit" which leads many people to feel that they owe themselves extra calories because they passed up food at normal mealtime hours.

For these reasons, it is important that you plan to have *three square meals per day.* At the start, you should plan to have these three meals *at the most conventional times of day,* starting with an early-morning breakfast. Even though you may not like the taste of food in the early morning, you can condition yourself to shift the inner cycle of your food interest and in doing so you can bring your eating under the normal conditions that will help you to limit both what and how much you eat. You may not like food at the start; if so, you can begin with a light breakfast and gradually build up. Eventually, consistency will help you to change what you may have regarded as an irreversible dislike of food at various times of day.

You may also plan to have snacks when you feel that they are important. Snacks must be within the range of foods and within the portions that are permitted by the food plan that you are following. When snacks are chosen, they must be taken with the same care that meals are eaten: eat them in the proper place, control access to seconds, and do nothing else while eating. You must also *schedule the exact time of your snacks just as carefully as you schedule your meals.*

You may vary the scheduled times of your meals or snacks by up to twenty minutes or so from day to day, *but greater variations defeat the purpose of the reconditioning program* that you have chosen to follow. Therefore, you will have to be prepared to discipline yourself on weekends as well as on weekdays, having breakfast, lunch, dinner, and any planned snacks at roughly the same time every day.

By now you may be wondering whether it is worth the bother to get up for breakfast at the same time on weekends as on work days, or to play havoc with your social schedule by insisting upon dinner at the same time throughout the week. Only *you* can decide. If freedom from persistent urges to eat is important to you, the effort necessary to retrain yourself to think of food *only at the times that you choose* will be a small price to pay.

Once you have reconditioned yourself to think of food at certain times only, you can go back to a more natural flexibility. As you will learn when you make this deconditioning effort, this urge-to-eat pattern develops a definite strength and resilience that can become strong enough to withstand a reasonable amount of variability.

If you are willing to make the effort, circle the hours of your planned three meals and snacks, if you choose them, on the Urge to Eat Self-Monitoring Chart and then record your success in eating at these times only.

As the weeks progress, data recorded on the chart will also give you a very good way to evaluate your success. You should find that your record fewer incidents in column 2 when your appetite is strong between scheduled meal hours. Demonstrating changes in your appetite in this way will help you to see just how well you are succeeding in this important self-retraining effort.

IN A NUTSHELL

Many of your most important biological processes follow a 24-hour cycle. While you cannot control the recurrence of the cycle, you can control the time that it begins and ends. This chapter has suggested that you choose times to eat and that you eat at these times only. After a matter of weeks you should find that your thoughts turn to food at preplanned hours only.

10/ Managing Appetite by Day and by Night

Man is one of the few species that enjoys the "privilege" of eating when not hungry and drinking when not thirsty.[1] This privilege is one of the banes of our existence because it lies at the root of our chronic overeating and overweight.

In theory, we should be hungry when our bodies have used up their available supply of nutrients and we should feel no hunger when our nutrient supply is adequate. In practice, however, even if our body's needs have been met, we feel "hungry" when:

1. We have not had a sufficient range of tastes and food textures to satisfy our need for these experiences;
2. We believe that we have not had enough to eat;
3. We are in contact with tempting foods; or
4. We turn to food to meet psychological needs.

At these times, our feeling is not hunger, but appetite, a major link in the problem eating chain.

Variety in Your Diet

During World War II, GIs ate tens of millions of cartons of K rations. This bland, dehydrated, and canned food provided all of their minimum daily nutrient requirements. But many soldiers complained that they could survive on these rations much longer than they cared to live.[2] Their hunger was appeased but their appetites remained unsatisfied. The reaction of these GIs demonstrated that "full" and "satisfied" are very different experiences.[3]

Recent lab studies have come to the same conclusion. Volunteers were allowed to drink their fill of a liquid diet that contained all of the necessary nutrients and calories, and yet the urge to eat was almost unabated: the subjects drank no more than they needed, but they were preoccupied with eating and longed for solid food.[4]

This has a very important implication for you.

IN ORDER TO LIMIT ONE SOURCE OF
"HUNGER" DURING OR BETWEEN MEALS,
MAKE CERTAIN THAT YOU EAT A VARIETY
OF FOODS WITH DIFFERENT APPEARANCES,
TASTES, AND TEXTURES.

Do not choose a diet in which the same foods turn up on your plate time and time again. You must *plan for variety: it will not happen by itself.* Vary the colors, tastes, and smells of your preselected foods so that every meal includes variety and so that few foods are repeated at less than three- or four-day intervals.

Be certain that you have a range of foods that require biting and chewing at no less than two of your three daily meals.

The failure to exercise the muscles of your mouth and

tongue can contribute to your feeling of not having had enough to eat.

Satiety Is in the Eye of the Beholder

The liquid diet studies have taught us other lessons as well. Lean and obese volunteers in these studies were given liquids with different caloric densities: sometimes the fluids looked rich, sometimes thin; regardless of their appearance, the liquids sometimes had high caloric value, sometimes low. The volunteers therefore did not know whether they were getting liquid that was rich or poor in calories. We have learned from these studies that:

1. Both the lean and the obese misjudged the caloric density of their meals, often thinking that high was low and that low was high;

2. Over time, both groups learned to adjust the caloric value of their intake to a constant level, requiring them to drink more on some days, less on others; and

3. When the volume of the drink was high, even if the caloric density was low, the volunteers reported feeling more satisfied than when the drink volume was low but the caloric value was high.[5]

In short, whether fat or thin, we tend to feel the urge to eat until we *think* that we have had enough to eat: actually having enough to eat is not enough to do the trick.

You can put these important observations to work for you at mealtimes by taking three very useful steps:

1. Plan to begin your noon *and* evening meals with a generous salad using vegetables that are permitted in comparatively large quantity according to the food plan you are following. This will help to increase the bulk of your meal.

2. Eat your meal on a 7-inch salad plate so that it appears to be larger in quantity.

3. Serve all foods in carefully measured portions and take second helpings only of those foods which are unlimited in the food plan you are following. That way you will know exactly when you have had your fill. To make this easier, serve "hotel" rather than "boarding house" style, with serving platters kept *off* the table.

By chewing vigorously at the start of your noon and evening meals, you are likely to feel satisfied sooner because your biting and chewing needs have been at least partially satisfied. If you eat your meal on a 7-inch salad plate rather than a 9-inch dinner plate, you increase the apparent size of your portion. The larger it looks, the more likely you are to feel satisfied. And by serving yourself your full portion at the start of the meal and not going back for seconds, you will learn to be satisfied with one measured helping.

Managing Nighttime Eating

Two out of three reducers interviewed by one eminent researcher reported that they did most of their eating at night.[6] Fifty percent of those who participated in a study conducted among members of Weight Watchers classes at the beginning of their weight-loss efforts reported that they, too, ate and ate and ate after the sun went down.

Night eaters have different food preferences. Some eat bread, others sweets. And they eat at different times. Some eat heavily between dinner and bedtime. Others rise after falling asleep and find their way to the kitchen. Some try valiantly to control their nocturnal eating. Others simply relax and enjoy it. But all have two things in common. First, they are nearly always breakfast avoiders and lunchtime nibblers. Their first hearty meal is very likely to be dinner. Second, they consistently report that early in the day they experience a strong aversion to the very foods which they find so irresistible at night.

Their skipping of meals early in the day paves the way for their nighttime eating. First, it creates hunger. These people are not necessarily physically hungry; their bodies have more than an adequate supply of energy in the form of convertible fat. But they have not had an opportunity to stimulate their taste buds, to exercise their chewing muscles, and to experience the sensation of food entering their stomachs. These are important physical sensations, the absence of which can be very disquieting.

The omission of meals early in the day also creates a "psychological caloric debt." Night eaters often feel that because they have been so "good" during the day, they owe themselves an extra treat at day's end. They may sometimes forget that they ate a particular food during the day, but their debit bookkeeping abilities are unsurpassed and they virtually never forget snacks which they have passed by.[7]

While there is a diabolical quality to their efforts to make up for lost treats, nighttime eaters may actually have a biological reason for enjoying their food more at night than during the day. The biorhythmic hormonal cycles mentioned in Chapter 9 affect the acuity of all of our senses at different times during each 24-hour period. For example, we may be bothered by the sounds of children's play at night but hardly notice it during the day. We may find bright lights glaring at night but walk about without sunglasses at high noon. We may feel sexually aroused in the evening by a person whom we hardly noticed during the day. We may also find the taste of some foods irresistible in the evening although we found them distasteful throughout the day.

Each of these sensory reactions could be influenced by secretions from various endocrine glands which shield us from strong reactions at some times of the day and intensify our reactions at others. Whatever the mechanism, there does appear to be good reason for believing that many foods taste better, at least to some people, after the sun goes down.[8]

In addition to hunger and heightened taste sensitivity, there is a third factor that makes nighttime eating a particular problem. There are usually fewer social and situational controls at night, controls that would help to put the brakes on problem eating. Nighttime eaters often eat alone because other members of their family are either occupied or asleep. They often feel let down at the prospect of long nighttime hours with little stimulation. In the morning, for example, they may anticipate the day's work and not feel the need to turn to food as a diversion. They may also find that they are particularly bored and lonely at night when there are fewer activities that can compete with food for their attention.

Whatever the personal combination of events, the end result is usually the same: the after-dark eater is likely to go beyond the limits of prudent eating. Careful steps must be taken to prevent this eating from getting out of hand.

Eating Before Bedtime

As a first step, all nighttime eaters must make it a hard and fast rule to *eat three full, planned meals at the appropriate times every day.* This rule must be followed *even if eating has occurred the night before.* Unfortunately, when people do eat at night, they attempt to "pay back" the extra calories the following day by skipping breakfast and possibly lunch as well. In so doing, they pass up nutritionally sound foods that could be eaten at times when control is strong. They then arrive at home in the evening overhungry and with weakened resolve. This sets the stage for a second night of eating foods with the lowest nutritional value.

When three meals have been eaten, the continuing urge to eat before bedtime must be considered *mood-motivated eating*. In other words, appetite after dark (it cannot be hunger if the three meals have been eaten) is *not* a sign that food is needed but a *signal* that you are bored, unhappy, angry, or anxious. As you will learn in Chapter II, the remedy for boredom is to find a stimulating alternative to eating. For unhappiness, the remedy is to seek constructive help from others. For anger, the remedy is assertion to correct a difficult situation. And meditation or other relaxation techniques are a more constructive response to anxiety than eating.

In addition to following one of the mood-management programs, it is also helpful to think of the evening as a series of thirty-minute, fifteen-minute, or even five-minute intervals that you believe you can successfully manage. Your goal then is to plan an activity that will get you through each time interval. When you plan activities in these small time units, you are always close to your next success—living through several more minutes without resorting to eating.

Use a chart like that in Figure 10.1. Write out your plan so that it is more concrete and specific. Whenever you write "No" on your chart, it is time for you to:

1. Analyze what has happened;
2. Plan a new activity for the next unit of time;
3. And go on with this next step *without dwelling* on your earlier mistake.

In other words, a slip-up in your behavior *is not an indication that you are a failure:* it merely means that the plan you

FIGURE 10.1

Breaking Long Evenings into Small Challenges

Time		What I will do	Did I do it?		Did I succeed in controlling my eating?	
(Choose the interval which works best for you)		(Naturally, you should choose activities which interest you)	*Yes*	*No*	*Yes*	*No*
From	To					
7:00	7:30	Watch evening news	Yes		Yes	
7:30	8:00	Do ironing, wash dishes, fix lunch for tomorrow	Yes		Yes	
8:00	8:30	Call Alice, Tom	Yes		Yes	
8:30	9:00	Complete math lesson plan	Yes		Yes	
9:00	9:30	Read novel	Yes		Yes	
9:30	10:00	Continue reading	Yes		Yes	
10:00	10:30	Shower, choose clothes for tomorrow	Yes		Yes	
10:30	11:00	Catch up on correspondence	Yes		Yes	
11:00		To sleep				

followed earlier was not equal to the task at hand. With more careful planning you should achieve greater success. In addition, the more times that you prove to yourself that you are controlling nighttime eating, the less you will be preoccupied with that danger in the future. You are building confidence for future nights.

Eating After Falling Asleep

People who get up in the night to eat have a tendency to hide their eating from those with whom they live. Eating when they are still drowsy after having awakened helps them further hide their eating from themselves. Many state that they cannot recall whether, if, and how much they ate. Unfortunately, however, it is all too obvious when a number of these late-night bouts have been fought and lost.

A five-step plan has proven to be highly effective in breaking the pattern of middle-of-the-night eating.

1. Early in the evening, prepare a small snack of an acceptable and nonpreferred food, like celery, lettuce, cauliflower, or other vegetable that you can bite and chew with no dip or dressing. Make sure that the food that you choose is not one of your favorite treats. In addition, the food should be low in caloric value and it should be a food that will not tax your resistance.

2. Drink no fluids for the six or seven hours before you retire, even if this means nothing to drink from as early as 4 P.M. on. The reason for this is that most middle-of-the-night eaters claim that their sleep is broken by the urge to void, with thoughts of eating coming *after* they have awakened for another reason.

3. Whether or not you wake up because you must go to the bathroom, pause a moment and remind yourself of the next step.

4. This step requires that you return to bed for a ten-minute wait. Practice meditation or another relaxation exercise (see page oo). If you fall asleep, good. If you do not fall asleep and find that your thoughts still turn to food, then you may go to the kitchen.

5. When you get to the kitchen, turn on the bright lights. Take the snack that you have prepared for yourself to the kitchen or dining room table. Use your own placemat and sit in your usual place. Eat the food slowly and concentrate on its taste and texture.

Each of these steps is important because each helps you to be aware of your eating, an awareness that can do much to build your control. Each step offers a means of breaking another link in the appetite chain. You have made it less likely that you will wake up. If you do awaken, you will try a primary line of defense by delaying your eating. If you still feel the urge to eat, that eating will be as much as possible under your conscious control. Finally, you will have demonstrated to yourself that you can have mastery over your eating impulses even when you are the weakest and your impulses the strongest.

If eating during the night is a problem for you, use the chart in Figure 10.2 to keep a record of your efforts and the results. You may have to experiment a bit with your own reactions in order to find the proper combination of techniques that is best for you.

FIGURE 10.2

Scorecard for Managing Nighttime Eating

	Mon.	Tues.	Wed.	Thurs.	Fri.	Sat.	Sun.
Prepared an acceptable snack							
Remembered to limit fluids before bedtime							
Did wake up to go to bathroom							
Did wait 10 minutes							
Did turn on kitchen lights, take prepared snack, and eat at my place at the table							
Did manage to eat only my prepared snack							

In A Nutshell

Management of daytime eating begins with variety in your diet. Research has shown that you must have taste and texture variety if you are to feel satisfied with what you eat. Because you are more likely to feel satisfied with your meals if you "think" you have had enough, you will also help to reduce your appetite for unnecessary food by making your portions appear larger and by making second helpings a thing of the past.

Night eating, before or after bedtime, is one of the most insidious habits faced by overeaters. Like a brush fire in a windstorm, once it begins there is much to keep it going and little to stop its spread. The most prudent approach to controlling night eating is to adopt a preventive approach. To control before-bedtime night eating, eat three meals daily and then plan short-duration activities that occupy your attention elsewhere. For after-bedtime eating, minimize the likelihood that you will awaken after retiring, but be prepared with an acceptable, nonpreferred snack and a definite plan of action that will make you very much aware of everything you do.

11 / Controlling the Moods Behind Your Urge to Eat

People's fancies turn to food when their emotional pitch is high. GIs in World War II who crouched in their foxholes awaiting an enemy attack would reach into their rucksacks for a bite to eat. Mourners eat to help themselves to cope with the loss of loved ones. And fans in the stands of closely contested (but not one-sided) ball games eat junk food by the pound. Throughout recorded history emotion and food have gone hand in glove.[1]

Although the data are by no means clear-cut on this important topic, most researchers believe that the overweight tend to be more emotional than the lean and also more likely to turn to food at times of stress.[2]

Irrespective of who does it more, the obese and the lean can and often do fall victim to the same vicious cycle:

1. Something in the environment triggers a strong emotion;
2. The person turns to a small amount of food;
3. The food is no match for the emotion; but
4. The eating itself sets off a secondary and often equally strong guilt reaction;
5. This guilt reaction leads to further eating of larger quantities of food.

Once this cycle begins, the more you eat the worse you feel; the worse you feel the more you eat—there's no way out until you're exhausted or the cupboard is bare.

Two emotions that often start this cycle are anxiety and depression. Anxiety is a feeling of tension that carries with it worries, inattention, distractibility, forgetfulness, heart palpitations, pounding pulse, sweating, headache, and stomach distress among many other symptoms. Everyone experiences some anxiety and each of us probably experiences at least mild anxiety almost every week. Anxiety is a dread of some feared experience but the threat that elicits anxiety is vague and amorphous while the threat which triggers fear is specific and focused. Because the threat in anxiety is not specific, the individual does not have a clear direction in which to respond. Nevertheless, the body becomes aroused as if to make a response. In effect, the individual is all geared up to take action but no action is available to take. The result is a kind of cognitive, physiological, and behavioral wheel-spinning in which all systems are highly active and utterly unproductive.

While anxiety is a fear of some unknown future event, depression is a reaction to unhappy past events. Depression is a feeling of despair, bringing with it pessimistic, melancholic, and self-depreciating thoughts with a slowness of speech, movement, and all activity. Sometimes depression is brought on by the loss of an important relationship or opportunity that leads to the withdrawal of support for familiar patterns of behavior.

For example, if you are accustomed to having morning coffee with a friendly neighbor and that neighbor moves away, you may undergo a midmorning depression without ever knowing it because your habitual routine is no longer possible.

Other times depression is the result of constant attacks—real or imagined—against which the individual is defenseless. And sometimes depression is an outgrowth of past failures that make the prospect of future successes seem all but nonexistent.

The common thread in both anxiety and depression is the frustration that the individual experiences whenever an effort is made to find a solution to the confronting problem. For the anxious person, everything is tried but nothing works because the threat has a thousand ever-changing faces. For the depressed person, nothing is tried because nothing can work, as "proven" by countless failures in the past.

Boredom and anger are the other two emotions that commonly trigger problem eating. Boredom is the result of living or working in an understimulating environment. In such environments our attention drifts aimlessly and painfully. Physical and psychological illness can result if we live for long in an environment that lacks the stimulation that we need to feed our tireless brains. When boredom becomes acute, we can panic. Because the overweight tend to be more sensitive to their environments (see page 79) boredom may affect their behavior more quickly than it does the lean.

While boredom arises when nothing happens in the environment, anger is provoked by something that either did happen or was believed to have happened. An injury, insult, or mistreatment can cause the person to strike out. Sometimes direct action is possible and the injured party will attack the provoker. But at other times direct action is not possible and aggression will be directed against innocent bystanders (who are guilty by association) or it may be self-directed. The fact that overweight children sometimes learn to cram food into their mouths as a means of expressing anger against their parents is an illustration of self-directed anger. Unfortunately, many learn to carry this same frustrated and self-defeating response into adulthood, making their overeating obvious, but sometimes being so timid that they must even hide their indirect, self-destructive counterattack.

In summary, anxiety and depression, boredom and anger are the four emotions which many overweight people cite as the emotional triggers of much of their impulsive eating. All four emotions have both thought and behavioral components that are summarized as follows:

	Thought Component	Behavioral Component
Anxiety	Something terrible is going to happen.	Fast and furious attempts to find something—anything —that will defend against the danger.
Depression	I have made errors in the past and am doomed to make the same mistakes again and again.	Inactivity because nothing helps.
Boredom	I have interests and I have needs but the environment does not support either.	Alternation between a frantic search for stimulation and resigned inaction.
Anger	My rights have been carelessly or intentionally violated.	Counter aggression against the provoker when possible, against the self at other times.

Each of the emotions has a belief system that may be accurate but which is usually incorrect. And all have behavioral

systems that frequently lead to unproductive actions that
only serve to compound the problem.

A Critical Choice

When one of these moods descends, three alternatives are
open to you:

1. You can do nothing, acquiesce, and suffer through;
2. You can take steps to change the offending situation; or
3. You can try to contain the emotion.

Acquiescence is tragedy because the suffering that results
is as unnecessary as it is real. *Changing the situation* gives
you the opportunity to nip the problem at its source. It is the
way for you to break the chain that leads to vicious-cycle
eating at its earliest links. Development of techniques for
emotion containment will equip you to deal with situations
that escape your control for some reason, without loss of
self-control. Even curbing your emotions is a way for you to
break the chain because, if you bring your moods under
control early, you may not be faced with food choices at the
kitchen door. Changing the situation will help to avoid the
problem in the future while containing the emotion can help
to escape from a very troubling situation.

Assertive Action

Because many of the provocations to troublesome emotions are social in nature, it is useful to develop assertive
skills that will help you to change these situations. Assertion
is any open expression in word or deed that leads others to

consider seriously your desires. *Assertive behavior* is emotionally honest, direct, self-enhancing, and expressive. It leads to feelings of self-respect and is most often greeted with respect by others. For example, if your teenage daughter announces that she has made a date on a night when you had asked her to babysit for the younger children you could assertively respond: "I had hoped that you would be able to stay home with Reggie and Tom as we agreed last week." *Nonassertive behavior* is indirect, self-denying, and dishonest communication. It is coupled with feelings of anxiety, despair, or anger, and leads the other person to feel either guilty, disgusted, or frankly superior. In response to your daughter's disclosure that she was planning to spend the evening with her friends you might nonassertively have replied: "You, ah, don't think that maybe you could, ah, put off the date until the next night?" Assertiveness is also different from *aggression* which is direct and may be honest, but which is coupled with self-righteousness on your part and leads to hurt, humiliation, and anger in the other person. Again, in response to your daughter you might have responded aggressively by saying: "You have no right to do that! I expect you to babysit and babysit you will!"[3]

It is important to be able to distinguish between assertive, nonassertive, and aggressive behavior. Assertion leads to positive change while non-assertion and aggression both tend to make matters worse rather than better. Dr. Patricia Jakubowski of the University of Missouri has developed a long list of situations which can be used to help people to make this important discrimination. Reprinted below are only ten of these situations and ten possible responses.[4]

Which of these responses do you think are Assertive (As), Nonassertive (Na), or Aggressive (Ag)?

	Situations	Responses
As Na Ag	1. Husband gets silent, instead of saying what's on his mind. You say,	I guess you are uncomfortable talking about what's bothering you. I think we can work it out if you tell me what's irritating you.
	2. A friend has asked you for the second time in a week to babysit for her child while she runs errands. You have no children of your own and respond,	You're taking advantage of me and I won't stand for it! It's your responsibility to look after your own child.
	3. You've been talking for a while with a friend on the telephone. You would like to end the conversation and you say,	I'm terribly sorry but my supper's burning, and I have to get off the phone. I hope you don't mind.

	Situations	Responses
As Na Ag	4. Your husband promised you that he would talk to your daughter about her behavior at school. The promise has not been carried out. You say,	I thought we agreed last Tuesday that you would have a talk with Barb about her behavior at school. So far there's been no action on your part. I still think you should talk to her soon. I'd prefer sometime tonight.
	5. Someone asks for a ride home and it is inconvenient because you're late, have a few errands and the drive will take you out of your way. You say,	I am pressed for time today and can take you to a convenient bus stop, but I won't be able to take you home.
	6. A good friend calls and tells you she desperately needs you to canvass the street for a charity. You don't want to do it and say,	Oh gee, Fran, I just know that Jerry will be mad at me if I say "yes." He says I'm always getting involved in too many things. You know how Jerry is about things like that.

	Situations	Responses
As Na Ag	7. Your husband expects dinner on the table when he arrives home from work and gets angry when it is not there immediately. You respond,	I feel awful about dinner. I know you're tired and hungry . . . it's all my fault. I'm just a terrible wife.
	8. Your husband wants to watch a football game on TV. There is something else that you'd like to watch. You say,	Well, ah, honey, go ahead and watch the game, I guess I could do some ironing.
	9. You're the only woman in a group of men and you're asked to be the secretary of the meetings. You respond,	I'm willing to do my share and take the notes this time. In future meetings, I'd like us to share the load.
	10. Your husband has criticized your appearance in front of your friends. You say,	I really feel hurt when you criticize my appearance in front of other people. If you have something to say, please bring it up at home before we leave.

The assertive statements are numbers 1, 4, 5, 9, and 10. The nonassertive statements are numbers 3, 6, 7, and 8. The only aggressive statement is number 2. If you correctly identified nine out of ten of the statements, you did quite well. If you missed two or more it is important for you to study the statements to be able to make these important discriminations.

There is a two-way street that connects our ideas and our actions. Irrational ideas lead to nonassertive defensive behavior or aggressive actions as attempts to show the other guy who's boss. Constructive ideas, on the other hand, are the basis for assertive action. If you replace your irrational ideas with constructive thoughts, you can increase the likelihood that you will think in terms of assertive behavior. If you think about yourself as acting assertively, you will also be able to replace irrationality with constructive thoughts because the action alternatives which are opened up by these thoughts will become clear to you.

Thinking assertively will help you to act that way. Assertive action is uncomplicated action. It involves three different dimensions:

1. Assertive behavior involves making requests rather than demands.
   Request: "Please help me with the dishes so that we can be ready to leave on time."
   Demand: "You must help me with the dishes."
2. Assertive behavior involves taking personal responsibility for your requests rather than starting from an accusatory position.
   Personal Responsibility: "I would very much like to go along on your next trip to San Francisco."
   Accusatory Approach: "You never take me on your business trips."
3. Finally, assertive behavior asks the other person to change overt behavior, not attitudes.
   Behavior Change: "I would like it if you would ask me

how I spent my day when you come home in the evening."

Attitude change: "I wish you would love me more."

None of these elements is complicated. A personal request for another's behavior change is all that you need to start you on your way.

Imagining yourself as taking assertive action can help to cue your assertive behavior. Did you know, for example, that one of the most successful techniques used for training athletic champions is instructing them to imagine their winning performance? Divers are trained to visualize their perfect completion of the dive before they leap into the air. Discus throwers visualize their complete spin and release as they hurl the weight toward a new world's record. Even runners visualize their movements every step of the way. To make the image complete, the athletes are also trained to imagine meeting obstacles in their performance and then to see themselves take the obstacles in their stride. You, too, should imagine yourself acting assertively toward your spouse, your children, your friends, your neighbors, your co-workers, your relatives—toward anyone important in your life. First see yourself easily successful, and then in your mind's eye imagine an initial negative reaction from the other person that you overcome by keeping your cool and acting assertively again.

The following illustration should make this process clear. Jane once valued Alice's friendship. But over the past year, the two women have spent little time together. Jane has been feeling hurt by the loss of Alice's friendship. She feels that she must have done something to offend Alice and is sure that Alice has found others with whom she would rather spend time.

One day the two women meet unexpectedly in the bank. In similar situations in the recent past, Jane had tried to avoid contact, fearing that Alice would reject her and confirm her fears. This time Jane imagines that she walks up to Alice and says: "Alice, I've really missed our lunches and shopping trips. I would very much like to meet you next week so we can pick up where we left off." In her mind's eye, Jane then imagines Alice saying: "I'd love to see you. You know, I've been very busy with Martha's wedding plans and a rest and time with you is just what the doctor ordered." Then she imagines Alice saying: "Well, frankly, Jane, I'm really very busy making plans for Martha's wedding so I'll have to take a raincheck." She imagines her pleasant feelings upon Alice's acceptance and her feelings of disappointment upon her imagined refusal.

Two things are important about the refusal: first, Jane sees herself accepting the unhappy news without falling through the floor; second, she comforts herself with the knowledge that she did all that she could to bring about a return of their friendship. These last points are very important. People do not dry up and float away when they are not successful in their efforts to reach out to others. And they gain from the experience of trying by knowing that they are being assertive. They are asking for what they want instead of passively accepting disappointment.

After going through this imaginary sequence for several different situations, the next step is to take action. What activities would you like to join? Imagine that you call the political party of your choice and volunteer to work in the campaign. See yourself being welcomed or being told that there is no further need for help. Imagine that you apply for a job and are told that your application arrived in the nick of time or that there is no need for someone with your experience. Imagine yourself proposing a block party to the neighbors and being told that the idea is wonderful or that it is a bomb. Make your own list of social assertiveness projects that you would like to complete and start with number one on the list.

Remember—*if you want to begin to feel differently about yourself, you will have to act differently. If you want to act differently, you will have to begin to think differently about yourself.* There is no better time to begin than the present. You will not succeed in every effort. But failure is not an unmixed blessing; you will feel better about yourself for trying even if you should happen to fail. Therefore, the personal payoff is far greater for trying many times over—even if you have a few extra failures—than in attempting to curb your losses by making few tries at assertive action!

A final point—many people have a tendency to put off until tomorrow things which should be done today. For example, you might have read through this chapter and decided that yes, there are areas of your life in which assertion could lead to the opening up of new experiences which would improve your ideas about yourself and help you to feel better about yourself and your life. "But," you might tell yourself, "I think that I should lose some weight first." Right? *Dead wrong! If you wait until you lose weight before you adopt a more assertive approach to life, you may have a very long wait ahead of you.* Assertive action now can give you better control over your life situation. That control can weaken the emotional pressure that leads you to overeat. Less problem eating can lead to better weight control. Don't take a wait-until-tomorrow attitude: start this change today!

Dropping the Other Shoe

Anxiety and depression, boredom and anger are all emotions that can trigger problem eating. Our best strategy is to adopt a *good offense,* to try to change our environments so these emotions are less likely to occur and are likely to be weaker when they do happen. But we must also have a *good defense,* a way to cope with these feelings when they do arise, as they inevitably will. Three good techniques are at your disposal.

Technique 1: A Break For R & R

Many of us lead unnecessarily pressured lives. We design schedules that are so tight that we have no preplanned time to relax. As a result, we suffer from the ill effects of mounting tension and are much more likely to overreact to the least frustration.

Playtime is not a luxury: it is a necessity for successful performance. Industry has increasingly recognized this fact by providing recreational opportunities at the sites of large factories and businesses. Large sums of money are being spent in the development of recreational opportunities that help workers to experience a change in pace through a break in routine. Relaxation of this sort discharges tension that interferes with creativity and productivity.

To keep within manageable bounds:

THINK THROUGH THE NORMAL ROUTINE
OF YOUR DAY TO FIND AN OPPORTUNITY
FOR AT LEAST ONE 30-MINUTE CHANGE OF PACE.

If your job involves sitting at a desk for eight hours, you might find a short walk invaluable. If you normally do physical jobs ranging from cleaning house to factory work, taking a sitting break to read a chapter from an interesting book, work on a crossword puzzle, chat with friends, or spend a little time on a hobby like macramé, knitting, whittling, or sketching can all help to recoup your energy and calm your nerves.

Planning your breaks ahead of time is much better than waiting until exhaustion forces you to take a rest. When you plan ahead, your energy is likely to be consistently high because you know that a break is coming. When you push yourself to the breaking point your spirits are likely to be low and your performance poor. When you finally do slow down, you are not likely to feel that you have done the job well, which builds your tension even more.

In addition to deciding in advance just when you will take your breaks, it is a good idea to plan what you will do for relaxation. Be realistic in choosing the time and the activity. If you have the job of pushing husband and children out the door with breakfasts under their belts and lunch boxes under their arms, planning a break before the school bus arrives is unrealistic. In the same vein, if jogging is your pleasure, don't plan to spend the time writing an essay.

To help you with your planning, use the chart in Figure II.I.

Technique 2: Meditation

Another way to cope with troublesome moods is meditation. This technique can help you to lower your general tension level and to exert control over many bodily processes. Armed with this control you can learn to relax as an alternative when you experience the urge to eat.

Meditation was first described in the Hindu *Vedas,* written

FIGURE 11.1

Planning and Monitoring Daily Rest Breaks

Day of Week	What are the times of your greatest normal strain?	When will you plan rest breaks to minimize your tension?	How will you use this time?
Monday			
Tuesday			
Wednesday			
Thursday			
Friday			
Saturday			
Sunday			

between 1,000 and 500 years before the birth of Christ. Since that time, virtually every major religion has included meditation in its recommendations to the faithful.[5] As a modern technique in mood control, meditation has burst onto the contemporary scene as a haven for serenity seekers because its techniques are easily learned, readily followed, and very likely to produce good results.[6]

Meditation can be defined as the focusing of attention upon a single target such as an idea, a sound, or an aspect of physical functioning. When meditators achieve complete concentration upon one feature of their immediate experience, they are cleansed of their concerns with all other features. A cliché that well describes the effect of meditation is: *out of mind, out of body.*

Meditation is believed to produce a fourth level of consciousness. Waking, sleeping, and dreaming are the three levels of consciousness that are part of our normal life experience. The meditator is awake but all of his or her bodily processes appear to slow down temporarily: heart rate slows, oxygen consumption decreases, blood pressure lowers or at least stabilizes, electro-conductance of the skin decreases, and even brain waves change, with a decrease in beta waves and an increase in alpha waves. All of these meditation-produced changes are the opposite of reactions that are observed in connection with the urges to fight or flee.[7]

Successful meditation is a kind of mental cleansing. It involves achieving freedom from ordinary daily concerns by focusing one's attention upon a single idea. There are many ways of achieving this result. In transcendental meditation one relaxes and simply repeats over and over the personal "mantra" that has been learned from a trainer. Less ritualized meditation instruction involves simply repeating a word such as "one" over and over. Zen meditation involves a noncritical reflection on the emotions and events that one has experienced during the preceding hours or day. This reflection must be "detached and nonevaluative," as it is intended not as a form of self-analysis but as a technique for achieving an important level of self-acceptance. This kind of nonevaluative self-reflection is difficult to achieve because one constantly evaluates the extent to which he or she is nonevaluative, a paradox that must be overcome if the fourth level of consciousness is to be achieved. Finally, meditators sometimes focus their attention on an external stimulus—they may focus their eyes on a candle or a flower, or close their eyes while listening to a quiet, repetitive sound such as a low hum or tick.

Would-be meditators would do well to try all of these techniques—a single-syllable word frequently repeated, nonevaluative review of recent experience, focusing on a visual object or a repetitious sound—in order to find the most comfortable means of purging their consciousness of troublesome concerns. There is no right or wrong in choosing one or more of these approaches; the only acceptable criterion is one's own feelings of emotional comfort and control.

Meditation is practiced for periods of approximately fifteen to twenty minutes in the most quiet and calm environment available. Choose a time each day and make an effort to practice every day. The meditator sits in a comfortable position with head and arms supported. The meditator breathes through the nose and begins by concentrating on the process of breathing by mentally repeating a word such as "one" with every exhale. When intrusive thoughts occur, the meditator simply retreats from them. There is no active fight against preoccupations: instead, there is simply a greater concentration upon the word, the effort to recount the day's experience, the point in space, or the sound in the air.

It is neither difficult nor easy to meditate. The achievement of the fourth level of meditative consciousness requires practice, and successful practice in turn requires routine. Therefore, it is important for each person to choose a time of day when meditation will be practiced and to make it a point to practice meditating at this same time every day.

Technique 3: Training Yourself So That Your Negative Thoughts Don't Get the Best of You

It has long been known that our emotional reactions have two components: an idea that is coupled with a physical reaction. Sometimes we can have an idea that passes without notice, but at other times that same idea can trigger a strong emotional response. If we can train ourselves to respond to troubling ideas without physical tension, we can protect ourselves from the ravages of uncontrolled emotion. As Dr. Joseph Wolpe of Temple University was to discover, this self-training is possible if we learn to relax our bodies at will and then to visualize thoughts while we are relaxed.[8]

Successful physical relaxation depends upon getting to know the way in which your body experiences tension. Sit in a quiet place or lie on a smooth surface. Begin by taking a few deep breaths and exhaling slowly. Think about the air passing into your lungs as you inhale. Then become aware of the feeling of the air slowly escaping through your nose as you exhale. Three or four deep breaths will prepare you for the process of bringing your muscles under control.

Close your eyes and concentrate all of your energy on one muscle group after another. If you are right-handed, begin always with your left hand and foot. If you are left-handed, begin with the right hand and foot. Start by pointing one toe and stretching your leg fully from the hip, tightening your thigh and calf muscles. You should feel a slight wedge sensation in the arch of your foot and a pulling of the muscles in your stomach and back as your leg stretches. Sense the complete feeling and then relax the tension. Focus all of your attention on the feeling of relaxation. Then repeat the exercise with the other foot.

Next make a fist with your nondominant hand while

stretching your arm and contracting the muscles in your forearm and biceps. Hold this position for a few seconds as you concentrate upon the sensation of tension, then try to have your consciousness enter the muscles of your shoulder, arm, and hand as they relax. Repeat this exercise with the other hand.

Then focus your attention upon your stomach and buttocks. Tighten all of the muscles in your lower body, hold them for a few seconds as you concentrate upon the sensation. Then relax the muscles slowly while you continue to study the feelings of relaxation.

Repeat the same sequence with your upper body muscles, "hunching" your shoulders as you contract your chest muscles. Notice the involvement of your upper arms and stomach as you feel the upper body tense. Then concentrate on the feeling of these muscles as they relax.

Finally, concentrate on the muscles of your lips, cheeks, and forehead. Screw up your face tightly and try to feel every wrinkle as you hold your tense expression for a few seconds. Then slowly release the tension.

When you have gone through a period of tensing each muscle group for about five seconds and then spent about fifteen seconds gradually relaxing the muscles and concentrating on the absence of tension, your limbs should feel heavier and you should experience a kind of sagging of your body onto the floor. If you still feel tension in any muscle group, repeat the exercise for that group and then each of the succeeding groups beginning with legs, then arms, lower body, upper body, and head, in that order.

When you feel fully relaxed, try to focus your attention on a specific area of your body at random: penetrate that area with your consciousness and fully experience the sensation of relaxation of that area. The goal of this relaxation exercise is to train you to be able to identify both tension and relaxation so that you can learn to instruct yourself to relax, wherever you are, when you begin to feel tension arising.

Once you have learned to relax, you are ready to begin to train yourself to induce this same calm feeling at times when you might otherwise respond with strong emotions. While you are relaxed, try to imagine yourself interacting with people who normally "make you feel tense." See yourself calmly responding first to meeting these people and then to interactions that involve increasing challenge. Any time that you experience the telltale sign of physical tension, back off, relax yourself again, and make a new attempt. *Never allow yourself to become tense while you are practicing relaxation training.* Eventually, you will have an imprint in your mind of you responding to would-be troubling situations with self-assurance and calm.

When you find yourself in these situations, summon up the image of the tranquil you and silently instruct yourself to relax those parts of your body that are your normal tension centers. You may still experience some emotion: that is only normal. You should, however, find that your emotions are now within your control and that you are free to handle the situation with assertive action.

In A Nutshell

Anxiety, depression, boredom, and anger are four emotions that very often trigger a vicious cycle of tension/eating/more tension/more eating. You can passively accept these emotions or you can actively attempt to deal with them. You can interrupt the cycle at an early point by assertively trying to change your interaction with others. You can also have a second line of defense by training yourself to plan rest periods that will keep your energy high, by learning to meditate to achieve a generalized tension control, and by learning to relax away interfering emotions when specific situations arise. All of these techniques can help to build your mastery over your moods and thereby cut back one source of the pressure that builds your urge to eat.

12 / Sleep Control: Another Mood-Management Technique

Sleep. You spend about one-third of your life doing it. You devote about one-third of your living space to it. You take it for granted until it goes awry and then it can destroy your functioning for days on end. Because it affects the way you feel, it can have a profound effect upon the way that you eat. But you have probably never thought of using sleep control as a means of gaining mastery over your urge to eat.

For the ancient Greeks, Sleep and Death were brother gods who dwelt in the regions of Hell. When a Greek passed into the realm of sleep, he entrusted himself to the gods, who might claim his soul for all eternity. Therefore, to sleep was to venture behind the mists of an awesome unknown.[1]

Some mystery still surrounds the nature and functions of sleep despite our use of fancy electronics to probe its every dimension. Many bodily functions slow down during sleep including muscular activity, heart rate, body temperature, and metabolic rate. We even consume about a fifth less oxygen when sleeping as opposed to being awake. While common sense tells us that sleep is a time to "recharge our batteries," the slowing down of all our functions would hardly permit this worthy chore to be accomplished.[2]

Laboratory researchers have shown that there are five

144

different stages of sleep. Brain waves differ at each of these stages. The first stage is closest to our waking brain-wave pattern, the fourth is the slowest and least like our waking pattern. We go from stage 1 to 2 to 3 to 4, then back to 2 again when we are undisturbed. From stage 2 we go into the fifth or Rapid Eye Movement (REM) stage, and it is during this stage that our dreams take place. Half of our sleep time is spent in stage 2 and about one-fifth is spent in the dream or REM stage. The rest of our sleep time is divided more or less equally between stages 1, 3, and 4. If our sleep is interrupted during the REM, third, or fourth stage, we seem to make up the difference during the nights that follow. Therefore it is not necessary for us to have the same amount of total sleep time every night: what we strive for is the proper amount of REM and deep sleep.[3]

Disturbances in sleep cycles appear to be more uncomfortable than changes in the absolute amount of sleep. Most people, if placed in a room in which cues that indicate the time of day are removed, adjust to a pattern that is very similar to their normal sleep cycle. When subjects are asked to go to sleep three hours before or after their normal bedtime, they show considerable behavioral and psychological disorganization. Performance of tasks which require concentration deteriorates markedly and mood generally turns toward irritability and depression. These are common experiences of air-travelers on transmeridian trips. Those flying three or more hours to the east have greater adjustment difficulties than those flying similar distances west because the deterioration associated with falling asleep earlier than usual is greater than that associated with falling asleep later.

Most travelers find that they require anywhere from one to seven days to readjust their sleep rhythms. Thus, even after a night or two of normal sleep following a night of sleep disruption, judgment may be poorer than normal. Therefore, it is a good idea to postpone the need to make important decisions for at least forty-eight hours following any long-distance flight.[4]

People with sleep disturbances often complain of difficulty in falling asleep at night. On the average they have been found to spend close to an hour awake in bed before falling asleep for the first time. They also report waking up an average of two or three times per night, and they are more likely than good sleepers to complain about restlessness through the night and waking up with the birds. Despite the fact that they spend fewer hours asleep at night, they sleep on the average only about an hour less than good sleepers, making up for some of their lost sleep by catnaps during the day. Also, as suggested earlier, they have about as much stage 3 and 4 and REM-stage sleep as good sleepers, giving up some time from the more shallow second stage of sleep.[5]

The major problem faced by insomniacs—those who sleep less than six and a half hours per night, who spend at least thirty minutes falling asleep, who are awake for at least half an hour during the night, and who experience great fatigue during the day—is not so much their lack of sleep as the fact that their sleep seems to be chronically *deregulated*. In other words, it is the unpredictability of when they will fall asleep and when they will wake up rather than the amount of sleep time lost during their twisting and turning episodes that contributes to their daytime problems.

Not surprisingly, their daytime problems are many. Insomniacs perform certain attention-demanding tasks more poorly than good sleepers. They also complain about emotional problems ranging from chronic tension and mild depression to exaggerated concern about bodily functions. Increased heart symptoms, elevated blood pressure, and regular and severe tension headaches are other common complaints among poor sleepers.[6] Unfortunately, many people turn to food as a means of coping with each of these stresses.

While a definite relationship between body weight and sleep irregularity has *not* been found,[7] there is good evidence that loss of sleep and overeating do go hand in hand. When sleep is irregular, mood changes for the worse. When mood is bad, many people turn to food for solace, as has been said. But when bad moods are coupled with fatigue that has been brought on by sleep loss, the resort to food is more likely still.[8]

It has been shown, for example, that many people turn to food as a replacement for sleep. It has also been shown that when sleep is very disturbed, individuals suffering from anorexia nervosa (a serious psychological problem in which people have been known to starve themselves to death) tend to eat less while overweight people tend eat more. Conversely, a return to normal sleep is likely to be coupled with weight gain by anorexics and weight loss by the obese.[9] Therefore, the regulation of disturbed sleep is an important step to be taken in any weight-management program.

Sizing Up Your Sleep Patterns

Many people overestimate the amount of difficulty which they have in sleeping while underestimating the amount of sleep which they get. Therefore, the best way to obtain a good measure of your sleeping pattern is to complete the data in Figure 12:1 for the next seven days. Getting into and out of bed at more or less the same time, whether for nighttime or nap sleep, helps to regulate your sleep. Therefore, assess-

FIGURE 12.1

A Sleep Evaluation Record

	Monday	Tuesday	Wednes-day	Thursday	Friday	Saturday	Sunday	Total Points
1. What time did you get into bed?								
2. Approximately what time did you fall asleep?								
3. How many times did you wake up long enough to check the time during the night?								
4. What time did you plan to wake up?								
5. What time did you actually wake up?								
6. What time did you get out of bed?								
7. In the morning after breakfast, did you feel well rested?								

8. Did you feel well rested midday?					
9. Did you feel well rested in the late afternoon?					
10. How many minutes did you spend napping during the day?					
11. Did you feel particularly tired before getting into bed for the night?					
TOTAL POINTS					

ment of these behaviors is important in adding up your sleeping quotient. Other important elements include limiting your fluid, coffee, and alcohol consumption, learning not to use the bed as a place for all manner of activities that could and should be done elsewhere, and making an attempt to be physically and psychologically relaxed before retiring. These are the kinds of behaviors that you will monitor in using Figure 12.1.

After seven days of recordkeeping you can add up your sleep score as follows:

For Question 1: Did you go to bed within the same one-hour range (e.g., between 10:30 and 11:30) at least six of the seven nights? If so, give yourself 10 points. If not, score nothing.

For Question 2: Did you fall asleep within fifteen minutes of going to bed at least six of the seven nights? If so, give yourself 5 points: if not, deduct 1 point for each night in which you tossed and turned for longer than fifteen minutes.

For Question 3: Did you manage not to look at the clock before daylight at least six of the seven nights? If so, give yourself 5 points: if not, deduct 1 point for each night that you checked the time before dawn.

For Question 4: Did you plan to wake up after the same number of hours of sleep at least six of the seven nights? If so, give yourself 5 points. If not, score nothing.

For Question 5: Did you wake up within thirty minutes of the same time on at least six of the seven days (e.g., between 7:00 and 7:30). If so, give yourself 5 points; if not, deduct 1 point for each morning more than one that you woke up at a time outside of your normal range.

For Question 6: Did you get out of bed within thirty minutes of waking up at least six mornings out of seven? If so, you have earned another 5 points. If not, deduct 1 point for each morning that you lingered in bed for longer than half an hour.

For Questions 7, 8, 9, 11: Score 1 point for each time that you could answer each of these questions "yes."

For Question 10: Score 5 points if you took no naps or if you took a nap for approximately the same amount of time at about the same hour every day. Deduct 1 point for each time that you took an unusually long or an unscheduled nap because you were overtired.

Sixty is a top score in this inventory, and it will be earned by good sleepers who do two things:

1. They determine how many hours of sleep they need per night; and
2. They get this sleep at highly regular hours.

Our need for sleep appears to be highly individual. A study in England showed that one in twelve people studied slept under five hours nightly, while 15 percent reported sleeping five to six hours, 62 percent for seven to eight hours, and 15 percent for nine or more hours per night.[10]

Americans sleep an average of 7.5 hours per night, we wake up once during the night about four nights out of ten, and we are efficient sleepers, snoring away for about 88 percent of our time in bed. However, the older we are, the less efficiently we sleep and women report more sleep restlessness than men.[11] Cases have been reported in which a single hour of sleep was sufficient for years on end,[12] while others may require nightly sleep of ten hours or more.

Only you can determine your own sleep needs and you can do this by keeping track of your sleep time at night and your energy and mood by day, eventually finding the proper balance. Once you know the amount of sleep you need to keep going, you must regulate the hours of sleep. Remembering that daily circadian rhythms influence everything that we experience during the day, you can appreciate the fact that sleeping regular hours can help you to achieve a well-regulated rhythm to your life. Therefore, 15 points or 25 percent of your total sleep inventory score can be earned through sleep regularity.

Another third of the points that you can earn in measuring the adequacy of your sleep results from your feelings of alertness or fatigue throughout the day (question 7, 8, 9, and 11). You may be "tired" at various times of the day because your work or play does not interest you or because your diet is inadequate. But if you find that you are tired at different times of the day throughout the seven days of the week, the chances are that you are experiencing the effects of inadequate sleep. Therefore, a score of 15 or less on these questions indicates a need for better sleep management.

Finally, difficulty in falling asleep (question 2) or in getting out of bed (question 6), and the taking of irregular naps (question 10), are all further indications of a sleep problem. Less than optimal scores on these three questions pose further evidence that you are undermining your own functioning by mismanaging your sleep.

Steps in Sleep Management

If you have a chronic sleep problem, it is a good idea to have a complete medical checkup. There are at least thirty-two different causes of sleep problems ranging from simply corrected difficulties such as a poor sleep environment to illnesses and serious diseases. It is important to make certain that your sleep difficulties are not caused by an untreated illness. Because of its interdependence with basic biological processes, disturbances in sleep can be a symptom of some underlying illness and this possibility should be eliminated before you take steps to improve the quality of your sleep.[13]

A Five-Step Program of Sleep Control

When you have a clean bill of health, make a decision about how you will approach your sleep problem. One approach would be to take a sleeping drug, generally termed a "hypnotic" drug. Use of these "sleeping pills" is very widespread. Americans spend $100 million for prescription drugs alone each year, with hundreds of millions more for over-the-counter drugs. Unfortunately, use of these drugs has been found to *increase rather than decrease* sleep problems. You feel tired so you take a pill. Over time, you develop a "tolerance" to the drug—your usual dose loses its effect—so you increase the dose you take. Higher doses of the drug cause disruption of your sleep rhythms so you feel chronically fatigued. That leads you to take higher doses still, to develop a dependence upon the drug, and to join the legions who have made sleeping pills one of America's most seriously abused drugs.[14]

Once the decision has been made to develop sleep control without the use of drugs, the next step is to reduce emotional and physical tension before you retire for the night. Managing your moods (Chapter 11) and increasing your physical activity (Chapter 14) can help you in this regard.[15]

Now you are ready to begin your sleep-control regime. How many hours of sleep do you need, as determined by your use of the sleep inventory? Because many people *overestimate* the amount of time that they spend trying to fall asleep and then *underestimate* the amount of time that they actually spend sleeping, adjustments in sleep time of thirty to sixty minutes are often sufficient.

Knowing how much sleep you should have, next decide that you will:

1. Go to bed at exactly *the same time of night,* seven nights each week.
2. Set the alarm to *wake up at exactly the same time every morning of the week,* no matter how long you tossed and turned before falling asleep the night before; and
3. Do not take naps if you can avoid them, but if you must nap, do so at *exactly the same time every day.*

This program offers the same gains and presents the same challenges as regulating the time of your urges to eat (Chapter 9). In both instances you will be attempting to retrain your body to move from chaotic to controlled biorhythmic functioning. As with your eating regulations, once you have gotten your sleep under control, you will be able to tolerate a little flexibility in your hours of retiring and waking. To achieve control of a process that has been deregulated for months or years requires close attention consistency. Therefore, in your initial efforts at sleep control, perfection should be your goal, as it is with retiming your urges to eat.

The second step of the program is another measure that you must take to help you sleep through the night. Very often people wake up at night because their bladders are full or because their bodies are reacting to signals from stimulants or depressants. Therefore:

1. Try to drink as little as possible after 4 P.M.;
2. Limit your consumption of coffee and tea as much as possible during the day, and have neither after 4 P.M.; and
3. Do not drink any alcoholic beverage, day or night.

As you will recall, these were some of the behaviors that you monitored in determining your sleep quotient. Curbing your fluid intake after 4 P.M. will help to make certain that your bladder is empty after you retire. Cutting down on coffee, tea, and alcohol will help you to relax more at bedtime. It is, of course, well recognized that coffee and tea are stimulants (tea has about half as much caffeine as coffee). But many people consider alcohol a "pick-me-up" by day and a drink to "calm me down" by night. In fact, the exact functions of alcohol are not fully understood but it is generally regarded as a central nervous system depressant. When alcohol enters the body, the nervous system steps up its activity to make up for alcohol's inhibiting effects. When the alcohol is burned off, the central nervous system is still overactive. This explains the tremors experienced by chronic drinkers when their intake slacks off. But even social drinkers experience this delayed arousal effect which can lead to sleep disturbance and tension that makes falling asleep again quite difficult.

The third step concerns management of the stimulus conditions of sleep.[16] In Chapter 7 it was pointed out that overeaters often condition themselves to feel hunger when they have linked eating and certain kinds of non-food-related activities such as watching television. In these instances, the television set, the reading matter, or the work project can become conditioned cues for the urge to eat. When poor sleepers use their beds for many different activities, it is possible that rather than cueing sleep, the bed can become a conditioned stimulus for other kinds of reactions. While it has been shown that good and poor sleepers both do about the same number of nonsleep activities, like reading or watching TV, even eating in bed, those with sleeping problems may be less able to tolerate this poor conditioning. Therefore it is important to:

TRY TO MAKE SLEEP ROUTINES
A "PURE EXPERIENCE"
JUST AS YOU DID WITH EATING.

For example, the television set should be turned around so that it cannot be watched from bed (or, better still, removed from the bedroom) and reading should be done in a chair rather than in bed. Activities such as sex which normally (but not necessarily) take place in bed should be given their own unique cues. For example, using a special light reserved only for sex, or lying with heads at the foot of the bed instead of in the normal sleeping position can both help to dissociate other activities from bed and allow the bed to become a pure stimulus for rest.

In addition to retraining yourself to associate only rest with bed, it is also important to *eliminate or lessen other distractors in the bedroom.* For example, controlling the level of light with room darkeners can be helpful. Use of an inexpensive "white noise" machine can help to mask distracting sounds. These are small devices which are sold by drug and department stores and they can be highly effective in muting the impact of sleep-disturbing sounds.

Another help is a program of muscle relaxation.[17] As you will recall, this program (described on pages 140–142) calls for tensing and relaxing major muscle groups beginning with the legs, then the arms, lower body, upper body, and head and neck. Because you cannot be tense and relaxed at the same time, training in relaxation can bring your bodily stress under control, and the method has been very effective in helping insomniacs to become more sleep-efficient.

Step five calls for thought control. The myriad thoughts that cross your mind as you try to fall asleep provoke emotional tension that bar the door to relaxing sleep. Therefore, efforts to break up the obsessional grip of such thoughts can go far toward overcoming this sleep-delaying tension.[18]

Thought purging can be accomplished by concentrating on neutral ideas. The familiar counting of sheep is not far from the mark. Recitation of a formula or concentration upon pleasing colors, sensations, and experiences can also do the trick, as can listening to soft music. However you focus your ideas, it is important to find a stimulus that is sufficiently strong to take your mind away from anxiety about whether or not you are falling asleep, and away from the major preoccupations of your life.

Follow the five-step program for a week. You may find it necessary to adapt one or more of the recommendations to your personal lifestyle. In adjusting the program to your individual needs, be certain to keep in mind the importance of consistency in all of your sleep rituals. This point cannot be overstated! The chart in Figure 12.2 is intended to help you keep track of your sleep-control efforts. Fill it out daily as a means of giving yourself feedback about what you have done and the jobs which still must be attended to. After a week, reassess your sleep adequacy by answering the questions in Figure 12.1 again. If you score higher on this second administration of the chart, you know that you are heading in the right direction. If you show no change, you should renew your efforts to find the proper combination of mood management, exercise (see Chapter 14), scheduling, stimulus control, and physical- and thought-control mechanisms so that you can enjoy the restorative sleep which we all need to function at our best.

FIGURE 12.2

Record of Success in the Sleep-Management Program

	Monday	Tuesday	Wednes-day	Thurs-day	Friday	Saturday	Sunday
1. Did you get into bed on schedule?							
2. Did you get out of bed on schedule?							
3. Did you schedule your naps and sleep only when planned?							
4. Did you reduce your fluid intake after 4 P.M.?							
5. Did you refrain from coffee or tea after 4 P.M.?							
6. Did you reduce your alcohol consumption?							
7. Did you remember to use the bed only for sleep (unless you associated another activity such as sex with a special set of cues)?							
8. Did you physically relax yourself upon getting into bed?							
9. Did you concentrate on neutral thoughts, avoiding preoccupation with falling asleep or with the							

IN A NUTSHELL

Many different factors affect our moods and our eating behavior. One of these factors is the level of our energy or, its opposite, our fatigue. If we suffer from irregular sleep, our moods are likely to be sour and our energy low. Sleep disturbance is very common in America and it is a self-made disorder. We can gain control of our sleep by retraining ourselves in regular sleep patterns and in actively managing our sleeping environment. Improve your sleep and you can improve your mood. Improve your mood and you can curb another source of your urge to eat more than you should.

13/ Hindrance and Help from Members of Your Family

If you see an overweight man on the street, what are the chances that he will be married to a heavy woman? Excellent, according to data collected in the Ten State Nutrition Survey. Dr. Stanley Garn of the University of Michigan has analyzed these data carefully and has found that whether or not heavy men and women marry one another, over the course of their lives together the leaner of the two will gradually put on extra weight to match the proportions of the heavier spouse. When Mother Goose observed that "Jack Spratt can eat no fat,/ His wife can eat no lean,/ And so between the two of them,/ They licked the platter clean," she naturally had in mind couples in the early days of their lives together. Because over the years, they would both lean toward the fat.[1]

Can the same be said of the fat child? What are the chances that a heavy child will have a heavy sibling? Dr. Garn found that if one child of two is heavy, there is a 40 percent chance that the other will be heavy as well. If the fat child is one of three, there is an 80 percent chance that one of the other two will also be fat. As you might expect by now, there is also about a 75 percent chance that the fat child, whom you single out on the street, will have at least one overweight parent.[2]

For many years it was believed that these findings of fatness similarities among family members meant that overweight was under the control of genetics. But an impressive array of findings has weakened this belief. It has been learned, for example, that genetically caused obesities are rare, and that when they occur they are usually accompanied by a variety of other anomalies such as skeletal malformations and mental retardation. Moreover, it has been learned that genes generally influence *body frame size* but they do not often directly influence *fat patterning per se.*[3]

While genetics play a factor in determining the predisposition to be heavy or lean, our genes receive important assistance in their mission from our experience after birth. This finding is supported by two groups of studies. In one it was shown that twins who are reared together are very similar in height and weight while twins who are separated at birth are similar in height but not in weight. In the second group of studies it was shown that foster and adopted children bear the same degree of resemblance to their new parents as do other children toward their natural parents.[4] Shared eating and exercise activities within the family thus seem to give the genes a major assist in making family members look-alikes.

Mothers are often signaled out as the arch-villains because they are believed to be the architects of their children's obesity. But the Ten State Nutrition Survey data indicted fathers as well. Families in the ten states were shown to have the following parent-child correlations:

Father-son	.25
Father-daughter	.20
Mother-son	.26
Mother-daughter	.19

Therefore, fathers and mothers seem to have about the same impact upon the eating and activity patterns of their children, although both have greater influence upon their sons than upon their daughters.

Mothers do have primary control over their newborn's feeding patterns. While some babies come into life with an above average number of cells in which fat can be stored, many babies who are overfed during the early weeks and months of their lives develop an unusually high number of these cells. As the child matures, these cells fill up with fat and increase in size. It is believed by many that the cells create a chemical need for fat and that if they are fat deprived, the body is "out-of-balance" and strives to correct the balance by excess food intake.[5] The evidence on this point is not at all clear, however, and it is probably safest to conclude that overfeeding infants can lead to a predisposition to fatness in childhood, adolescence, and later life, but that this predisposition requires a helping hand from weight-related learning later on along the line.

It has been estimated that about 70 percent of the infants under one year range from being overweight to being obese. And yet only about 49 percent of the 10 year olds are overweight or obese. About one-third of those who were very heavy babies are still very heavy at the age of seven while 60 percent of the seven-year-olds who are very heavy were overweight at birth. Therefore, some children whom one would expect to be genetically doomed to obesity at birth have a different experience in life. Interestingly, these tend to be children in larger families. As one researcher put it, "A mother with only one child is more concerned with persuading that one child to eat and grow than is a mother with several children."[6] Of course, it is also possible that with more than one mouth to feed there may simply not be enough food to go round to fatten all of the family's young.

When the dust settles, it becomes clear that, as the animal husbandry experts have learned, it is possible to breed animals for fatness. But the fattening process can be helped along by overfeeding the cultured animals and by keeping them as inactive as possible. There is no reason to believe that humans are any different. Some people have an inherited predisposition to fatness. But the effects of this predisposition can be mitigated to some extent by careful dietary management and by concerted attempts to increase the rate of energy expenditure.

The Forces That Fatten Children

Unfortunately, the false idea that "one cannot overfeed an infant" dies as slowly as the utterly foolish belief that "a fat baby is a healthy baby."[7]

In infancy the mother clearly has control of what the baby eats. During childhood, the youngster can become a co-conspirator with his or her mother but still the mother calls most of the nutritional shots. By adolescence, however, the teenager has an opportunity to make many independent eating decisions. Some of these decisions may not be wise. It is a fact that overweight teenagers are far more likely than their normal-weight classmates to have highly erratic eating patterns. Overweight adolescents are the ones most likely to report skipping breakfast and lunch and to have ill-defined mealtimes in general. Their food intake is also most likely to vary significantly in content and quantity from one day to the next.[8]

Overweight children are also more likely than their normal-weight peers to come from families in which there is some interpersonal disturbance that may or may not involve the use of food directly. For example, mothers of the overweight have been shown to have been more likely to use food as rewards for good behavior and the families of the overweight were much less likely to use mealtimes as times of family closeness. In addition, family and marital strife which often led to temporary or permanent parental separations was also the more common lot of the overweight. Finally, whether the family stresses were overt or covert, the nutritional practices of the teenagers tended to be quite poor if family tension was high and good if family interaction was positive.[9]

Unfortunately, it is not known whether family stress came before or after the development of adolescents' weight problem. Moreover, it is very important to point out that some, but by no means all of the families of overweight adolescents displayed these stressful reactions. In fact, some of the families of heavy teenagers can be considered to be among the better or even best functioning of families.

A third difference found between overweight and normal-weight teenagers is the *amount and intensity of their physical activity.* In every study to date, normal-weight adolescents were found to exercise longer and more vigorously than their heavier classmates. While it has been observed that most Americans spend far more time eating than exercising, overweight adolescents seem to use what little time they spend exercising quite inefficiently. For example, slow-motion movies of girls at a summer camp found slim campers were 150 percent more active than overweight campers while playing volleyball and 250 percent more active while swimming.[10] These frequently reported results stand in sharp contrast to the studies of teenage eating habits showing that overweight teenagers consume about the same amount of food as their

slender classmates. One significant key to the control of teenage obesity, therefore, is a carefully planned increase in the
level of physical activity, step by step.

It is by no means clear whether inactivity or overweight
comes first. However, there is evidence that activity patterns
are learned along with eating habits early in the young child's
life and, of course, their parents and siblings are the unwit-
ting teachers. Whether inactivity or overeating comes first,
it is clear that by definition the overweight take in more
energy than they burn, and they store their excess energy as
fat.[11] The longer this problem persists for children and
adolescents, the stronger will be the habits that can lock the
child into a lifelong pattern of excess weight. Because 80
percent of the adolescents who are overweight face obesity
in adulthood,[12] prudence demands that, whenever possible,
the chain which leads to obesity must be broken at its very
earliest possible point.

In many households this requires rethinking decisions
about infant feeding practices, decisions about early-child-
hood activity patterns, decisions about the family's social use
of food, and decisions about the food and exercise options
offered to adolescents.[13]

Some Very Important Considerations

Decades of research have led to the following conclusions
about the role of family experience in promoting and maintaining obesity:

1. For a small number of individuals, genetic and metabolic
   factors do create a predisposition to above average fatness;
2. For most people, however, the foundation for fatness is laid
   down after birth;

3. Infant overfeeding, childhood inactivity, erratic food habits in adolescence, family tension, and spousal influence all contribute to a situation in which the overweight simply consume more food energy than they burn, even though their eating may not be excessive in the least.

Therefore, *social learning* plays a major role in the development of obesity, a role which may be far more important than that of biological factors which have received so much attention in the past.

It is reasonable to assume that few people in this culture choose to be fat. This fatness must be viewed as a consequence of the interaction between biology and experience, neither of which were under the direct control of the overweight person during the most important early, formative years. This leads to the further assumption that *no person who has been heavy since birth or early childhood was the architect of his or her own obesity. But it is also essential to realize that, in the final analysis, it is only the overweight person who can decide that corrective action is necessary. While he or she did not choose fatness, it is the overweight person who must choose thinness.* Failure in weight loss is the only reasonable expectation when others attempt to make this most important decision. In fact, when parents or spouses attempt to impose this decision, relationships can become so strained that greater weight gain results.

Let's see how this might look in real life. Jenny is fifteen. When she was born she was a "bouncy baby." As an infant she was covered with soft and cuddly "baby fat." She was "plump" as a child, "husky" as a preteen, and "on the heavy side" in mid-adolescence. Through most of this time she has weighed about 25 percent more than she should. Her mother is "on the stout side" and her father is slowly moving from a size 36 to a size 38 belt. Both parents know that Jenny's weight is a problem. Her father becomes angry when he sees her overeat, her mother feels a sting of pain when she sees Jenny reach for extra cake or cookies. Both parents bring sweets into the house, "for company," "to celebrate this or that," or "just to keep Jenny happy." Both also eat the sweets that they bring home.

Jenny feels hopeless about her weight. She used to be made fun of by the other children on the block, but now she is accepted although not warmly welcomed into their activities. She tried to play the active games the others play but had a hard time keeping up, so she spent much of the game time alone. She does not like to see her body in the mirror, although she does like her pretty face and smooth complexion. She feels hassled by her parents about her weight and resists their attempts to make her thin. Basically, she resents their efforts to control her weight because she is struggling to find her own boundaries for her own sense of self and she feels their efforts to be encroachments on her personal life space. Although she has never said anything about it, she also doubts their sincerity: "If weight control is so important, why are they so fat? and why do they eat the junk they do?"

What, then, is the role of Jenny's parents? Whether or not they contributed to the development of her inactivity and overeating, they can play an important role in her development of more constructive patterns of behavior. Jenny will have to come to her own decision about whether or not to lose weight. Her parents can help her to identify the problem and the possible solutions, but she alone must make the commitment to change.

Once she has made the decision, her parents, her brothers

and sisters, and even her friends, can all cooperate to make her weight change possible. This help begins from the realization that all family members have an important impact upon each other's behavior:

1. They set examples for each other;
2. They *prompt* each other's actions; and
3. They selectively *pay off* each other's efforts.

Everything that is said or done in a family serves as an example for others. If Jenny sees Dad take a third helping of spaghetti, she learns that three is not too many servings of Mom's pasta. When Dad sees Mom take a modest first portion and decline seconds, he learns that she values moderation. When Mom sees Jenny take an apple instead of a cupcake for dessert, that, too, is an object lesson. We always display our values to others by what we do rather than by what we say!

Family members also prompt each other's actions both by word and deed. Mom reminds Junior to drink his milk —that's a verbal prompt. She also keeps the freezer well supplied with Junior's favorite flavor of ice cream—that's a prompt by deed. When we are not busy demonstrating the kind of behavior which we expect, we are usually occupied with promoting its occurrence, directly or indirectly.

Finally, family members also follow one another's actions with some kind of response which may either strengthen or weaken chances that the same action will be repeated another time. The most powerful and also the most common kind of payoff is attention. Attention is a universally powerful way of strengthening behavior. People will imperil their lives to gain attention, and children would rather be punished than be ignored. Therefore, any response made to another's action will make that action more likely to be repeated.

Everything that members of the family do has an impact upon everything done by the others. Sometimes the impact is exactly what is expected; sometimes the predictions are proven dead wrong. Right or wrong, positive or negative, family members cannot *not* influence one another.[14]

Therefore, in order to be as helpful as possible:

1. Every member of the family must set the best *example* possible;
2. Each must take responsibility for *prompting* the actions which he or she considers important; and
3. Each must consistently *pay off the others* for their constructive actions.

How Parents Can Help a Teenager Lose Weight and Maintain the Loss

The typical adolescent doubles in weight during the teenage years. This growth is obviously a time of great importance for a healthy adulthood. Important, too, is the fact that much of the weight gain of teenagers is attributable to an excess of food intake over energy expenditure, and not simply the result of overeating. Taken together, these observations require that:

1. Goals of very gradual weight loss be established for teenagers;
2. The nutritional needs of developing bodies be met completely; and
3. A well-balanced food plan be combined with a gradual increase in activity.

Rapid weight loss due to excessive cuts in the minimum food requirements and radically increased exercise can create greater problems than they could possibly solve. The name of the game for both children and adults is *weight loss through small steps.*

Parents can start the ball rolling by developing some very important attitudes. They must give up the idea that fat children are healthy children. They must also give up the belief that the average, healthy child suffers injury through overheating and fatigue after vigorous exercise. In addition, they must give up the time-honored cliché that "parents know best." Such thinking is a red flag to the emerging adolescent.

Attempts of parents to hold the reins too tightly generally lead to rebellion. For example, parents who peer over their child's shoulder at the readout on the bathroom scale every day are likely to find the numbers growing ever worse. A sensible weight-management program for teenagers must fully credit the child's independence and capacity to take responsibility.

Parents should openly discuss the caloric facts with their children. For example, it is a fact that just two extra cookies per day (e.g., chocolate chip or fig bars) can add up to 700 extra calories per week and to over ten unwanted pounds per year. It is also true that a half-hour walk can burn about 150 calories per day, 4,500 per month, or 54,000 calories per year—enough to slough about fifteen extra pounds.

Children and teenagers can both be asked to use the resources available in their schools and communities to collect similar important information. Early in the program, it is wise to ask children to keep close records of what they eat and what they do. These can be the same records that are kept by adults, those shown on pages 27 and 214.

Using the data from these records, plans should be made for increasing activity. Adolescents should be encouraged to have as much social contact as possible and to use this contact as a means of building social skills. Because overweight adolescents are self-conscious and many have been the victims of ridicule by their classmates, they are shy and inhibited. But all have a strong desire to make and to maintain friendships. The way to friendship is through progressively more varied activities. Good choices for activities are those that require intelligence, creativity, and interpersonal abilities, as well as those which build physical skill and dexterity.

A second important activity is self-care and grooming. Because overweight adolescents often feel that they do not compete successfully in the contest for good looks, many have a tendency toward carelessness in dress and grooming. Unfortunately, a careless appearance advertises self-disdain and invites social rejection. Therefore, efforts to improve personal tidiness are rarely wasted.

In addition, and most importantly, adolescents should be encouraged to increase their level of physical activity. Overweight people, in general, have a tendency to find energy-saving rather than energy-expending ways of using their bodies. Therefore, overweight children must begin to recondition themselves to stand rather than to sit, to move about rather than to stand, to walk rather than to ride, and to move quickly rather than slowly.

When the adolescent has identified weight as a problem worth concerted effort, parents can help by using the three tactics of social influence which have been described. The following table gives but a few illustrations:

	Moderate eating	Greater social activity	Better grooming	More physical activity
Example	Eat moderate meals	Engage in skill-building family activities	Attend to own personal appearance	Go for walks, begin physical activities
Prompt	Ask how much the adolescent plans to eat at the start of the meal	Arrange for other sitters to stay with younger sibs so that teenager can be with friends	Provide an adequate clothes budget	Provide easy access to sports facilities
Payoff	Warmly recognize moderate eating	Express interest in outside activities.	Notice improved appearance	Allow teen to keep bus or cab fare if he or she walks

Finally, because the normal relationship between parents and teenagers is fraught with difficulties, excessive involvement of the parent in the weight loss program may be a source of considerable strain. Therefore the teenager's participation in a self-chosen weight-loss program, whether through a clinic or a responsible weight-control organization such as "Weight Watchers," can often spell the difference between success and failure. While data on the subject are scarce, one study did show that obese teenagers who participated in a weight-loss group had half the number of personal problems as were reported by those who were nonparticipants.[15] Such participation has the advantages of offering professionally supervised program planning and group support from people who are clearly *not* involved in the resolution of identity growth crises at home.

How Spouses Can Help

Have you or your spouse gained weight since you married? Have you changed your eating habits in any important ways? Has your activity increased or decreased significantly? Has the role of food in your life altered significantly—that is, are you more or less likely to turn to food as a means of meeting a crisis? Many couples make these and more changes following their marriages. Read on, and meet some people who have had these experiences.

Tom and Roni have been married for six years. Before they were married, each held jobs in the plant, Tom as a relief foreman and Roni as a lab technician in the plastics department. Both were on the go much of the time and their meals were quick and light. The only times they had complete meals were at the family dinners they felt they had to join. Tom played catcher on a semi-pro softball team and Toni was a figure skater. Both were Class A bowlers in a mixed Tuesday-night bowling league.

After they were married, Tom traded softball for night school and Roni gave up figure skating for pregnancy. They did continue to bowl on Tuesday nights but they cut out practice sessions to save money. Meals, which had been hasty affairs before marriage, became important times. Roni felt that she had to compete with Tom's mother for culinary honors and she therefore learned to bake bread and pies and became a skilled gravy and sauce chef. Both paid closer attention to Roni's cuisine than to their swelling waistlines. Their problem: a sudden gain in the amount of food that they ate coupled with a drop in the level of their physical activity.

Al and Zena (known to their friends as the "A to Z" kids when they were courting) live next door to Tom and Roni. They were both plump when they were married. They have had four children and with each pregnancy Zena gained thirty pounds before delivery and lost only ten pounds afterward. Al is a solicitous husband who pays careful attention to Zena's every desire. He knows that she has a "sweet tooth" so he often surprises her with treats from her favorite bakery. Zena feels that Al is very sensitive and tries hard never to hurt his feelings. Therefore, even though she knows that the sweet treats are a problem for her, she heaves to when the bakery box arrives. For Al and Zena the problem is that each sees food as love: to give food is to express love and to eat food is to accept a loving offering.

Sid and Marcy who live farther down the block have a different problem. When all three families first moved onto the block they were quite friendly. But over the years, Sid and Marcy made their fights ever more public until the others began to shy away from them. Marcy's father had a drinking problem and she had a morbid dread and dislike of alcohol. As if to spite her, Sid began to drink and has now reached the point at which three doubles every evening are the minimum necessary "fuel for his burners." Sid has made clear to Marcy that he finds slender women attractive and heavy women gross. As if out of spite, Marcy has taken to eating up a storm whenever Sid takes a drink or does anything which she considers to be an insult. Sid uses alcohol as a weapon and Marcy uses food as a weapon. Their problem is that both work hard at destroying themselves instead of making a frontal assault on their relationship difficulties.

These are three common patterns—activity is allowed to decline while food intake rises, food is used as a means of expressing love, and eating is used as a form of expressing anger. There are many others. In each, food is permitted to become something which it is not. If food is used to placate the spouse, if it is used to pay for indulgence, if it is used instead of social contact, or if it is used as an arena in which to try unsuccessfully to resolve other marital stresses, eating can only cause more problems than it resolves.

Using the three tools of social influence—example, prompting, and paying off—these problem interactions can be reversed. It will naturally be easiest for Tom and Roni to set things straight in their home, but even Sid and Marcy can gain greatly from a few simple changes.

Set a Good Example

This means that each partner should eat the proper amounts of well-selected foods and shun overeating at mealtimes and problem treats between meals. It also means that each should get as much physical activity as is healthful and practical. This can be done in small ways by looking for opportunities to take extra steps instead of saving steps, and in larger ways by walking or planning some other activity every day.

Each partner should also set an example by acknowledging the positive things which the other does. There is strong evidence for the maxim that "Positive Input is Needed in Order to Change Relationships."[16] Negative exchanges help to fix behavior at its current level while positive exchanges make things better. For example, when Sid shouts "Stop that" at Marcy as she reaches for a second helping of dessert, he tells her that he will pay attention when she makes a mistake. "Stop that" shouters ignore positive behavior when it occurs and their negative communications tend to be the only attention which others receive. If when Marcy refuses a second helping of a tempting dish Sid said, "Marcy, that's great! I'm really impressed with what you're accomplishing!" —then Marcy would learn that she could earn Sid's attention through positive actions. Then and only then would she be in a position to make a strong run at achieving a major change. If Marcy wants Sid to treat her in this way, she must set an example by offering her praise when he curbs his drinking!

Prompt the Kind of Action That You Would Like to Have Happen

When one person decides to develop new eating patterns, that is an important change for the family. All behavioral patterns develop a certain momentum. Others in the family expect certain actions and respond to these actions in predictable ways. Many times family members inadvertently work to keep things as they have been; for example, they telegraph negative expectations: "Since you didn't get your way, Sid, I suppose you're going to hit the bottle again." With these words Marcy casts a role which Sid will find very difficult not to follow.

When new patterns emerge, readjustment is necessary. Even if the change is one which all in the family desire, others will have the tendency to keep acting as though the new behavior had not occurred. Therefore, each time that one person decides to make a change, it is very important that he or she announce what is planned and what help is desired. For example, Zena might say, "Al, I have been having some really bad feelings about myself and I have decided to start to lose weight. You could help me a lot by taking me to a show, asking me to go for a walk, or just sitting close to me to tell me that you care, and by helping me to keep sweets out of the house." That way Al can hear Zena's message loud and clear and it will be his choice whether to help or to hinder her efforts.

Marcy found from her self-monitoring chart that her problem eating tended to occur at three different times: while she prepared meals, when she ate alone because Sid stayed late at the store, and when she was angry. Sid used the Keep Track chart to get a fix on his drinking. He found that he downed half of his liquor before dinner every night and the other half when he felt alone and annoyed later in the evening.

When they compared notes, Sid and Marcy found that they could make some pleasant changes. Marcy realized she felt rejected when Sid came home in the evening, took his drink into the living room, and read the paper while she finished dinner. She asked Sid to keep her company and even to pitch in as one way to help her overcome her late-afternoon depressions. For his part, Sid liked this early-evening contact and he was able to lessen his before-dinner drinking. Marcy asked Sid please to let her know at least a day in advance when he planned to stay late at the store so that she could prepare her dinner ahead of time and have only the proper portions ready. That way she avoided cooking for two and having extra food readily available when she felt lonely. Sid and Marcy also agreed to spend at least an hour together every evening after dinner. Whether they just talked, played cards, read, or watched television together, each felt a kind of closeness during this time. It cut down Marcy's feelings of anger and Sid's feelings of isolation. Each thus prompted the other to make a change that could go far toward creating a positive climate, as well as breaking early links in the problem-eating chain.

There are hundreds of other prompts which may be useful. One wife asks her husband to serve her portions of food, knowing that he will not make the mistake of giving her a little extra. Another wife asks for her husband's company while she cleans up after dinner, knowing that when he is with her she will be able to resist the temptation to eat table scraps. Still another wife asks her husband to phone her at exactly 12:30 every day: she begins her lunch at about ten past twelve and uses his call as a signal to leave the kitchen and get started with her afternoon activities. A husband asks his wife to make lunch for him so that he can avoid the temptations of going past the cafeteria food displays, while another husband prompts his wife to have apples instead of peanuts available for snacks.

To find the kind of prompts that will help you, look over your eating record carefully and identify the times when eating is a problem.

Discuss these times with your partner and work together on a suggestion list which will serve as his or her prompts for your new eating routine.

Pay Off the Behaviors Which You Wish to Have Continued

There are two common problems in the payoff department. First, we all have a tendency to pay more attention to negative behavior than to positive. We tend to react to negatives as if they were intentional wounds while we respond to positives as though they were our perfect right. In order to set this situation straight, considerable attention must be paid to offering strong and unambiguous payoffs for constructive behaviors.

The second problem in managing payoff properly is that we all have an inclination to act inconsistently. Inconsistency can lead to confusing double messages. For example, after Zena asked Al to find ways other than food gifts to express affection, he did make an effort to be inventive. After a time, however, he passed a shop with marzipan fruits in the window. He knew that Zena had a passion for marzipan, so he decided to bring home a real surprise—"to show what a good job he thought she was doing." As soon as Zena saw the candy, she felt two very strong conflicting emotions: she did love marzipan, but she knew how terrible she would feel if she gave in to temptation. If she smiled warmly and accepted the candy, in effect she would have told Al to disregard her earlier prompt and go back to the candy-as-usual routine. If she accepted the candy, she would undermine her own good efforts. What she had to do is:

1. Relate to the underlying positive feeling in the offer;
2. And then consistently refuse.
3. Suggest a nonfood alternative.

Zena might say, "Al, I know that you want to do something special for me and you know that marzipan used to be my passion. But now it is really important for me to get myself under good control and I'd love it if you would offer to take me to the movies instead of buying sweets when you want to tell me that you care." That way Al knows that Zena has heard the important message—he loves her—but he also knows the way in which he can help her best. Zena is then faced with the difficult task of setting the marzipan aside and not taking even a single taste of this or any future treat.

Very often painful choices must be made. In the long run, everyone's interests are best served when alternatives to food are sought and used as a means of expressing affection, coping with strong emotions, relieving boredom, and the like. As Zena begins to feel better about herself, she will have much more to offer Al and he will then be richly rewarded for his efforts to help her succeed. Therefore, while it may be difficult, *absolute consistency* is required in paying off others for helpful changes, whatever they may be.

IN A NUTSHELL

Some important points have been made in this chapter. First, it was pointed out, through a review of the scientific literature of the past four decades, that obesity is a family affair. Whether or not families create problems of overweight in their members, families certainly help to maintain overeating and inactivity. By the same token, families can be invaluable resources in meeting the challenge of developing better eating and activity patterns. Once the overeater/underexerciser has reached the decision that change is needed—and it must be his or her personal decision—help from other family members can be carefully planned using the three techniques of social influence. The steps are simple:

1. Working from your Self-Monitoring Chart, identify times when problem eating occurs and times when physical activity can be expanded;
2. For each time decide:
   a. Which family member will set what good example?
   b. Which family member will offer which prompts? By word? And/or by action?

c. And finally, which family member will offer what kind of payoff?

Plans should be made by all members of the family working as a team. The plans should be simple in order to be realistic. They must call for positive interactions only—*no negative prompts, no negative payoff.* And they must include an opportunity for each person to keep track of what he or she does pursuant to the plan.

If Dad and Jenny agree that Jenny should walk to school each day, and that Dad will walk with her and take the bus from her school to his office, then Dad should keep track of the days on which he sets this good example. If Al agrees to serve Zena's portions and to keep the serving dishes near the stove rather than on the table so that Zena is not tempted to take seconds, then he should keep track of the times that he remembers to do so. Finally, if Sid agrees to spend fifteen minutes with Marcy in the kitchen each evening, as a way of paying her off for curbing her urge to eat during the late afternoon, then he, too, should keep track of his efforts. The form which can be used for these records is illustrated in Figure 13.1.

None of these steps has to be complex. For example, it was found that one woman consumed 1,251 calories in three night-eating bouts when she was alone, and 185 calories in three other bouts when her husband was present.[17] Therefore, the mere presence of a family member can act as a prompt for prudent food selection and portion control.

FIGURE 13.1

A Chart for Keeping Track of How Some
Family Members Help Others

Who? Will set what Example? Will offer which Prompts? Will Pay Off good behaviors in what way? It was done the following times on the following days:							

	MONDAY	TUESDAY	WEDNESDAY	THURSDAY	FRIDAY	SATURDAY	SUN
Example							
	MONDAY	TUESDAY	WEDNESDAY	THURSDAY	FRIDAY	SATURDAY	SUN
Prompt							
	MONDAY	TUESDAY	WEDNESDAY	THURSDAY	FRIDAY	SATURDAY	SUN
Pay Off							

14 / Working Down an Appetite While Working Spirits Up

There was a time when the sidewalks of Everytown, U.S.A., were crowded: now strollers are the exception and not the rule. Our ballfields were once jammed with eager sportsmen of all ages: now most of us spend our Sundays as TV jocks and the parks are the province of "health nuts" and the young. We used to sharpen our own pencils, chop ice for our own martinis, and open our own cans by hand: now these and dozens of other minor jobs have become the work of our electronic slaves. We have refined the art of doing nothing to such a point that we even have machines to rub our backs when they ache from inactivity. In short, we will spare no expense and apply the heights of our ingenuity to any task that will allow us to push a button rather than move an arm, to sit instead of stand, or to ride rather than walk. We have reached that unhappy moment when no task is too slight to warrant calling upon a machine to do the job for us, and no trip too short to hold us back from climbing into the family car.

The result of this energy-sparing way of life is serious. We have become a nation of heavy-limbed, stiff-jointed armchair dwellers. As a result, our bellies have broadened and our stamina has waned.

I'm Heavy Already: What Good Can Activity Do Me Now?

It is not at all unusual to read statements like the following: "Overweight? Forget exercise. You'd have to climb to the top of the Empire State Building three times in a row to lose one single pound," or "If you're trying to walk your weight off, forget it! You have to walk from dawn to dusk to get rid of one pound of fat."

While some authorities question the role of activity in weight control, the Food and Nutrition Board of the National Research Council clearly recognizes its importance. In its Recommended Dietary Allowances, *the* authoritative statement of minimum nutritional needs, the Council considered activity to be the "dominant factor leading to variability in energy needs."[1] Specifically, the Council recommends that men and women who engage in moderate activity consume 300 more calories per day than those whose activity is light, and that those who engage in heavy activity take in 600 to 900 calories more to meet their extra energy needs. It therefore stands to reason that anyone who holds caloric intake constant and increases the level of activity would have to burn fat stores to fuel this extra effort.

Let's look at what happens with a 125-pound woman and a 150-pound man. The sleeping woman burns approximately 1.0 calories per minute and the man 1.1. Sitting or standing, the woman burns up to 2.0 calories, the man up to 2.5. Walking slowly on a level surface, the woman burns up to 3.9 calories per minute, the man up to 4.9. Walking briskly on a level surface accounts for up to 5.9 calories per minute for women and 7.4 calories for men. And walking up a hill while carrying a load can account for 10.0 and 12.0 calories per minute for a woman and man respectively. In other words, vigorous activity requires over five times the calories burned while sitting still.

What does this mean for Joe and Jane who think about activity as a way of trying to burn off their extra fat? Assuming that they each weigh 150 pounds, they would have to spend about seventeen minutes walking or four minutes running to burn up the calories in an extra banana. Getting rid of the extra calories in a donut would require about twenty-nine minutes of walking or eight minutes of running. An ice cream soda is worth a forty-nine-minute walk or a thirteen-minute run. And a generous helping of strawberry shortcake would keep them on the sidewalk for seventy-seven minutes or on the track for twenty-one.[2]

All of this seems like a large effort for a small reward, but we get a different picture when we take a closer look. Our 150-pounder burns about 5.2 calories per minute while walking. If he or she goes for a thirty-minute stroll this would burn up about 150 calories. If the walk were taken five days each week for a year, and *if food intake stayed the same* throughout the year, 39,150 extra calories would be burned or enough to shed over eleven pounds in twelve months, twenty-two pounds in two years. What is more, if Joe or Jane weighed more than 150 pounds, their rewards would be even greater because it takes greater energy to move heavier bodies through space. For example, a small, lean man running a mile in about ten minutes will use 121 calories, but a 220-pound man running the same mile will burn 219 calories in the same amount of time.[3] Therefore the more you work, the longer you spend at it, and the heavier you are, the more calories you will burn for the effort.

Finally, as an added bonus, it is important to note that the weight-related benefit of exercise extends long after the exerciser sits down to rest. In one controlled experiment, resting metabolism four hours after a vigorous workout was from 7.5 to 28 percent *higher* than it was at the same time on days when no exercise took place.[4] That means that hours after activity ends, our bodies still burn extra fat. Clearly, then, an increase in activity can be of considerable value in using up unwanted calories.

The value of increased activity goes far beyond its impact upon weight. It can improve the health of the heart and circulatory system in several different ways, not the least of which is by preventing the buildup of extra cholesterol in the bloodstream and by cutting down the amount of fat that's already there.[5] It can also improve your state of mind in six important ways; even a small increase in the amount of physical activity can help to:

1. Reduce the level of tension and stresses which you experience;
2. Help you to rest more comfortably and to sleep better;
3. Help to improve your concentration and enthusiasm for work and play;
4. Help to improve your mood;
5. Help to reduce your appetite; and
6. Help to improve your self-confidence.[6]

Increased activity can help to reduce tension because tension is, at its root, a physical experience. As you learned in Chapter II, helping muscles to relax, the cues that trigger the psychological experience of stress can be minimized. When you feel less tension, you are likely to find relaxation easier and sleep deeper and more satisfying. Feeling better rested, you are almost certain to find it easier to concentrate on your work and to meet the challenges of everyday living. This, in turn, can give rise to more positive experiences in work and play, both of which logically help you to feel positive as well. Then your lowered tension, greater rest, concentration, enthusiasm, and improved mood all combine to help *reduce your urge to eat.* Instead of working *up* an appetite, research has clearly shown that *light to moderate activity works appetite down.*[7] Repeat: *Research has shown that food intake decreases when work load moves from light to moderate.*

Moderate increases in activity appear to cut the urge to eat and help to burn stored fat in the bargain. With all of these systems "go," it is small wonder that increased activity can help you to feel better about yourself and more confident in the future.

Increased activity feeds into improved self-esteem in two other ways. First, when you do something active you are doing something for all the world to see. You know, and others can know too, that you have taken action to help yourself. This is different from those dozens of good decisions that you make not to eat this or that: they are nonactions, they can't be seen. They are very important decisions but they do not offer you the same opportunity to stand up and be counted as does taking the bold step into increased activity.

Second, increased activity has a very important symbolic value. When you follow through on your commitment to yourself in this specific way, you know that you have finished a job well done. This can go far toward building your motivation to meet other challenges throughout the week. Activity, then, seems to be as good for your spirit as for your body, and it is clear that you can gain a lifetime of benefit from a little extra effort every day.

A Caution

An increase in activity should not be undertaken without specific medical approval by anyone who has suffered any cardiovascular stress, including hypertension and heart at-

tacks. Those who have diabetes, electrolyte imbalances, ane-mia, varicose veins, and various other medical problems must also plan any activity with great care. [8]

If you are very much overweight or very much out of shape, a rapid increase in activity could lead to joint prob-lems or other forms of physical stress. Therefore, it is impor-tant to rule out these or other kinds of potential dangers (rare though they may be) by *consulting with your doctor before you start to move about.*

Activity Won'ts

Several assumptions lead people to steer clear of healthful physical activity. We have already knocked out the excuse that activity has to be avoided for fear of working up an appetite. But "committed passives" have many other lines of defense against becoming active. For example, many people think that "physical activity" means "vigorous exercise" of the smelly sweatsuit variety. This is not necessarily the case! Physical activity means any effort to move your body around more than is your normal pattern. You can be physically active without getting out of breath, without getting over-heated, and without changing from your everyday street clothes. In fact, the kind of exercise for which you do suit up may not suit you at all. It usually implies toe touching and knee bending, exercises which can be useful but which are often so uncomfortable that they are rarely pursued long enough to be of benefit.

Another excuse offered by people who won't increase their activity is that exercise is dull. Here, we run into semantics again. Perhaps stretching the same muscle for count after count is dull. Perhaps going through the same routine won't hold your interest. The fact is, though, that there are dozens of activities that can be useful to you, and you certainly can vary them to hold your interest every single day.

Some people won't exercise because they do not want to call public attention to themselves. But many activities can be done in the privacy of your own home and others can be done in unobtrusive ways in public places. For example, climbing stairs in your own home or office several extra times a day can be very useful.

Another activity "won't" stems from the belief that any useful program requires too much planning or too many people. Sure, if baseball is your number, you need seventeen others to help you out, or if jai alai is your choice, you'll have to find a court. But you can also choose from numerous solo ventures (e.g., swimming, bicycling, ice skating, rope jumping, or hitting a tennis ball against a wall) and activities that require neither companions nor equipment, such as walking, jogging, and climbing stairs.

Finally, the most basic unrealized excuse for avoiding exercise is simply that it involves change. Increasing activity means using muscles that may have been in mothballs for years, and it means getting in touch with your body in ways that you may not have experienced before. Above all, it means that you must develop some new attitudes and this may be the most difficult change of all.

Activity Choices

Once you have overcome your excuses for not becoming more active, you are faced with the challenge of deciding what to do. As a general rule:

1. You want to change your lifestyle in as many small and large ways as possible to

2. Increase the amount of energy that you spend in doing what you do all day long.

To do this you will have to:

1. Find ways to use more energy in your everyday activities; and
2. Choose new activities to build onto the things that you do.

At home, if you normally sit while talking on the telephone, try standing. If you normally ask others to bring the plates to you so you can wash the dishes, get the dishes yourself. If you normally sit and do nothing after dinner, plan a twenty-minute stroll. If you normally leave the heavy cleaning to someone else, think about doing more of it yourself. If you clean the basement and the garage once each year, think about bringing them up to snuff more often. In other words, change your daily routine so that during the time that you are at home your body is much more active.

You can also change your style on the job. If you normally ride the bus to work, try boarding the bus a stop or two farther from your home and then plan to get off a stop or two before your office. If you drive to work and park next door, park several blocks away instead. If you normally use the elevator in the building, think about using the stairs instead. If you normally sit at your desk or in the staff cafeteria for breaks, think about using the time to walk through the halls around the building, or walk to a more distant place to eat. If you eat lunch in the staff cafeteria, try walking several blocks to a sandwich shop instead. If you rely upon others to bring work to you, see if you can't find ways to fetch the supplies yourself. Again the watch word is: *do as much as you can yourself, relying as little as possible on others.*

The caloric differentials for each one of these small

changes are not large, although they all can add up to a sizable energy expenditure over time. For example, if you stand instead of sitting you burn 1.5 instead of 1.3 calories per minute. If you walk instead of stand, your caloric use jumps from 1.5 to 3.1 per minute. If you walk downstairs instead of riding the elevator, you use 7.1 calories per minute instead of 1.5. And if you walk upstairs, it's 10.0 per minute instead of 1.5. Moreover, you can raise the ante 10 percent for each fifteen pounds that you weigh above 150, so that a 225-pound man burns 15 calories to the 150-pounder's 10 calories for each minute of stair climbing, or 150 in ten minutes as against the thin man's 100.[9] Because the increases in energy expenditure are cumulative—that is, every little bit counts—you do not have to exert yourself all at once. For instance, the 225-pounder who normally makes four trips each day up and down five stories in an elevator can use up a significant amount of energy by using the stairs instead as often as possible.

Beyond these frequent and small increases in physical activity, it is wise to plan a once-a-day larger activity as well. You might plan a walk each day. Choose an amount of time that you would like to spend and plan a gradual increase in the distance you travel during this time. That way, you will build up your stamina and, naturally, the farther you go per unit of time, the more energy you will spend in the effort. Many people find a twenty-minute walk both pleasurable and beneficial.

You can also choose a sport. You may follow your sport once or more each week, and you may choose more than one sport in any week. Rowing, skating, and cycling slowly can take care of 5 calories per minute, while doing any of them at a faster clip can be worth up to 15. Ping-Pong is worth 5 to 7 calories per minute, tennis 7 to 11, and dancing 5 to 8.

Running a mile in twelve minutes is a 120-calorie effort, while running two miles in the same time burns twice the energy. And once again, the more you weigh, the greater will be your caloric loss.[10]

In working out a plan for personal activity, it is a good idea to follow five specific rules, after having your doctor's okay:

1. Choose an activity that is natural for you, not one which you think that you "should" select.
2. Plan specific activity times for every single day.
3. Make activity a daily rather than a sometime commitment.
4. If you can, find someone to join in your activities, but always be prepared to go it alone.
5. Start small, work your way up.

Choosing to do things that come naturally is important because you are obviously less likely to follow through on programs which "put you out of joint." Planning to follow through on your activity at specific times each day will increase the chance that the activity gets done. You do not have to choose the same time every day. For example, after work on weekdays and early morning on the weekends might be one person's choice, while another might take the early mornings during the week and afternoons on weekends. Just as you individualize the choice of which activity you will pursue, so, too, should you individualize when you plan to follow through.

You also have to make the decision to follow through with an activity that can be done every single day. If you allow the weather to be a factor, you'll risk breaking the activity habit. If you depend upon others to fire you up, their unavailability can stand in your way. Therefore, just as you have backup plans for each step in breaking your eating chain, have backup plans for foul weather and solo days. For example, if you walk/jog for twenty minutes a day, be ready with a stair climb in bad weather. If you plan a tennis game, be ready for a brisk walk around the park if your partner fails to appear.

Now that you know the essentials, the next move is yours. Make that move now! The longer you wait, the less likely it is that you'll act. Use the chart in Figure 14.1 to plan your program. And then follow through with your plans to the best of your ability. Your rewards will be higher spirits, fewer urges to eat, and a gradual reduction in your excess weight.

IN A NUTSHELL

Many people believe that activity builds appetite. The fact is, however, that increased activity can *lower* your urge to eat. It can also improve your spirits and your health. To become more active you must overcome the tendency to equate activity with work. You can increase your activity by adding energy to the things that you normally do every day. You can also increase your activity by planning some kind of mild or moderate exercise for a short time every day. By changing your lifestyle to include more use of energy, you can do yourself inestimable good.

FIGURE 14.1

My Activity Planner

Day	Exactly what time will I begin and end?	What's my first-choice activity?	What's my backup if the weather is bad or I'm alone?
Monday			
Tuesday			
Wednesday			
Thursday			
Friday			
Saturday			
Sunday			

15/ Heading Off Binges at the Pass

B inge eating poses the same threat to the person seeking weight control that tornadoes do to the plains dweller, typhoons do to the South Sea islander, and blizzards do to the people of the Arctic: they threaten to destroy a lifetime of effort. But binges, unlike forces of nature, are controllable, psychologically motivated events. And even though binges might not be prevented from beginning, some precautions can help to lessen their ravages.

Binges are different things to different people. Some people regard a slight extra indulgence as a binge, but others do not feel that they have binged unless they have eaten madly for hours or even days. Binge eating usually begins with a combination of moods such as boredom and anger. Binges start small and build up rapidly, and they are more likely to occur on days when regular meals have been skipped. Members of Weight Watchers classes were asked to describe the binges that they experienced before becoming members. One person in eight reported binging on days when they had eaten all three meals, one in four reported binging on days that they had skipped breakfast, and three out of five of those who skipped breakfast and lunch reported binging as a major problem. Therefore, negative moods and omitted meals can set the stage for binging.

Members of Weight Watchers classes also reported that: these binges tended to begin at night, although they might extend into the following day; the binging almost always took place at home; they almost always hid binge eating from others; these binges often began with small or moderate amounts of a preferred food but then went on to include larger amounts of almost anything; and they rarely knew how much they ate either during or after a binge. These observations have helped to form a five-step program for binge control:

1. When you feel the need to eat a between-meal snack, try distraction first by turning to something other than food.
2. Wait at least ten minutes before you eat, after you experience the urge to eat.
3. When you do eat, choose a food that is *not* on your "much preferred" list.
4. Take the smallest possible quantity of the food that you eat. If you go back for more, again take the smallest possible helping.
5. Consider anything that you have eaten to be water over the dam. Don't dwell on it. Begin immediately to follow your original eating plan.

Distraction can help to break your preoccupation with eating. You can distract yourself by making a change in your environment and your activity. If you are sitting in the living room and the urge to eat strikes, move to the basement, the bedroom, or the backyard—go anyplace where you will not be in contact with food. If you are watching TV when the urge to eat strikes, turn the TV off and put on your favorite music. If you are reading, try TV. If you are cleaning, turn to a hobby. Do anything that will change your environment and occupy your mind. In changing both environment and activity, you take into account the fact that your urge to eat is a response to your present situation: *change the situation and you can limit the urge to eat.*

The ten-minute wait will give you time to think. It can help to break the grip of your preoccupation with food, giving you an opportunity to become interested in other things. Waiting the ten minutes can also *give you proof that you are still in control.* This renewed self-confidence can help you to limit your eating at this time. Use a kitchen timer that sounds a bell to time the ten-minute interval. When the bell rings, if you have it in you to wait ten minutes more, set the time and see what you can do.

Choosing a *nonpreferred* food is a very important link in this urge-control chain. Research has shown that while the obese are not more sensitive to the taste of food than are the lean,[1] many overweight people do have difficulty in limiting the foods they prefer.[2] Because your resistance is low when you are set to binge, you may experience a tendency to eat far too much of your favorite foods. Moreover, if you eat your favorite foods at these times you are, in effect, rewarding yourself for allowing your eating to get out of hand.

Make a list of the foods that you particularly like as snack foods (using the spaces below), and a second list of nonpreferred foods that are generally on hand. For example, you might like cookies, nuts, and chocolate as snacks—they would go on your "Preferred: To be Avoided" list. On the other hand, your refrigerator could always be stocked with carrots, celery, radishes, or pepper strips: they can be added to your "I Don't Like These As Well So They're Okay" list.

Preferred: To Be Avoided	I Don't Like These As Well So They're Okay
1.	1.
2.	2.
3.	3.
4.	4.

Many dieters take an all or nothing approach to their food management. As suggested on page 37, they are "dichotomous thinkers." It has been shown, for example, that when dieters in a research setting were given an opportunity to have a snack, those who thought they had broken their diets ate more than those who believed they had eaten only what they should. In actual truth, both had eaten exactly the same amount before they had been given a chance to snack. The message is this:

DO ALL YOU CAN TO MAKE CERTAIN
THAT EVERY TIME YOU EAT
YOU HAVE GIVEN YOURSELF AN OPPORTUNITY
TO DRAW THE FINAL LINE.

If you plan to eat a slice of bread and know that you should eat only one slice, take it, close the package, return it to its proper place, and go to the table where you will sit and eat it. Go back, if you must, to take a second, but repeat the same routine. If you take the package to the table with you, you are likely to eat "automatically," you will lose track of how much you eat, and you will not stop yourself before the damage is done.

Finally, after you have started to snack and realize that you are deviating from your eating plan, it is essential that you give yourself constructive messages. Many binge eaters tell themselves that they have done a "terrible thing" and have proven that they have "no willpower." These are self-indulgent statements that merely set the stage for further problem eating. Instead, you should treat management of your urge to eat as a challenge. Ask yourself the question: "How can I keep my eating within bounds?" instead of making self-derogatory statements. Because your thoughts guide your actions, directing your thoughts constructively can help you to keep your actions in check.

In A Nutshell

Managing binge eating, then, begins with controlling your moods and planning your meals wisely. It also means that you should have a strategy ready that will allow you to break the chain of binge eating early and often so that you have the greatest possible number of opportunities to keep your eating within reasonable bounds. Panic is the greatest single threat about an eating binge. Preplanning and a realization that binging only means that the first set of limits was ineffective so a second line of defense is needed can both help to control the panic and to contain the damage that binges can do. Above all, when binging slows down your weight-control efforts, take the binge in your stride and continue with your self-management program at the earliest possible moment. Binging does not create disaster: overreaction to binges is the major villain.

16/ Planning What to Eat

Up to this point, you have been taught how to manage your urge to eat. Now it is time to talk about what to eat.

Weight is maintained when the body takes in just enough energy in the form of food to keep its vital processes going and its muscles active. Weight is gained when more energy is taken in than is needed for these two purposes, and weight is lost when energy consumption falls below energy need. In other words, *weight is a simple product of supply and demand.* When the supply and demand of energy are in balance, weight is maintained. When supply exceeds demand weight is gained, and when demand is greater than supply weight is lost.

When we take in more energy than we need at the moment, our bodies burn what they need and store most of the rest. Later, if energy demands become greater than outside energy supply, our bodies turn to their stores and burn some of their supply. When we gain weight we store energy against future needs, and when we lose weight we literally burn up some of this supply.

When we store extra energy for future needs, we do to ourselves the same thing that we do to our cars when we put gas in the tank. The average gas tank holds enough fuel to allow the car to cruise from 200 to 400 miles between filling stations. If the car's gas tank were enlarged so that it could hold 200 gallons instead of 20 gallons, it would have a greater cruising range. But 20 gallons of gasoline weighs under 200 pounds and 200 gallons weighs close to 2,000 pounds. To handle that added weight the car would have to be built much more sturdily, it would have to lose considerable maneuverability, and it would get fewer miles to the gallon. The same is true for humans. If we normally store enough energy for five or six days of life, but add to our supplies enough for fifty or sixty days, we strain our body structures, we curtail our mobility, and we get sharply reduced mileage from the food that we consume.

The energy balance equation is universal but it does not apply with equal efficiency to all people. Some overweight people eat more than some of the lean, as found when their behavior is observed in public eating places.[1] But many others eat as little or even less than the lean, with the major difference being not how much energy goes in, but how much energy goes out in the form of physical activity.[2] The balance between intake, output, and fat storage is not one of a simple two-plus-two-equals-four mathematics. Somewhere in the process, some people seem able to "waste" some calories: they eat a lot, do little, and still don't gain very much weight. Other people are very efficient and for them every calorie counts. For all, however, the basic weight-control formula is the same: cut intake relative to output to lose weight, and reverse the process to put weight on.

Our bodies store energy in three forms. Some energy is stored as *carbohydrates* (actually glycogen and sugar) in the bloodstream, muscles, and liver. This energy supply is very important because it is the immediately available fuel for the organs and it sustains life. A feeling of faintness can result when this supply falls below the necessary life-supporting level. Therefore, the body works hard to keep an adequate supply of glycogen or blood sugar at all times.

Energy is also stored as *protein,* which is the building block of its muscles and organs. The conversion of protein to energy could seriously weaken the body because tissue loss from any of its muscles, the heart, brain, and liver, or other organs can impair its ability to survive. Moreover, protein is a poor source of fuel. Protein supplies only 4 calories of energy per gram. (A calorie is the amount of heat—i.e., energy—needed to heat one gram of water, one degree centigrade.) And because protein is about 80 percent water, one pound of it would net only 450 calories or about one-sixth of the daily energy need of a typical young man. Because the body seems to have an inner wisdom, it turns to protein as an energy supply only after it has exhausted the energy that has been stored as fat.

Fat is the best of the body's energy supplies. It yields 9 calories per gram and, because fat is only 15 percent fluid, *one pound of fat yields 3,500 calories.* This is the critical number for all weight losers because, within small variations, the average man or woman who takes in an extra 3,500 calories—over a period of hours, days, or weeks—gains close to one pound of fat while the person who takes in 3,500 calories less than he or she burns—again over a period of hours, days, or weeks—will lose one pound of fat, give or take a little.

We can see the importance to reducers of the number 3,500 in the following illustration taken from the medical literature. Mrs. "Green" is a thirty-year old housewife who is five feet four inches tall. She weighs 225 pounds. We can assume for the purpose of this illustration that she normally needs 2,600 calories to keep her vital life-sustaining processes going and to supply the energy which she needs to go on about her business. If she cuts her daily food intake to approximately 1,200 calories, and if she maintains her usual level of activity, she would draw upon her energy reserves for 1,400 calories daily. In two days this would mean that she would burn up 2,800 calories' worth of fat tissues, in three days 4,200 calories' worth, and so on. Every day that she registers a 1,400-calorie deficit she could lose 0.4 pounds of fat, although this loss will not register on the scale every day. If her goal weight is 125 pounds she has 100 pounds to lose, losing 0.4 pounds per day, it should take her 250 days to reach her goal weight.[3]

Because the body can do nothing with extra energy other than to store it, taking in even a few extra calories every day can lead to a large aggregate weight gain. For example, eating one small extra cookie or one large extra apple per day (70 calories) would lead to the gain of an extra pound of fat every seven weeks, or between seven and eight pounds per year. Carried over a period of four or five years, this very small indulgence can lead to a very significant weight problem. Fortunately, however, the same pattern works in reverse. Eliminating one cookie or one extra fruit from your daily diet can lead to a very satisfying weight loss at year's end.

Because most of us are impatient, we are dissatisfied with the prospect of taking 250 days to achieve any goal, even one as important as losing 100 pounds. Some people try to speed up the process by using mechanical reducing aids. Others take pills with or without their doctor's prescription. Still others try to eat as little as possible, often without medical supervision.

There are three problems with all of these schemes. First, it is often either unhealthy or impossibly uncomfortable to follow them for very long. Second, during the process of losing weight no new constructive habits are learned. Therefore, maintaining the loss of weight is all but impossible. Indeed, research done on many of the tested quick-loss schemes (and most have not been researched) nearly always shows that weight lost in a hurry is regained just about as fast. This sets the stage for the third problem with rapid weight loss: if it leads to quick regains it can be quite bad for your health.

The chief of the Heart Disease Control Program of the United States Public Health Service has suggested that the "yo-yo" pattern of weight loss and gain may be worse for your health than just staying as overweight as you were in the first place.[4] He pointed out, for example, that (1) laboratory animals that are allowed to stay thin live longer than those that are allowed to overeat, underexercise, and therefore become fat; but (2) that those staying fat lived longer than those whose weight fluctuated between thinness and fatness. He also pointed out that cholesterol or fat deposits build up in the bloodstream while weight is being gained, and that there is no evidence that these deposits are lost when excess pounds are shed. Crushed self-esteem and the very real possibility of major problems in blood chemistry are just two of the unwelcome consequences of attempts to lose too quickly and too easily. Therefore, you will do well to pass by those wonder diets, devices, and drugs that may have been promoted by people who claim to have "discovered nature's long-buried secret."

What you need instead is a program that will lead to the loss of from one to two pounds per week, unless you are very much overweight and under a doctor's care.[5] Any program that brings you down too quickly is likely to bump you back up just as fast, and you'll be much the worse for wear.

Diets of from 1,100 to 1,400 calories per day for women, and of 1,500 to 1,800 calories per day for men, are likely to offer the opportunity for just such a gradual loss of weight. The lower end of the calorie range would be best for you if you are less active or are in the lower weight range for your sex and height, and you will need the higher end of the range if you are more active than most and if you are on the husky side compared to your peers.

The diet that you choose must have these four important characteristics beyond offering gradual loss of weight:

1. It must provide all of your minimum daily food requirements;
2. It must give you enough to eat so that you are not faced with constant hunger;
3. It must give you enough variety every day so that your desire for different tastes and textures is satisfied; and
4. Following the weight-loss program must provide you with an education for lifelong changes in what you eat.

If the program that you choose does not meet your body's daily nutritional needs, you will run the risk of suffering one of several serious nutritional inadequacies that could seriously impair your health. This will cause true hunger and malnutrition. If you eat so little that you are always hungry, you are likely to experience a tormented existence and quickly give up your diet. Your appetite will never rest. If you eat the same few foods day after day, the monotony will cause you to stray from your program. Again, your appetite will rear its nasty head. And if the diet that you follow is eccentric because it gives you little choice or requires you to eat foods that are not normally available, you will have little chance of following the program in the years after your weight goal has been reached.

To find a food plan that meets these requirements—gradual loss, nutritional balance, prevention of hunger, satisfaction to your appetite, and maintenance for life—you can go to many different sources. The nutrition clinic of your local hospital or public health department can offer advice. So, too, can your family doctor. You could also consult a responsible weight-control organization like "Weight Watchers," being sure that its food program was developed under professional supervision. You do not have to be a nutritional expert in order to plan your own program, but in choosing the plan you should have the benefit of professional advice.

A Sample Menu for the Week

Medical authorities recommend that 35 percent of the calories in our daily diets should come from fat, 45 percent from carbohydrates, and 20 percent from protein.[6]

Fats are our most concentrated source of energy. They also serve as carriers for certain vitamins and they contribute to the health of our blood, arteries, nerves, and skin.[7] We eat two kinds of fats. Saturated fatty acids are essential to our diets, but when we take in too many, we can suffer from the problem of unhealthy buildup of fats in our hearts and circulatory systems. Saturated fats are found in whole milk, butter, eggs, and the "hard" fat of red meats. Polyunsaturated fatty acids are also essential to our diets and they can be found in vegetable oils, nuts like almonds, pecans, and walnuts, and skim milk, among other sources. Our fat intake should be balanced between saturated and polyunsaturated fatty acids.

Carbohydrates are a source of energy and they help to regulate the metabolism of fats and protein. Carbohydrates come in three different forms. In one form they are simple sugars like those in honey and fruit, or so-called double or refined sugars. In another form they are starches found in grains. Their third form is cellulose, available in the skins of fruits and vegetables. Sugar is an energy source but when sugar is taken in, blood sugar levels rise. When the sugar intake has been utilized, the body feels a need for more sugar and so more and more sweet food is eaten. Starches are also an energy source but because they are chemically more complex than sugars, their digestion takes longer and they are therefore a slower acting energy supply. Cellulose is important because it provides bulk to our diets and bulk helps to regulate intestinal and bowel functions.

Some carbohydrates have been termed "empty calories." These include the refined sugars and starches that contain food energy but none of the vitamins, minerals, and trace elements that are essential to good health. Other carbohydrates like fruits and vegetables provide calories along with these health-sustaining elements.

Protein is the building material of our muscles, blood, skin, hair, nails, and organs. Aside from water, it is the most plentiful material in our bodies. The building blocks of protein are the twenty-two amino acids. Few natural proteins like a single kind of meat, fish, or poultry contain all of the amino acids that our bodies need. Therefore we must build into our diet a rich variety of proteins so that our amino acid needs are met.

Unfortunately, foods that are high in protein are also often high in saturated fat. Prime meat with marbleized fat is a good example. Therefore, it is important to buy the leanest meat possible and to trim the visible fat from it. It is also important to include at least three to five fish meals in your diet for the week; fish is a protein source with a lesser amount of saturated fat. Poultry, also high in protein, is low in saturated fat.

Figure 16.1 presents a *sample* seven-day menu plan that might be reported by a member of a Weight Watchers class. Notice that the basic allowances shown are those for women, with additional allowances of certain foods for adolescents and men. The following week, this member would be encouraged to follow set guidelines learned in class for preparing a menu plan with some different foods. This food plan:

- Does provide all of the essential nutrients;
- Does offer enough food to control hunger;
- Does provide sufficient variety so that food interest can be sustained; and
- Does offer a program that permits reeducation of lifelong eating habits.

This is the kind of plan that you must learn to develop with professional assistance.

FIGURE 16.1

A Sample Seven-Day Menu Plan*

	Monday
Breakfast	Grapefruit, 1/2 medium Poached Egg, 1 Whole Wheat Bread, 1 slice Skim Milk, 4 fl. oz. *Youth:* Add: Skim Milk, 8 fl. oz.
Luncheon	Tuna Fish, 3–4 oz. Mayonnaise, 2 tsp. Lettuce Tomato, 1 medium Peach, 1 medium

*Basic allowances are for women. Adjustments for Men and Youth are indicated. In addition to those shown, men and youth can add one or two fruit servings daily, and youth can add 8 fl. oz. of skim milk.

Sample 7-Day Menu Plan © Weight Watchers International, Inc., 1978

Beverage
Men and Youth: Add: Bread, 2 slices

Snack   Unflavored Yogurt, 4 fl. oz.

Dinner   Roast Chicken, 4–6 oz.
Baked Potato, 3 oz.
Margarine, 1 tsp.
Carrots, 1/2 cup
Apple, 1 medium
Beverage
Men: Roast Chicken 6–8 oz.

Snack   Skim Milk, 4 fl. oz.

Tuesday

Breakfast   Banana, 1/2 medium
Ready-to-Eat Cereal, 1 oz.
Skim Milk, 4 fl. oz.
Beverage
Men and Youth: Add: Bread, 1 slice

Luncheon   Camembert Cheese, 2 oz.
Rye Bread, 2 slices
Fresh Spinach and Mushroom Salad
Vegetable Oil, 1 tsp.
Beverage
Youth: Add: Skim Milk, 8 fl. oz.

Snack   Pear, 1 small

Dinner   Mixed Vegetable Juice, 8 fl. oz.
Broiled Fish, 4–6 oz.
Asparagus, 10 spears
Baked Butternut Squash, 4 oz.
Margarine, 1 tsp.
Green Salad
Vegetable Oil, 1 tsp.
Skim Milk, 4 fl. oz.
Beverage
Men and Youth: Add: Bread, 1 slice
Men: Broiled Fish, 6–8 oz.

Snack   Buttermilk, 6 fl. oz.
Strawberries, 1 cup

Wednesday

Breakfast   Orange Juice, 4 fl. oz.
Cottage Cheese, 1/3 cup
Cracked Wheat Bread, 1 slice

Skim Milk, 4 fl. oz.
Beverage

Luncheon   Salmon, 3–4 oz.
Tomato Wedges
Shredded Cabbage, 1/2 cup
Mayonnaise, 1 tsp.
Cucumber Slices
Pineapple, 1/4 medium
Beverage
Men and Youth: Add: Bread, 2 slices
Youth: Add: Skim Milk, 8 fl. oz.

Snack   Skim Milk, 8 fl. oz.

Dinner   Broiled Veal, 4–6 oz.
Enriched Rice, 1/2 cup
Margarine, 1 tsp.
Zucchini, 1/2 cup
Romaine Salad
Vegetable Oil, 1 tsp.
Applesauce, 1/2 cup
Skim Milk, 4 fl. oz.
Beverage
Men: Broiled Veal, 6–8 oz.

Snack   Bouillon, 1 packet

Thursday

Breakfast   Honeydew Melon, 2" wedge
Boiled Egg, 1
Enriched White Bread, 1 slice
Margarine 1 tsp.
Beverage
Youth: Add: Skim Milk, 8 fl. oz.

Luncheon   Tomato Juice, 8 fl. oz.
Sardines, 3–4 oz.
Pumpernickel Bread, 1 slice
Pickle, Celery and Carrot Strips
Nectarine, 1 medium
Skim Milk, 4 fl. oz.
Beverage
Men and Youth: Add: Bread, 1 slice

Snack   Buttermilk, 6 fl. oz.

Dinner   Broiled Liver, 4–6 oz.
Onions, 4 oz.

Cauliflower, 1/2 cup
Lettuce Wedge
Vegetable Oil, 2 tsp.
Beverage
Men and Youth: Add: Bread, 1 slice
Men: Broiled Liver, 6–8 oz.

Snack   Skim Milk, 4 fl. oz.

Friday

Breakfast   Grapefruit Juice, 4 fl. oz.
Hard Cheese, 1 oz.
Raisin Bread, 1 slice
Unflavored Yogurt, 4 fl. oz.
Beverage

Luncheon   Mushroom Omelet (2 eggs)
Green Salad
Vegetable Oil, 1 tsp.
Grapes, 12 medium or 20 small
Beverage
Men and Youth: Add: Bread, 2 slices
Youth: Add: Skim Milk, 8 fl. oz.

Snack   Mixed Vegetable Juice, 8 fl. oz.

Dinner   Broiled Pork Chop, 4–6 oz.
Broccoli, 1/2 cup
Corn, 1/2 cup
Margarine, 1 tsp.
Endive Salad
Vegetable Oil, 1 tsp.
Tangerine, 1 large
Beverage
Men: Broiled Pork Chop, 6–8 oz.

Snack   Skim Milk, 8 fl. oz.

Saturday

Breakfast   Blueberries, 1/2 cup
Uncooked Cereal, 1 oz.
Skim Milk, 4 fl. oz.
Beverage
Men and Youth: Add: Bread, 1 slice

Luncheon   Frankfurter, 3 oz.
Frankfurter Roll, 1
Sauerkraut, 1/2 cup

Cucumber Salad
Vegetable Oil, 1 tsp.
Orange, 1 small
Skim Milk, 4 fl. oz.
Beverage

Snack   Tomato Juice, 8 fl. oz.

Dinner   Shrimp, 4–6 oz.
Brussels Sprouts, 4 oz.
Margarine, 1 tsp.
Eggplant, 1/2 cup
Tossed Salad
Vegetable Oil, 1 tsp.
Skim Milk, 8 fl. oz.
Beverage
Men and Youth: Add: Bread, 1 slice
Men: Shrimp, 6–8 oz.

Snack   Plums, 2 medium
Youth: Add: Skim Milk, 8 fl. oz.

Sunday

Breakfast   Raspberries, 1/2 cup
Semi-Soft Cheese, 1 oz.
Rye Bread, 1 slice
Skim Milk, 4 fl. oz.
Beverage

Luncheon   Roast Turkey, 3–4 oz.
Baked Acorn Squash, 4 oz.
String Beans, 1/2 cup
Margarine, 2 tsp.
Skim Milk, 4 fl. oz.
Beverage
Men and Youth: Add: Bread, 2 slices

Snack   Fresh Fruit Salad, 1/2 cup

Dinner   Broiled Steak, 4–6 oz.
Sliced Tomatoes on Lettuce
Mayonnaise, 1 tsp.
Wax Beans, 1/2 cup
Whole Wheat Bread, 1 slice
Cantaloupe, 1/2 medium
Beverage
Youth: Add: Skim Milk, 8 fl. oz.
Men: Broiled Steak, 6–8 oz.

Snack   Unflavored Yogurt, 4 fl. oz.

Monitoring What You Eat

Once you have decided on what you should eat, it is a good idea to monitor your success in following the program that you have selected. For some purposes, keeping a complete "diary" of your food intake is important. For example, many members of Weight Watchers classes record their eating during a complete week from time to time in order to receive feedback from their lecturer about the appropriateness of their food choices. In general, however, a simple "yes/no" record can give you a great deal of information, enough to plan successful changes in your efforts to manage what you eat.

Figure 16.2 provides a useful simple record. Notice that it includes the same information about eating urges and behavior that you were asked to collect in Chapter 2 (Figure 2:1) but adds two additional columns.

In column 5 check:

"Yes" if you ate a food that is included in the food plan that you are following;
"No" if the food that you ate is *not* included in the food plan that you are following; and
"None" if you ate nothing at all.

In column 6 check:

"Yes" if you ate an allowable portion of the food that you selected;
"No" if you ate more than the allowable portion of the food that you selected; and
Leave blank if you did not eat during this hour.

If you eat nothing during any given hour, check the "None" box when the hour is over. If you eat something, check the "Yes" or "No" box for choice and for portion size

FIGURE 16.2

Expanded Personal Self-Monitoring Chart

Circle Day (1) Time	Sunday	Monday (2) Level of Your Urge to Eat	Tuesday	(3) Did You Eat? Yes	Wednesday No	Thursday	(4) Planned Action	Friday	(5) Did You Choose an Allowable Food? Yes	Saturday No	(6) Did You Take The Proper Amount? Yes	No
7:00–8:00												
8:00–9:00												
9:00–10:00												
10:00–11:00												
11:00–12:00												
12:00–1:00												
1:00–2:00												
2:00–3:00												
3:00–4:00												

4:00–5:00									
5:00–6:00									
6:00–7:00									
7:00–8:00									
8:00–9:00									
9:00–10:00									
10:00–11:00									
11:00–12:00									
12:00–1:00									
1:00–7:00									

before you eat the food that you have chosen. Research has shown that by doing your recording before you eat, you can provide yourself with one additional choice point and may give yourself a chance to stop your problem eating before it begins.[8] In this way, recording what you eat can help you to control your food intake and work toward improving your chances for success.

In evaluating information from the chart, it is important to make note of many different kinds of information, including the following:

1. How many hours on which days did you eat nothing at all?
2. How often did you manage to eat nothing even though your urge to eat was strong (e.g., "3" or "4")?
3. How many hours did you eat the correct portions of well-chosen foods?
4. How many hours did you choose the proper foods but choose portions that were a bit too generous?
5. How many hours did you choose the wrong foods and eat too much of these?

Data about your successes is *more* important than data about your mistakes. Use these data to build your confidence about your strengthening self-control. Data about your mistakes is information that you can use not as a cue for self-reproach but rather as a stimulus for creative action.

For example, if you learn that you make constructive food choices throughout the day, but have difficulty during the evenings, try to identify the daytime strengths that can help at night as well. If you find that you have difficulty in managing your eating with others but do very well alone, try to think of ways in which you change the social eating conditions so that you can make use of some of the strengths that you draw upon when you are alone.

In A Nutshell

Many people look for magic in the pantry. They look for special foods that will "absorb the calories" from other foods that they eat. They look for one or two foods that meet all of their needs so that they do not have to make decisions about what to eat. They look for very light diets and depend upon pills to blunt their appetites, fool their bodies into believing that they got more food than they actually have, or disrupt the digestion and absorption of the foods that they eat. Or they look for the severest of diets to take pounds off fast. All of these are short-range solutions—if they are solutions at all.

If you do not satisfy your basic needs for food, you will have difficulty following a program and are not likely to lose much weight.

If you do not re-educate yourself to chose food wisely as you lose weight, you will have little hope of maintaining your weight loss.

Therefore you must look at your weight-loss program as a time of personal renewal. Eat enough to feel satisfied and teach yourself how to choose food wisely while you motivate yourself with weight loss. This is the only safe way for you to take pounds off and have a reasonably good chance to keep them off.

Once you have chosen the food plan that you will follow, keep a record of your efforts from time to time. Evaluate your successes so that you can learn how to build on your strengths, and learn what you can from your mistakes so that you can build plans for greater self-mastery as your skills develop.

17/ Setting Your Sights

Most people have a goal weight in mind for themselves. Perhaps you remember how much you weighed when you last felt fit and looked trim. Or perhaps you have failed the mirror test (found those pounds you thought you'd lost), the belt test (gasped for breath when you closed the belt of your favorite pants or dress), or the pinch test (found too much meat when you took a pinch of your midriff), and then made a "guess-timate" of how much fat you saw or held. Believe it or not, there is a good chance that your guess is more right than wrong.

Despite decades of research on the subject, experts still seek a reliable and efficient means of evaluating weight.[1] Everyone who has ever stepped on a penny scale or been examined in a doctor's office is familiar with tables of weight by height and sex. Some of these tables show the average weight of people with different characteristics. Other tables show desirable weights—those measures of pounds per inch of person that insurance companies tell us correlate with average or better life expectancy. The problem with both tables is that the average person is heavier than the insurance companies tell us he or she should be, and even many with desirable weights can actually be obese. For obesity is a

218

condition that exists when people have more than a normal load of fat—about 20 percent of body weight for men, 30 percent for women. Unfortunately, weight and fat are not the same; for example, during World War II some navy recruiters were embarrassed to learn that they had rejected as too heavy some of the foremost football players of the day even though they had hardly an ounce of fat on their well-toned bodies.[2]

Tables 17.1 and 17.2 represent the best compromise that the Weight Watchers medical experts could find between average versus desirable weights, and between measures of bulk versus proportion of fat. Notice that for men and women, a range of weights is given for people of different ages and different heights. The charts are used at Weight Watchers classes in the following way:

1. Find the weight range for people of your sex, age, and height.
2. Plan to lose weight until you reach the upper limit of the range for people in the group to which you belong.
3. When you have reached this upper limit of your goal weight range, you can decide whether this weight is acceptable to you or whether you should go on losing some or all of the pounds that would bring you to the lower limit of your goal weight range.

It is not possible to pick an exact weight for yourself before you begin to lose weight. People differ in the proportions of their bodies that are made up of bone and muscle. If you have more of either, your most desirable weight may be a bit higher than would be true for others who have less bone and muscle but whose age and height are the same as yours.

If you have any doubt about how much you should weigh, it is a good idea for you to consult your family doctor. You can do this at the start of your efforts to lose weight, when

Table 17.1

Weight Range for Men

| Height Range Without Shoes | Age in Years | | | | 25 |
| | 18 | 19–20 | 21–22 | 23–24 | & Over |
Feet Inches	Weight in Pounds				
5 0 (60)	109–122	110–133	112–135	114–137	115–138
5 1 (61)	112–126	113–136	115–138	117–140	118–141
5 2 (62)	115–130	116–139	118–140	120–142	121–144
5 3 (63)	118–135	119–143	121–145	123–147	124–148
5 4 (64)	120–145	122–147	124–149	126–151	127–152
5 5 (65)	124–149	125–151	127–153	129–155	130–156
5 6 (66)	128–154	129–156	131–158	133–160	134–161
5 7 (67)	132–159	133–161	134–163	136–165	138–166
5 8 (68)	135–163	136–165	138–167	140–169	142–170
5 9 (69)	140–165	141–169	142–171	144–173	146–174
5 10 (70)	143–170	144–173	146–175	148–178	150–179
5 11 (71)	147–177	148–179	150–181	152–183	154–184
6 0 (72)	151–180	152–184	154–186	156–188	158–189
6 1 (73)	155–187	156–189	158–190	160–193	162–194
6 2 (74)	160–192	161–194	163–196	165–198	167–199
6 3 (75)	165–198	166–199	168–201	170–203	172–204
6 4 (76)	170–202	171–204	173–206	175–208	177–209

Table 17.2

Weight Range for Women

Height Range Without Shoes	Age in Years				
	18	19–20	21–22	23–24	25 & Over
Feet Inches	Weight in Pounds				
4 6 (54)	83–99	84–101	85–103	86–104	88–106
4 7 (55)	84–100	85–102	86–104	88–105	90–107
4 8 (56)	86–101	87–103	88–105	90–106	92–108
4 9 (57)	89–102	90–104	91–106	92–108	94–110
4 10 (58)	91–105	92–106	93–109	94–111	96–113
4 11 (59)	93–109	94–111	95–113	96–114	99–116
5 0 (60)	96–112	97–113	98–115	100–117	102–119
5 1 (61)	100–116	101–117	102–119	103–121	105–122
5 2 (62)	104–119	105–121	106–123	107–125	108–126
5 3 (63)	106–125	107–126	108–127	109–129	111–130
5 4 (64)	109–130	110–131	111–132	112–134	114–135
5 5 (65)	112–133	113–134	114–136	116–138	118–139
5 6 (66)	116–137	117–138	118–140	120–142	122–143
5 7 (67)	121–140	122–142	123–144	124–146	126–147
5 8 (68)	123–144	124–146	126–148	128–150	130–151
5 9 (69)	130–148	131–150	132–152	133–154	134–155
5 10 (70)	134–151	135–154	136–156	137–158	138–159
5 11 (71)	138–155	139–158	140–160	141–162	142–163
6 0 (72)	142–160	143–162	144–164	145–166	146–167
6 1 (73)	146–164	147–166	148–168	149–170	150–171
6 2 (74)	150–168	151–170	152–172	153–174	154–175

© Weight Watchers International, Inc., 1975

you reach the upper limit of your goal weight range, or at any point before you reach the lower limit.

Putting Your Weight into Perspective

After you have established your starting weight, and know your goal weight, you should start a graph that you will use to keep your weight in a lifetime perspective. Figure 17.1 shows the graph that Mrs. Green had used. It will teach you some very important lessons about weight control.

Mrs. Green weighed 180 pounds on Day 1 of her weight-loss effort. She is thirty-eight years old and is five feet five inches tall, so her goal weight range is 118–139 pounds. Realizing that loss of one and one-half pounds per week would be optimal for her, she estimates that she should reach the upper limit of her goal weight in approximately twenty-eight weeks (180 − 138 = 42 ÷ 1.5 = 28). Therefore she counts twenty-eight weeks and makes a dot at 138 pounds. Now she draws a very light line from 180 to 138 to give her expected rate of loss.

On the same day during each of the next twenty-eight weeks, Mrs. Green weighs herself at the same time of day, wearing the same clothing, on the same scale. She then puts a dot opposite the number of pounds that is appropriate, in the column for the current week. Going to a class for her weekly weighing or sharing her chart with a relative or friend can help to build her motivation to persevere.

Notice that Mrs. Green's actual experience differs somewhat from the line of her expected rate of loss. *This is true for everyone: our bodies are not perfect machines and they respond with some irregularity.*

First, it is clear that she lost more than three and one-half

FIGURE 17.1

Mrs. Green's Weight Chart

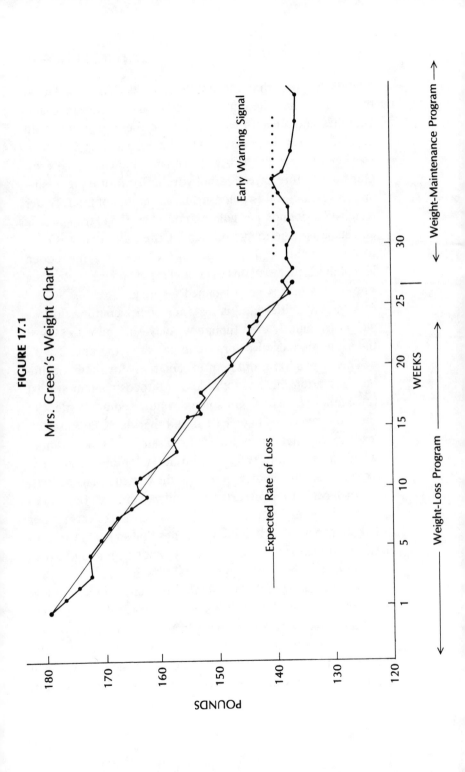

pounds during each of the first three weeks. This is explained by the fact that she cut back her intake of carbohydrates (starches and sugars), eating some of these physically and psychologically important foods but consuming less than was her style before she began to change her eating patterns. Our bodies store excess carbohydrates for future processing and this storage takes place in a large amount of fluid. Water weighs 8.2 pounds per gallon and, when the extra starches and sugars are no longer consumed, the water that was used to store the old supply is voided by the body. It is this sudden loss of fluids that explains the initial rapid and very satisfying rate of loss that is not sustained for long.

After this initial fluid is lost, our bodies continue to lose weight irregularly even though we may eat food with almost the same number of calories one day after the next.[3]

There are several different explanations for these inevitable fluctuations in the rate of loss. All foods contain at least trace amounts of salt. On some days the sodium content of the foods we eat is higher than on other days. Because salt leads to the retention of fluids, more salt means more liquid, which means more weight. Another salt–fluid problem is experienced by women prior to their menstrual periods. Women begin to retain extra salt midway through their menstrual cycles, and the salt leads to the retention of extra water (which explains the "bloated" feelings that so many premenstrual women experience), with the fluids beginning to pass a day or two before the menstrual flow begins.[4]

Another cause of the predictable fluctuation in weight loss is any change in the reducer's level of physical activity. Remember that weight is gained when energy intake is greater than energy utilization, and weight is lost when we use more energy than we consume; any change in physical activity will have an effect when food consumption is fairly constant.

Because many people tend to ignore physical activity as a factor in weight management, it would be wise to take a moment to consider what the scientists have taught us. A review of just two studies can set our thinking straight.

In the first study, a team of researchers at the University of Vermont made an attempt to have normal-weight young men gain weight by eating as much as three times their normal daily diet for periods of from three to five months. At the end of that time the men gained an average of only 10 percent of their body weight. But when the experiment was repeated in a prison setting, the inmate subjects gained as much as 25 percent of their body weight. The researchers concluded that restricted activity in the prison settings prevented the inmates from increasing their energy output to use up at least some of the extra calories, a feat that the lean subjects apparently accomplished as a means of keeping down their weight gain.[5]

The second study was the work of Dr. George Bray of the University of Southern California. He kept careful track of the food intake and energy output of patients participating in his weight-management program. As seen in Figure 17.2, his patients cut their energy utilization as soon as they reduced their caloric intake. In other words, when they started to take in fewer calories, they also began putting out fewer calories in the form of activity. The result was that *they undid much of the benefit they might have realized from their dietary efforts.*

Taken together, these studies show that many lean people gain weight slowly because they increase their activity in order to burn up the extra calories they consume. Heavy people, on the other hand, have a tendency to lose weight slowly because they cut down their activity in keeping with their reduced rate of energy consumption.

FIGURE 17.2

Activity Rate and Caloric Intake

Among Weight-Losing Adult Women*

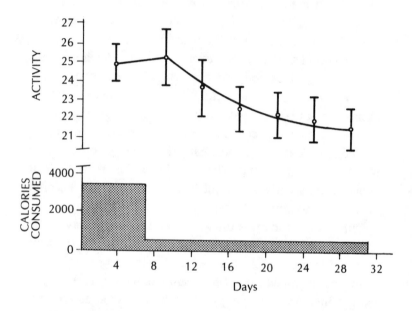

*Adapted from George A. Bray, Effect of caloric restriction on energy expenditure in obese patients, *Lancet*, 1968, *2*, 397–398.

In other words, when lean people consume more calories than their bodies need they seem spontaneously to increase the rate of their activity as a means of burning the extra calories rather than converting them to fat. Meanwhile, overweight people seem spontaneously to cut the rate of their activity when they eat less, making it more difficult for them to have a deficiency of the 3,500 calories which would allow them to lose each pound of fat. Knowing this can help weight-conscious people to focus their attention on how much they do as well as on what they eat while trying to lose weight.

Any gains in weight which are occasioned by salt intake will be lost when the salt and resulting fluid retention are dissipated. This might take a matter of weeks. The scale might show no weight change whatever, despite the best possible eating discipline, because the scale cannot differentiate between fat and fluid. But eventually the fluids must be sloughed and a dramatic weight loss will vindicate the weeks of hard work. However, when the plateau in weight loss is due to inactivity, the body is left with a surfeit of calories that it can only handle by conversion into fat.

Weight losers are very sensitive to the numbers recorded on their scales. When a weight loss is expected and the scale shows a plateau or a small gain, the reducer can become discouraged and decide that the diet plan is not paying off. Discouragement such as this can lead to the abandonment of highly successful weight-loss programs. When the scale shows a weight gain in a week when the reducer knows that overeating *has* occurred, an effort should be made to analyze how to overcome the obstacle that produced the overeating. It is very important that the reducer avoid the trap of "catastrophizing," of deciding that all is lost because of overindulgence for a moment, a day, or even a week. Instead, it is important to apply the principles that have been learned to gain control of the troublesome situation.

It is also possible for a weight *loss* to occur during a week in which overeating has taken place. Many people take this as a sign that they can lose weight without paying strict attention to what they eat. Unfortunately, they are making a tremendous error, an error that often leads to dramatic and disappointing diet failures. Such weight loss following overeating should be considered a temporary and unearned parole, not a reprieve. Again, it is very important to analyze the circumstances that brought on problem eating and to take steps to develop a more effective self-control strategy for the future.

When weight has not been lost despite the fact that there has been no overeating during the week, this disappointing result must be understood as a common and by no means fatal occurrence. The weight loser should be comfortable with the knowledge that fat is being burned as long as food intake is reduced and activity levels are maintained. Therefore, a larger than normal weight loss can be anticipated a few weeks hence if the reducer merely continues to follow the weight-loss program. Look carefully at Figure 17.1 and you will see the peaks and valleys that brought joys and sorrows to Mrs. Green as she worked on developing ever-higher levels of self-control.

Looking Ahead

Once Mrs. Green reached the upper level of her goal weight range, she felt that another ten-pound loss was needed. She persevered and lost those pounds, much as she expected. Then she entered a new phase of her weight-management program. She realized that her weight gains in the past always began one pound at a time. Even though she would have liked to think that she suddenly woke up one bleak morning twenty pounds heavier than when she had gone to bed, she had to reckon with the fact that this was never the case: she had had dozens of chances to reverse the process of weight gain before it got out of hand. Therefore, she decided to plan to keep her weight within a manageable range for the rest of her life.

Many people who succeed in maintaining the weight loss

through monthly attendance at Weight Watchers classes do this very thing. A study of those who maintained and those who failed to maintain their losses led to the observation that *maintainers permitted themselves a very narrow channel of weight fluctuation while regainers waiter longer to sound the warning bell.*

Those who maintained their losses felt that the time for action came when they strayed some two to five pounds above their goal. Regainers, on the other hand, did not believe that the time for action was upon them until their weights had risen twelve or more pounds. Unfortunately, the task of losing twelve pounds is far more formidable than that of losing five. Moreover, in the time that it took to gain back twelve pounds, many former bad habits could be strongly reestablished. For this reason, it is vitally important for you to add an *early warning system* to your weight chart. Then you will know it's time to act when taking action is still a simple matter. On Mrs. Green's chart, the dotted line at 130 pounds is such a signal. Any time that her weight moves above this warning line, she makes a special effort to regain her self-control and in that way is never far from her desired weight. Most people should work within a range of from two to five pounds.

IN A NUTSHELL

It is important for you to have a goal weight, but to realize that when you near your goal you may wish to adjust your goal slightly down. It is also wise for you to project the rate of your loss of weight, estimating your losses at between one and two pounds per week. Be prepared, however, to find greater losses at the beginning and plateaus or small gains once you are underway. These are natural events that may be due to salt–fluid retention or to changes in your rate of physical activity. However, if you continue to follow your food plan as you should, your fluid gains will eventually be lost. In addition, if you regain your normal pattern of activity after a brief rest brought on by illness, bad weather, or the pressure of work, this plateau, too, can be overcome.

After you reach your goal weight, you will slowly be able to add more food to your diet because you will no longer need the caloric deficit that produced your weight loss. These foods should be reintroduced slowly and you should learn just how much you can add and still maintain your weight.

Finally, when you do reach your goal weight, you should establish for yourself an early warning system. You should allow yourself a range of a few pounds within which your weight will fluctuate, and you should be ready to reestablish your weight-loss program whenever these limits are approached.

While you can add calories when you are at goal weight, you must still be as careful in meal planning during weight maintenance as you were during weight loss. Whether you are striving to reach or to maintain goal weight, you must be equally careful in managing your eating behaviors. All of the techniques mentioned in this book are useful in losing weight and in maintaining weight, and all should become your constant companions throughout your weight-maintenance efforts.

18 / Is Weight Maintenance Worth the Effort?

M any people concern themselves with weight control only when they worry about how they will look in a bathing suit or when they struggle to shed enough pounds to fit into their party clothes. Once the summer sun has set or the party's over, they relax into their weight-gaining ways until the next cosmetic crisis. Unfortunately, this "yo-yo" pattern of weight gain and loss is as harmful to their health as to their egos.[1] The risks of carrying excess weight are so great as to make weight management anything but a matter to take lightly. If you are even just a little overweight, there is a good chance that you suffer in several different ways without your necessarily knowing what is happening.

Health Risks

The most obvious risks are the ways in which those extra pounds pose a burden for your health. Despite the fact that few of us believe that the worst could happen to us, the worst does, in fact, happen to an alarming number of men and women in the prime of their lives. For every 100 average-weight men who die in their twenties and thirties, only 72 underweight men will die young. On the other hand, as opposed to the 100 average-weight men, 141 moderately overweight and 212 severely overweight men will give up many of the best years of their lives.[2] Not very many of the seriously overweight escape life-shortening illnesses.[3] Men who are as little as 20 percent overweight have more than ten times the normal chance of becoming hypertensive. Hypertension, in turn, can lead to heart disease and death.[4] Diabetes is another life-shortening disease and one that can cause misery along the way. Overweight women have a 450 percent greater than normal chance of becoming diabetic, but their risk returns to normal when they lose their excess weight.[5]

Hypertension and diabetes are only two of the many illnesses associated with excess weight. The list also includes nephrosis or kidney disease, gout, premature ovarian failure, the shortness of breath which is known as the "Pickwickian syndrome" (named for the red-faced, bloated, gasping character from the Dickens novel), and crippling muscle and bone injuries brought on by saddling the hollow bones and thin muscle fibers with the need to support far more weight than they were designed to carry.[6]

Some very heavy people do manage to live out their lives without suffering from any of the common medical complications of obesity. But most overweight people suffer from at least some of these illnesses and they worry about falling victim to others. And for every overweight person who escapes physical ill effects, scores of others feel the effect of excess weight on their vigor and vitality.

Psychological Risks

If the health risks of obesity are pandemic, so, too, are the psychological risks. Because it is believed that fewer than one in twenty obesities involve identifiable physiological causes,[7] many researchers have tried to explain obesity as the result of psychological defects. For these researchers, some emotional problem is construed as the chicken, and those extra pounds are viewed as the egg.[8]

Early observations were dominated by the work of psychoanalytic writers who speculated that the obese have a personality defect arising from early life experiences.[9] However, hypotheses about rejecting mothers and children's turning to food for solace have not withstood the test of research. Moreover, it was learned that many events found in the families of the obese beset the lean as well.[10]

Later researchers tried to isolate some feature of the personalities of the obese that could account for their distress. Here again, any trait found among the obese was found in the lean as well, and the net result of decades of research has been the conclusion that the obese are *not more*—and may even *be less*—neurotic than the lean.[11]

There is, of course, the possibility that future research will show that the obese start life with a different emotional makeup from the lean. But the chances that any such difference will separate the tens of millions of the obese from the tens of millions of the lean is small indeed: psychology is just not that powerful and profound!

If there is no intrinsic psychological difference between the obese and the lean, how, then, can we explain the fact that the overweight are heavy without necessary physiological cause? The problem is *learning, not neurosis*. The overweight *learn* to eat more food than they need to keep themselves going and they *learn* to be less active than is desirable for their health and happiness. They learn other things as well: to surround themselves with the wrong kinds of food; to permit their eating to come under the control of many different kinds of environmental events that should have no relationship to food; to mismanage the timing and behavioral dynamics of their eating; to allow potential pleasures in their lives to remain untapped so that food plays too central a role; and to turn to food as a means of coping with troubling emotions.

The overweight are likely to have *less than normal stimulation* from social, vocational, and avocational activities, *more than normal self-consciousness* about food intake and body size, and *less than normal satisfaction* with what they achieve and how they manage their lives. Just as food is allowed to play too central a role in their active lives, so, too, do the overweight allow their management of eating to become *the* way that they evaluate their own performance as they go from day to day. This can lead to hypersensitivity, lessened self-satisfaction, and lowered productivity. Therefore, just as weight loss can help you to lead a longer and healthier life, it can also help you to lead a happier life as well.

Social Risks

The social risks of obesity are more subtle than the health and psychological risks. The social risks stem mainly from the stereotypes with which many people—fat and thin alike —regard the overweight.

Stereotypes are a convenience: they offer us prepackaged ideas about other individuals and groups without our having to expend the effort to form our own ideas. They are self-serving: they usually help us to feel good about ourselves, often at the expense of others. They are powerful because they guide our behavior toward others and thereby set up self-fulfilling prophesies. They are also pernicious because they often result in lost opportunities for our personal development and in cruelty toward others.

Most people have stereotyped ideas about themselves, their relatives, their friends and enemies, members of their church and of other churches, residents of their city, state, and country as opposed to those who live in other cities, states, and countries, people of their own race as opposed to those of other races, and people of their social class and occupation as opposed to those in other classes and occupations. Most people also have stereotyped beliefs about others who look different in some way. Some people tend to be suspicious, afraid, and at the same time condescending to those who have orthopedic handicaps, who are blind, or who show some outward sign of illness or injury. Unfortunately, even a little extra visible flab around the midsection can also trigger stereotyped reactions.

It has been found, for example, that overweight children are often rejected by their peers and do not receive equal treatment from their counselors at school: they are viewed as less capable than the lean. It has been found that college entrance officials tend to consider overweight applicants as less bright prospects than those whose weight is in the normal range. In the same vein, employers tend to expect lightweights to be better workers than heavyweights. Whether any of these expectations is true—and research does *not* bear them out—doors are often closed to the overweight, who only seek equal opportunity with the lean.[12]

Often without ever knowing the cause, the overweight

experience prejudice at school, on the job, in the playground, and in every social situation. Their reaction can be disappointment and a turning against themselves; they feel that they have somehow brought about their own misfortune. To be painful, these experiences do not have to be gross: indeed, more subtle prejudice can cause the greatest level of self-questioning precisely because it is so difficult to pin down. Therefore the social risks of being overweight carry an importance equal to the risks of health and psychological weight-related stress.

In A Nutshell

Even a few extra pounds can pose a more serious problem than you have realized. Extra weight may not be a direct cause of mortal illness. However, it has been shown to set the stage for some life-shortening illnesses and for other illnesses that can cause considerable discomfort. Overweight can also bring on psychological stress if you are confronted day in and day out with a tangible reminder that you failed to meet your own expectations. Finally, overweight can cause you to be closed out socially and it can prevent you from enjoying many of the opportunities that might otherwise be yours.

Weight control involves some work; it's not all play. But even the work brings with it the pleasure of achievement as you succeed in one objective after another. Moreover, the effort that you expend in learning how to manage your urge to eat can pay further dividends. You are learning ways to control your behavior in other areas of your life. When these dividends are added to the major benefit—reduction in the risks of being overweight—the reward for weight control is great indeed, and surely enough to justify a year-round effort.

19/ There Is an Answer

Y ou know the risks of staying heavy and you have made a choice to work at being thin. Throughout this book you have been shown methods to improve many different aspects of your behavior. Behind these lessons has been a simple basic assumption:

PEOPLE ARE OVERWEIGHT
BECAUSE THEY DO NOT KNOW
HOW TO STAY AT THEIR DESIRABLE WEIGHT.

Obesity therefore equals misinformation and misguidance, not necessarily genetic bad luck or a weak character.

Many people rely upon diets to turn their weight around. But knowing what to eat is only part of the answer. Indeed, most weight-conscious people have a reasonably good idea of what goes into a healthful, weight-controlling diet. Therefore, it is as important to learn how to follow a food plan as to learn which plan to follow. Any effective weight-management system must train you to change your eating behavior, so that your food intake is what it ought to be. But the system must go further: it must also train you to minimize your urge to eat so that you are not bombarded by constant thoughts of food. This requires changes in far-reaching aspects of your lifestyle.

Because many programs focus only on food and not behavior, or because they focus on behavior in the narrowest sense and do not reprogram the urge to eat, many suffer from the so-called dieters' depression. This is a reaction to weight loss that includes feelings of disorganization, unhappiness, and tension. The people in whom these feelings are strongest are usually those who have been removed from their natural surroundings for weight loss, who were unusually depressed and anxious at the outset, and who follow crash programs that offer little behavioral retraining.[1] Under these conditions, adverse reactions are just what one would expect.

On the other hand, when fairly stable people attempt to lose weight in their natural environments, by following moderate dietary restrictions in a program that includes reeducation, they enjoy weight loss and positive mood change as well.[2] As an example, members attending a random sample of Weight Watchers classes across North America were less happy than their typical neighbors before they began their weight-loss efforts. Within five weeks of experiencing new levels of self-management success, however, their tested mood reactions were *better* than the norm.[3] So it is safe to assume that as you achieve control over your urge to eat, you will take new pleasure in many other aspects of your life as well.

Lest the wrong impression be given, weight loss is not without its stress. All changes create a certain amount of uncertainty and anxiety. We all take comfort in familiar aspects of our behavior and our life situations. Changes in our actions or in our environments almost always lead to a certain level of discomfort. For example, accepting a promotion with a higher level of pay and more interesting work can be a mixed blessing. With the greater rewards will come increased responsibilities: it is not uncommon for a person to wonder whether he or she will measure up. A party where there are many strangers is likewise a mixed blessing: it offers a chance to meet new people, but it also brings the risk of being rejected or ignored.

In the same way, developing new eating patterns means an important change. We are accustomed to the ways in which we use food, sometimes as a crutch and other times as a stimulus. When starting out on a new program, the weight loser has no assurance that the new patterns will be as satisfying as the old. We also develop patterns of social interaction that are influenced by our bodily dimensions. A very heavy person, for example, may be excluded from certain kinds of social interactions. Weight loss can open new doors but behind any of the doorways is the potential for failure. Therefore, shedding extra pounds can mean walking away from a convenient rationalization for inactivity—for some, a risky venture.[4]

You can expect to experience some tension: this is a natural consequence of your effort to learn new behaviors. And there may be times when you will be uncertain what to do as you seek new ways to handle old situations that triggered eating in the past. At times like these you will need imagination and support. Imagination will help you to see solutions to problems that appear to be irresolvable. Support will help you to take the actions that are necessary.

What is the best way for you to assure success in losing weight and maintaining weight? Some people are self-starters: they have the ability to stand aside from their normal routines and to find innovative solutions to their problems. They are able to risk change to reach an important goal. With the suggestions in this book, they can make a new beginning.

Other people work well with a partner. They can pair up with a relative or friend and share the mutual process of self-discovery and change. They can follow through on these suggestions and adapt them to their specific needs.

Most of us, however, are reluctant to reach out for new ways to meet old challenges. And most of us cannot sustain our motivation to change for more than a short time. We know that the development of new behaviors is a long and difficult process and our best bet may be to secure the support of more than one other person.

Those who have trouble going it alone, and who value group support rather than the support of a single individual, turn to groups for help in losing weight. However, all groups are not alike, and the differences significantly affect the quality of the services that they offer. In many respects, Weight Watchers is the standard-setter for weight-loss groups and you would do well to find a group that offers each of the following services, all of which are included in the Weight Watchers approach:

1. A food plan developed under professional supervision so that you can be certain that your basic nutritional requirements will be met while you lose weight and work to maintain your loss;

2. A food plan that can be adapted to the various stages of weight control—initial loss, any plateau experienced during weight loss, and the maintenance of your loss—so that you have guidance in food choice as your needs change through the progress that you make;

3. A socially constructive and positive interaction during meetings so that you receive the kinds of encouragement that you need in taking each successive step toward greater self-management;

4. Meetings that are clearly structured so that you know from

week to week exactly what you are expected to do in an effort to build your self-control;

5. A behavior-change program that helps you to alter many aspects of your eating-related behavior including the change of those aspects of your environment that contribute to over-eating;

6. A private weigh-in so that you get independent feedback each week about your progress; and

7. An approach that is taught to you in a manner that helps to build your understanding of the reasons behind each recommendation so that you can, if you wish, build upon the recommendations and personalize the program to meet many of your own needs.

Whether you go it alone, choose a partner, or join a responsible group, you are starting out on a new road that leads to self-discovery and new ways to manage your behavior. Treat each challenge that you face as an opportunity for new learning. Meet each challenge through a series of small, well-chosen steps. Realize that for every challenge you face you must choose one strategy that will help you break the behavior chain at a very early link, and a second strategy to call upon if the first fails to meet the test. Finally, be willing to hold *nothing* sacred in your life—be ready to change wherever change is needed. Do these things and the joy of self-control awaits you!

Notes

Chapter 1

1. A. P. Burdon, Obesity: A review of the literature stressing the psychosomatic approach, *Psychiatric Quarterly,* 1951, *25,* 568; R. I. F. Brown, The psychology of obesity, *Physiotherapy,* 1973, *59,* 216; A. J. Stunkard, Obesity and the denial of hunger, *Psychosomatic Medicine,* 1959, *21,* 282; A. J. Stunkard and S. Fox, The relationship of gastic motility and hunger: A summary of the evidence, *Psychosomatic Medicine,* 1971, *33,* 123; J. Hirsch, Discussion, *Advances in Psychosomatic Medicine* (Basel, Switzerland: Karger, 1972), *7,* 229; S. Lepkovsky, Fundamental problems of appetite control, in Nancy L. Wilson (ed.), *Obesity* (Philadelphia: F. A. Davis, 1969); D. J. McFarland, Recent developments in the study of feeding and drinking in animals, *Journal of Psychosomatic Research,* 1970, *14,* 229; N. E. Miller, C. J. Bailey, and J. A. F. Stevenson, Decreased 'hunger,' but increased food intake resulting from hypothamic lesions, *Science,* 1950, *112,* 256; O. W. Wooley, S. C. Wooley, and R. B. Dunham, Can calories be perceived and do they affect hunger in obese and nonobese humans? *Journal of Comparative and Physiological Psychology,* 1972, *80,* 250; P. T. Young, Physiologic factors regulating the feeding process, *American Journal of Clinical Nutrition,* 1957, *5,* 154.

2. See, too, G. R. Leon and K. Chamberlain, Emotional arousal, eating patterns, and body image as differential factors associated with varying success in maintaining weight loss, *Journal of Consulting and Clinical Psychology,* 1973, *40,* 474; and G. R. Leon and K. Chamberlain, Comparison of daily eating habits and emotional states of overweight persons successful or unsuccessful in maintain-

ing a weight loss, *Journal of Consulting and Clinical Psychology,* 1973, *41,* 108.

Chapter 2

1. Daniel Cappon, Review article: Obesity. *Canadian Medical Journal,* 1958, *79,* 568.
2. J. E. Meyer and V. Pudel, Experimental studies on food intake, *Journal of Psychosomatic Research,* 1972, *16,* 305.
3. J. Rodin, Effects of distraction on performance of obese and normal subjects, *Journal of Comparative and Physiological Psychology,* 1973, *83,* 68.
4. O. W. Wooley and S. C. Wooley, Short term control of food intake, in G. Bray (ed.), *Obesity in perspective* (Washington, D.C.: U.S. Government Printing Office, 1975).
5. A. S. Bellack, R. Rozensky, and J. Schwartz, A comparison of two forms of self-monitoring in a behavioral weight reduction program, *Behavior Therapy,* 1974, *5,* 514; R. G. Romanczyk, Self-monitoring in the treatment of obesity: Parameters of reactivity, *Behavior Therapy,* 1974, *5,* 531; R. B. Stuart, Behavioral control of overeating, *Behaviour Research and Therapy,* 1967, *5,* 357; R. B. Stuart, A three dimensional program of the control of overeating, *Behaviour Research and Therapy,* 1971, *9,* 177.

Chapter 3

1. W. H. Sebrell, Metabolic aspects of obesity: Facts, falacies and fables, *Metabolism,* 1957, *6,* 411.
2. Aaron T. Beck, *Cognitive Therapy and the Emotional Disorders* (New York: International Universities Press, 1962).
3. D. Meichenbaum, Toward a cognitive theory of self-control, in G. Schwartz and D. Shapiro (eds.), *Consciousness and self-Regulation: Advances in Research* (New York: Plenum Press, 1975).

Chapter 4

1. F. C. Shontz, Body image and its disorders, *International Journal of Psychiatry in Medicine,* 1974, *5,* 461.

2. John R. Buchanan, Five year psychoanalytic study of obesity, *American Journal of Psychoanalysis,* 1973, *33,* 30–35; A. Stunkard and M. Mendelson, Disturbances of body image of some obese patients, *Journal of the American Dietetic Association,* 1961, *38* 328; A. Stunkard and M. Mendelson, Obesity and the body image: I. Characteristics of disturbances in the body image of some obese persons, *American Journal of Psychiatry,* 1967, *123, 364;* A. Stunkard and V. Burt, Obesity and the body image: II. Age at onset of disturbances of body image, *American Journal of Psychiatry,* 1967, *123,* 1143.

3. P. F. Secord and S. M. Jourard, The appraisal of body cathexis: Body cathexis and self, *Journal of Consulting Psychology,* 1953, *17,* 343.

4. Myron L. Glucksman, Psychiatric observations on obesity, *Advances in Psychosomatic Medicine* (Basel, Switzerland: Karger, 1972), *7,* 194–216; M. L. Gluckman and J. Hirsch, The response of obese patients to weight reduction, *Psychosomatic Medicine,* 1969, *31,* 1–7.

5. P. Balch and A. W. Ross, Predicting success in weight reduction as a function of locus of control: A unidimensional and multidimensional approach, *Journal of Consulting and Clinical Psychology,* 1975, *43,* 119; D. W. Reid and E. E. Ware, Multi-dimensionality of internal versus external control: Addition of a third dimension and non-distinction of self versus others, *Canadian Journal of Behavioral Science,* 1974, *6,* 131; J. B. Rotter. Generalized expectancies for internal versus external control of reinforcement, *Psychological Monographs,* 1966, *80,* No. 1 (Whole No. 609).

6. V. Hays and K. J. Waddell, A self-reinforcing procedure for thought stopping, *Behavior Therapy,* 1976, *7,* 559.

Chapter 5

1. U.S. Bureau of the Census, *Statistical Abstract of the United States* (Washington, D.C.: U.S. Government Printing Office, 1975).

2. C. Lerza and M. Jacobson, *Food for People, Not for Profit* (New York: Ballantine, 1975), p. 165.

3. U.S. Bureau of the Census, *Statistical Abstract of the United States* (Washington, D.C.: U.S. Government Printing Office, 1975).

4. Ibid.

5. R. Choate, The sugar coated children's hour, in Lerza and Jacobson, *Food for People, Not for Profit.*

6. David M. Gardner, Deception in advertising: A conceptual approach, *Journal of Marketing, 39,* 40–46.

7. U.S. Bureau of the Census, *Statistical Abstract of the United States* (Washington, D.C.: U.S. Government Printing Office, 1975).

8. G. Tom and M. Rucker, Fat, full and happy, *Journal of Personality and Social Psychology,* 1975, *32,* 76–766.

9. P. Taylor, Packaging: The costs add up, *Environmental Action,* August 10, 1974.

Chapter 6

1. R. E. Nisbett and S. Gurwitz, Weight, sex and the eating behavior of newborns, *Journal of Comparative and Physiological Psychology,* 1970, *73,* 245.

2. S. Schachter and J. Rodin, *Obese Humans and Rats* (Washington, D.C.: Erlbaum/Halsted, 1974); D. Singh and S. Sikes, Role of past experience on food motivated behavior of obese humans, *Journal of Comparative and Physiological Psychology,* 1974, *86,* 503.

3. R. Goldman, M. Jaffa, and S. Schachter, Yom Kippur, Air France, dormitory food, and the eating behavior of obese and normal persons, *Journal of Personality and Social Psychology,* 1968, *10,* 117; L. S. Levitz, The susceptibility of human feeding behavior to external controls, in G. Bray (ed.), *Obesity in Perspective* (Washington, D.C.: U.S. Government Printing Office, 1975), p. 53; J. Mayer, L. Monello, and C. Seltzer, Hunger and satiety sensations in man, *Postgraduate Medicine,* 1965, *37,* 97; G. Tom and M. Rucker, Fat, full, and happy: Effects of food deprivation, external cues, and obesity on preference ratings, consumption, and buying intentions, *Journal of Personality and Social Psychology,* 1975, *32,* 761.

4. J. Rodin, Effects of distraction on performance of obese and normal subjects, *Journal of Comparative and Physiological Psychology,* 1973, *83,* 68; J. Rodin, The relationship between external responsiveness and the development and maintenance of obesity, in D. Novin, W. Wyrwicka, and G. Bray (eds.), *Hunger: Basic Mechanisms and Clinical Implications* (New York: Raven Press, 1976);

P. Pliner, Effect of external cues on the thinking behavior of obese and normal subjects, *Journal of Abnormal Psychology*, 1973, *82*, 233.

Chapter 7

1. S. C. Wooley, Physiological versus cognitive factors in short term food regulation in obese and nonobese, *Psychosomatic Medicine*, 1972, *34*, 62.
2. A. M. Isen and P. F. Levin, Effect of feeling good on helping: Cookies and kindness, *Journal of Personality and Social Psychology*, 1972, *21*, 384; I. L. Janis, D. Kaye, and P. Kirschner, Facilitating effects of "eating-while-reading" on responsiveness to persuasive communications, *Journal of Personality and Social Psychology*, 1965, *1*, 181.

Chapter 8

1. S. W. Hill, Eating responses of humans during dinner meals, *Journal of Comparative and Physiological Psychology*, 1974, *86*, 652.
2. D. J. Gaul, W. E. Craighead, and M. J. Mahoney, Relationship between eating rates and obesity, *Journal of consulting and Clinical Psychology*, 1975, *43*, 123; J. E. Meyer and V. Pudel, Experimental studies on food-intake in obese and normal weight subjects, *Journal of Psychosomatic Research*, 1972, *16*, 305; M. Wagner and M. I. Hewitt, Oral satiety in the obese and non-obese, *Journal of the American Dietetic Association*, 1975, *67*, 344.
3. A. R. Marston, P. London, L. Coiper, and N. Cohen, In vivo observation of the eating behaviour of obese and non-obese subjects, in A. Howard (ed.), *Recent Advances in Obesity Research*, vol. 1 (London: Newman Publishing Company, 1975).
4. O. W. Wooley, S. C. Wooley, and K. Turner, The effects of rate of consumption on appetite in the obese and non-obese, in A. Howard (ed.), *Recent Advances in Obesity Research*, vol. 1 (London: Newman Publishing Company, 1975), p. 212.
5. H. A. Jordon, Physiological control of food intake in man, in G. Bray (ed.), *Obesity in Perspective* (Washington, D.C.: U.S. Government Printing Office, 1975).

Chapter 9

1. G. G. Luce, *Biological Rhythms in Human and Animal Physiology* (New York: Dover Books, 1971).

2. H. Strughold, *Your Body Clock* (New York: Scribners, 1971).

3. S. Schachter and L. P. Gross, Manipulated time and eating behavior, *Journal of Personality and Social Psychology*, 1968, *10*, 98.

4. J. Rodin, Causes and consequences of time perception differences in overweight and normal people, *Journal of Personality and Social Psychology*, 1975, *31*, 898.

5. E. Wick, Overeating patterns found in overweight and obese patients, in M. E. Kline, L. L. Coleman, and E. K. Wick (eds.), *Obesity: Etiology, Treatment and Management* (Springfield, Ill.: Charles C. Thomas, 1974).

6. C. S. Chulouverakis, Facts and fancies in weight control: (1) Nibbling versus gorging, *Obesity and Bariatric Medicine*, 1975, *4*, 52.

7. G. A. Bray, Lipogenesis in human adipose tissue: Some effects of nibbling and gorging, *Journal of Clinical Investigation*, 1972, *51*, 537; P. S. Wadhwa, E. A. Young, K. Schmidt, C. E. Elson, and D. Pringle, Metabolic consequences of feeding frequency in man, *American Journal of Clinical Nutrition*, 1973, *26*, 123; C. M. Young, D. L. Frankel, S. S. Scanlan, V. Simko, and L. Lutwak, Frequency of feeding, weight reduction, and nutrient utilization, *Journal of the American Dietetic Association*, 1971, *59*, 473.

8. P. Fabray, J. Fodor, Z. Hejl, and T. Braun, The frequency of meals: Its relationship to overweight, hypercholesterolemia and decreased glucose tolerance, *Lancet*, 1964, *2*, 614; F. Fabray, *Feeding Patterns and Nutritional Adaptations* (London: Butterworths, 1969); P. Fabray, J. Fodor, Z. Hejl, H. Geizerova, and O. Balcarova, Meal frequency and ischaemic heart-disease, *Lancet*, 1968, *2*, 190.

9. Editors, Feeding patterns in resistant obesity, *Food and Nutrition Notes and Reviews*, 1974, *31*, 34; J. F. Munro, D. A. Seaton, and L. J. P. Duncan, Treatment of 'refractory obesity' with a diet of five meals a day, *British Medical Journal*, 1966, *3*, 950; D. A. Seaton and L. J. P. Duncan, Treatment of 'refractory obesity' through a diet of two meals a day, *Lancet*, 1964, *2*, 612; C. M. Young, S. S. Scanlan, C. M. Topping, V. Simko, and L. Lutwak, Frequency of feeding, weight reduction, and body composition, *Journal of the American Dietetic Association*, 1971, *59*, 466.

Chapter 10

1. J. A. Brilat-Savarin, *The Physiology of Hunger* (New York: Dover, 1960).

2. S. Lepkovsky, Fundamental problems of appetite control, in N. L. Wilson (ed.), *Obesity* (Philadelphia: F. A. Davis, 1969).

3. P. H. Linton, M. Conley, C. Kuechenmeister, and H. McClusky, Satiety and obesity, *American Journal of Clinical Nutrition,* 1972, *25,* 386.

4. R. G. Campbell, S. A. Hashim, and T. V. Van Italie, Studies of food intake regulation in man, *New England Journal of Medicine,* 1972, *25,* 1402; J. M. Price and J. Grinker, Effects of degree of obesity, food deprivation, and palatability on eating behavior of humans, *Journal of Comparative and Physiological Psychology,* 1973, *85,* 265; H. A. Jordon, W. F. Wieland, S. P. Zebley, E. Stellar, and A. J. Stunkard, Direct measurement of food intake in man: A method of objective study of eating behavior, *Psychosomatic Medicine,* 1966, *28,* 836.

5. B. C. Walike, H. A. Jordon, and E. Stellar, Preloading and the regulation of food intake in man, *Journal of Comparative and Physiological Psychology,* 1969, *68,* 327; O. W. Wooley, S. C. Wooley, and R. B. Dunham, Can calories be perceived and do they affect hunger in obese and nonobese humans? *Journal of Comparative and Physiological Psychology,* 1972, *80,* 250; J. E. Meyer and V. Pudel, Experimental studies on food intake in obese and normal weight subjects, *Journal of Psychosomatic Research,* 1972, *16,* 305; O. W. Wooley and S. C. Wooley, The experimental psychology of obesity, in J. J. Silverstone (ed.), *Obesity: Pathogenesis and Management* (Acton, Mass.: Publishing Sciences Group, 1975); J. LeMagnen, Peripheral and systematic actions of food in the caloric regulation of intake, *Annals of the New York Academy of Science,* 1969, *157,* 1126; Henry A. Jordon, Physiological control of food intake in man, in G. Bray (ed.), *Obesity in Perspective* (Washington, D.C.: U.S. Government Printing Office, 1975).

6. A. J. Stunkard, Eating patterns and obesity, *Psychiatric Quarterly,* 1959, *33,* 284.

7. R. J. McKenna, Some effects of anxiety level and food cues on the eating behavior of obese and normal subjects: A comparison of the Schachterian and psychosomatic conceptions, *Journal of Personality and Social Psychology,* 1972, *22,* 311; S. Schachter and L. Gross, Eating and the manipulation of time, *Journal of Personality and Social Psychology,* 1968, *10,* 98.

8. G. G. Luce, *Biological Rhythms in Human and Animal Physiology*

(New York: Dover Books, 1971); J. M. Price and J. Grinker, Effects of degree of obesity, food deprivation and palatibility on eating behavior of humans, *Journal of Comparative and Physiological Psychology,* 1973, *85,* 265.

Chapter 11

1. G. A. Devos and A. E. Hippler, Cultural psychology: Comparative study of human behavior, in G. Lindzey and E. Aronson (eds.), *The Handbook of Social Psychology* (Reading, Mass.: Addison-Wesley 1969); S. Staurfer, A. Jundsain, R. Williams, M. Smith, I. Janis, S. Star, and L. Cottrell, Jr., *The American Soldier: Combat and Its Aftermath,* vol. 2 (Princeton, N.J.: Princeton University Press, 1949); E. J. Webb, R. Campbell, D. Schwartz, and L. Sechrest, *Unobtrusive Measures, Nonreactive Research in the Social Sciences* (Chicago: Rand McNally, 1966).

2. E. E. Abramson and R. A. Wunderlich, Anxiety, fear and eating: A test of the psychosomatic concept of obesity, *Journal of Abnormal Psychology,* 1972, *70,* 317; E. H. Conrad, Psychogenic Obesity: The Effects of Social Rejection Upon Hunger, Food Craving, Food Consumption, and the Drive-reduction Value of Eating for Obese vs. Normal Individuals (Ph.D. dissertation, New York University, 1969); C. P. Herman and J. Polivy, Anxiety, restraint and eating behavior, *Journal of Abnormal Psychology,* 1975, *84,* 666; J. McKenna, Some effects of anxiety level and food cues on the eating behavior of obese and normal subjects: A comparison of the Schachterian and psychosomatic conceptions, *Journal of Personality and Social Psychology,* 1972, *22,* 311; S. Schachter, R. Goldman, and A. Gordon, Effects of fear, food deprivation, and obesity on eating, *Journal of Personality and Social Psychology,* 1968, *10,* 91.

3. A. J. Lange and P. Jakubowski, *Responsible Assertive Behavior* (Champaign, Ill.: Research Press, 1976).

4. P. Jakubowski, A discrimination measure of assertion concepts (unpublished manuscript, University of Missouri, St. Louis, 1975; reproduced with the author's permission).

5. H. Benson, Your innate asset for combatting stress, *Harvard Business Review,* 1974, *52,* 49.

6. G. A. Marlatt and J. K. Marques, Meditation, self-control and alcohol use, in R. B. Stuart (ed.), *Behavioral Self-Management: Tactics and Outcomes* (New York: Brunner/Mazel, 1977).

7. D. J. Goleman and G. E. Schwartz, Meditation as an intervention

in stress reactivity, *Journal of Consulting and Clinical Psychology,* 1976, *44,* 456; D. H. Shapiro and S. M. Zifferblatt, Zen meditation and behavioral self-control: Similarities, differences, and clinical applications, *American Psychologist,* 1976, *31,* 519; R. K. Walace and H. Benson, The physiology of meditation, *Scientific American,* 1972, *226,* 85.

8. J. Wolpe, *The Practice of Behavior Therapy.* (New York: Pergamon Press, 1969).

Chapter 12

1. I. Karacan, R. L. Williams, P. J. Salis, and C. J. Hursh, New approaches to the evaluation and treatment of insomnia, *Psychosomatics,* 1971, *12,* 81; A. McGie and S. M. Russel, The subjective assessment of normal sleep patterns, *Journal of Mental Science,* 1962, *108,* 642.

2. R. J. Berger, Bioenergetic functions of sleep and activity rhythms and their possible relevance to aging, *Federation Proceedings,* 1975, *34,* 97; W. B. Webb, Sleep as an adaptive response, *Perceptual and Motor Skills,* 1974, *38,* 1023.

3. L. C. Johnson, Are stages of sleep related to waking behavior? *American Scientist,* 1973, *61,* 326; M. A. Sackner, J. Landa, T. Forrest, and D. Greeneltch, Periodic sleep apnea, *Chest,* 1975, *67,* 164; J. M. Taub and R. J. Berger, Acute shifts in the sleep-wakefulness cycle: Effects of performance and mood, *Psychosomatic Medicine,* 1974, *36,* 164; W. B. Webb, Sleep behavior as a biorhythm, in W. P. Colquhoun (ed.), *Biological Rhythms and Human Performance* (New York: Academic Press, 1971); L. J. Monroe, Psychological and physiological differences between good and poor sleepers, *Journal of Abnormal Psychology,* 1967, *72,* 255.

4. J. M. Taub and R. J. Berger, Performance and mood following variations in the length of timing of sleep, *Psychophysiology,* 1973, *10,* 559; J. M. Taub and R. J. Berger, Acute shifts in the sleep-wakefulness cycle, loc. cit.; J. M. Taub and R. J. Berger, The effects of changing the phase and duration of sleep, *Journal of Experimental Psychology: Human Perception and Performance,* 1976, *2,* 30; J. M. Taub, P. E. Tangua, and D. Clarkson, Effects of daytime naps on performance and mood in a college student population, *Journal of Abnormal Psychology,* 1976, *85,* 210; R. T. Wilkinson, After effect of sleep deprivation, *Journal of Experimental Psychology,* 1973, *66,* 439.

5. M. W. Johns, T. J. A. Gay, J. P. Masterton, and D. W. Bruce, Relationship between sleep habits, adrenocortical activity and personality, *Psychosomatic Medicine,* 1971, *33,* 499; I. Karacan, R. L. Williams, R. C. Littell, and P. J. Salis, Insomniacs: Unpredictable and ideocyncratic sleepers, in *Sleep: Physiology, Biochemistry, pharmacology, clinical implications: First European Congress on Sleep research* (Basel, Switzerland: Karger, 1973); I. Karacan, R. L. Williams, P. J. Salis, and C. J. Hursch, New approaches to the evaluation and treatment of insomnia, loc. cit.; L. J. Monroe, Psychological and physiological differences between good and poor sleepers, loc. cit.

6. R. D. Coursey, M. Buschbaum, and B. L. Frankel, Personality measures and evoked responses in chronic insomniacs, *Journal of Abnormal Psychology,* 1975, *84,* 239; W. C. Dement and C. Guilleminault, Sleep disorders: The state of the art, *Hospital Practice,* 1973, *8,* 57; S. N. Haynes, D. R. Follingstad, and W. T. McGowan, Insomnia: Sleep patterns and anxiety level, *Journal of Psychosomatic Research,* 1974, *18,* 69; A. McGhie, and S. M. Russell, The subjective assessment of normal sleep patterns, loc. cit.

7. A. H. Crisp and E. Stonehill, *Sleep, Nutrition and Mood* (New York: Wiley, 1976).

8. J. M. Taub, P. R. Tanguay, and D. Clarkson, Effects of daytime naps on performance and mood in a college student population, loc. cit.

9. A. H. Crisp and E. Stonehill, The relationship between weight change and sleep: A study of psychiatric outpatients, in *Sleep: Physiology biochemistry, psychology, pharmacology, clinical implications: First European Congress on Sleep Research* (Basel, Switzerland: Karger, 1973); A. H. Crisp and E. Stonehill, Sleep patterns, daytime activity, weight changes and psychiatric status: A study of three obese patients, *Journal of Psychosomatic Research,* 1970, *14,* 353; V. T. Karadzic, Physiological changes resulting from total sleep deprivation, in *Sleep: Physiology, biochemistry, psychology, pharmacology, clinical implications: First European Congress on Sleep Research* (Basel, Switzerland: Karger, 1973); P. Naitoh, R. O. Pasnau, and E. J. Kollar, Psychophysiological changes after prolonged deprivation of sleep, *Biological Psychiatry,* 1971, *3,* 309; O. Petre-Quadens and J. D. Schlag, *Basic Sleep Mechanisms* (New York: Academic Press, 1971); M. A. Sackner, J. Landa, T. Forrest, and D. Greeneltch, Periodic sleep apnea, loc. cit.

10. G. S. Tune, Sleep and wakefulness in normal human adults, *British Medical Journal,* 1968, *2,* 269.

11. L. J. Monroe, Psychological and physiological differences between good and poor sleepers, loc. cit.

12. Ibid.

13. U. J. Javonovic, Suggestions for the treatment of sleep disturbances and conclusions, *Sleep: Physiology, biochemistry, psychology, pharmacology, clinical implications: First European Congress of Sleep Research* (Basel, Switzerland: Karger, 1973).

14. A. McGhie and S. M. Russel, The subjective assessment of normal sleep patterns, loc. cit.; R. Spiegel, A survey of insomnia in the San Francisco Bay area, cited in C. E. Thoresen, and T. J. Coates, Behavioral treatments for insomnia: A promise to be fulfilled, *Psychological Bulletin*, 1975, *83*, 340; I. Karacan, R. L. Williams, P. J. Salis, and C. J. Hursch, New approaches to the evaluation and treatment of insomnia, loc. cit.; I. Oswald, L. Adamson, and R. Norton, EEG, sleep and dependence studies of hypnotics, in *Sleep: Physiology, Biochemistry, Pharmacology, Clinical Implications: First European Congress on Sleep Research* (Basel, Switzerland: Karger, 1973).

15. F. Baekeland and R. Lansky, Exercise and sleep patterns in college atheletes, *Perception and Motor Skills*, 1966, *23*, 1203; J. Hobson, Sleep after exercise, *Science*, 1968, *162*, 1503; J. Matsumoto, T. Hihisho, T. Suto, T. Sadahiro, and M. Miyoshi, Influence of fatigue on sleep, *Nature*, 1968, *218*, 177.

16. S. N. Haynes, D. R. Follingstad, and W. T. McGowan, Insomnia: Sleep patterns and anxiety level, loc. cit.; S. N. Haynes, M. G. Price, and J. B. Simons, Stimulus control treatment of insomnia, *Journal of Behavior Therpay and Experimental Psychiatry*, 1975, *6*, 279.

17. T. D. Borkovec and D. C. Fowles, Controlled investigation of effects of progressive and hypnotic relaxation on insomnia, *Journal of Abnormal Psychology*, 1973, *82*, 153; T. D. Borkovec and T. C. Weerts, Effects of progressive relaxation on sleep disturbance: An electroencephalographic evaluation, *Psychosomatic Medicine*, 1976, *33*, 173; J. H. Geer and E. S. Katkin, Treatment of insomnia using a variant of systematic desensitization, *Journal of Abnormal Psychology*, 1966, *71*, 161; E. Jacobson, *Progressive relaxation* (Chicago: University of Chicago Press, 1938).

18. R. D. Coursey, M. Buschbaum, and B. L. Frankel, Personality measures and evoked responses in chronic insomniacs, loc. cit.; D. Evans and I. Bond, Reciprocal inhibition therapy and classical conditioning in the treatment of insomnia, *Behavior Research and Therapy*, 1969, *7*, 323; M. Kahn, B. Baker, and J. Weiss, Treatment

of insomnia by relaxation training, *Journal of Abnormal Psychology,* 1968, *73,* 556.

Chapter 13

1. S. M. Garn, The origins of obesity, *Arcchives of American Journal of Diseases of Children,* 1976, *130,* 465; S. M. Garn and Dianne C. Clark, Trends in fatness and the origins of obesity, *Pediatrics,* 1976, *57,* 4431.
2. J. Bauer, *Institution and Disease* (New York: Gruen and Stratton, 1949); S. M. Garn and Dianne C. Clark, Trends in fatness and the origins of obesity, loc. cit.; Matsuki and Yoda, Familial occurrence of obesity: An observation about height and weight of college women and their parents, *Keio Journal of Medicine,* 1971, *20,* 135.
3. L. H. Newburgh, Obesity, *Archives of Internal Medicine,* 1942, *70,* 1033.
4. S. M. Garn, Personal Communication, June 24, 1976; Matsuki and Yoda, Familial occurrence of obesity, loc. cit.; R. H. Osborne and F. W. DeGeorge, *Genetic Basis of Morphological Variation* (Cambridge, Mass.: Harvard University Press, 1959); I. R. Shenker, V. Fisichelli, and J. Lang, Weight differences between foster infants of overweight and underweight foster mothers, *Journal of Pediatrics,* 1974, *84,* 715.
5. J. Hirsch, J. L. Knittle, and L. B. Salans, Cell lipid content and cell number in obese and nonobese human adipose tissue, *Journal of Clinical Investigation,* 1966, *45,* 1023; J. Hirsch, Adipose cellularity in relation to human obesity, *Advances in Internal Medicine,* 1971, *17,* 289; D. Brook, J. K. Lloyd, and O. H. Wolf, Relation between age of onset of obesity and size and number of adipose cells, *British Medical Journal,* 1972, *2,* 25; B. Salans, S. W. Cushman, and R. E. Weismann, Studies of human adipose tissue, *Journal of Clinical Investigation,* 1973, *52,* 929; P. Bjorntrop and L. Sjostrom, Number and size of adipose tissue fat cells in relation to metabolism in human obesity, *Metabolism,* 1971, *20,* 702.
6. R. D. G. Creery, Infantile overnutrition, *British Medical Journal,* 1972, *23,* 727; R. O. Fisch, M. K. Belek, and R. Ulstrom, Obesity and leanness at birth and their relationship to body habits in later childhood, *Pediatrics,* 1975, *56,* 521; A. G. L. Witelaw, The association of social class and sibling number with skinfold thickness in London schoolboys, *Human Biology,* 1971, *43,* 414.

7. T. R. Collins, Infantile obesity, *American Family Physician*, 1975, *11*, 162; L. S. Taitz, Overfeeding in infancy, *Proceedings of the Nutrition Society*, 1974, *33*, 113; Erica F. Wheeler, The problem of obesity in children, *Nursing Times*, 1972, *68*, 711.

8. R. L. Huenemann, Food habits of obese and nonobese adolescents, *Postgraduate Medicine*, 1972, *51*, 99.

9. S. L. Hammar, M. M. Campbell, V. A. Campbell, N. L. Moores, C. Sareen, F. J. Gareis, and B. Lucas, An interdisciplinary study of adolescent obesity, *Journal of Pediatrics*, 1972, *80*, 373; M. A. Hinton, E. S. Eppright, and H. Chadderdon, Eating behavior and dietary intake of girls 12 to 14 years old, *Journal of the American Dietetic Association*, 1963, *43*, 233; E. J. Kahn, Obesity in children: Identification of a group at risk in a New York ghetto, *Journal of Pediatrics*, 1970, *77*, 771; E. J. Stanley, H. H. Glaser, D. G. Levin, P. A. Adams, and I. L. Coley, Overcoming obesity in adolescents, *Clinical Pediatrics*, 1970, *9*, 29.

10. B. A. Bullen, R. B. Reed, and J. Mayer, Physical activity of obese and nonobese adolescent girls appraised by motion picture sampling, *American Journal of Clinical Nutrition*, 1964, *14*, 211; R. I. Huenemann, L. R. Shapiro, and M. C. Hampton, Teenagers' activities and attitudes toward activity, *Journal of the American Dietetic Association*, 1967, *51*, 433; M. L. Johnson, B. S. Burke, and J. Mayer, Relative importance of inactivity and overeating in the energy balance of obese high school girls, *American Journal of Clinical Nutrition*, 1956, *4*, 37; P. A. Stefanik, F. P. Heald, and J. Mayer, Caloric intake in relation to energy output of obese and non-obese adolescent boys, *American Journal of Clinical Nutrition*, 1959, *7*, 55.

11. P. A. Stefanik, F. P. Heald, and J. Mayer, Caloric intake in relation to energy output of obese and non-obese adolescent boys, loc. cit.; R. L. Huenemann, Food habits of obese and non-obese adolescents, *Postgraduate Medicine*, 1972, *51*, 99; J. B. G. A. Durnin, M. E. Lonergan, J. Good, and E. Ewan, A cross-sectional nutritional and anthropometric study, with an interval of 7 years on 611 adolescent school children, *British Journal of Nutrition*, 1974, *32*, 169; E. M. Hutson, N. L. Cohen, N. D. Hunke, R. C. Steinkamp, M. H. Rourke, and H. E. Walsh, Measures of body fat and related factors in normal adults, *Journal of the American Dietetic Association*, 1965, *47*, 179; M. C. McCarthy, Dietary and activity patterns of obese women in Trinidad, *Journal of the American Dietetic Association*, 1966, *48*, 33; G. A. Rose and R. T. Williams, Metabolic studies on large and small eaters, *British Journal of Nutrition*, 1961, *15*, 1.

12. S. Abraham and M. Nordsieck, Relationship of excess weight in children and adults, *Public Health Reports,* 1960, *75,* 263; F. P. Heald and M. A. Khan, Teenage obesity, *Pediatric Clinics of North America,* 1973, *20,* 807; J. K. Lloyd, O. H. Wolff, and W. S. Sheland, Childhood obesity: Long term studies of height and weight, *British Medical Journal,* 1961, *2,* 45.

13. F. P. Heald, Treatment of obesity in adolescence, *Postgraduate Medicine,* 1972, *51,* 109.

14. Richard B. Stuart and William J. Lederer, *Caring Days: Techniques for Improving Marriages* (New York: W. W. Norton, in press).

15. D. H. Karpowitz and F. Zeis, Personality and behavior differences of obese and non-obese adolescents, *Journal of Consulting and Clinical Psychology,* 1975, *43,* 886.

16. Richard B. Stuart and William J. Lederer, *Caring Days.*

17. L. S. Levitz, The susceptibility of human feeding behavior to external controls, in G. Bray (ed.), *Obesity in Perspective* (Washington, D. C., U.S. Government Printing Office, 1975).

Chapter 14

1. Food and Nutrition Board, National Research Council, *Recommended Dietary Allowances* (Washington, D.C.: National Academy of Sciences, 1974).

2. F. Konishi, Food energy equivalents of various activities, *Journal of the American Dietetic Association,* 1965, *46,* 186.

3. D. L. Costill and E. L. Fox, Energetics of marathon running, *Medicine and Science in Sports,* 1969, *1,* 81.

4. H. A. deVries and D. Gray, After effects of exercise upon resting metabolic rate, *Research Quarterly,* 1963, *34,* 314.

5. J. N. Morris, J. A. Heady, P. A. B. Raffle, C. G. Roberts, and J. W. Parks, Coronary heart disease and physical activity of work, *Lancet,* 1953, *2,* 1053; H. L. Taylor, E. Lepetar, A. Keys, W. Parlin, H. Blackborn, and T. Puchner, Death rates among physically active and sedentary employees of the railway industry, *American Journal of Public Health,* 1962, *52,* 1967; W. B. Kannel, P. Sorlie, and P. McNamara, The relation of physical activity to risk of coronary heart disease: The Framingham study, in O. A. Larson and R. O. Malmborg (eds.), *Coronary Heart and Physical Fitness* (Baltimore: University Park Press, 1971); E. R. Buskirk, Cardiovascular adaptation to physical effort in health men, in J. R. Naughton and H. R.

Hellerstein (eds.), *Exercise Testing and Training in Coronary Heart Disease* (New York: Academic Press, 1973); S. M. Fox and J. L. Boyer, Physical activity and coronary heart disease, in H. H. Clarke (ed.), *Physical Fitness Research Digest* (Washington, D.C.: The President's Council on Physical Fitness and Sports, 1972); R. H. Rochelle, Blood plasma cholesterol changes during a physical training program, *Journal of Sports Medicine and Physical Fitness,* 1961, *1,* 63; H. L. Taylor, Relationship of physical activity to serum cholesterol concentration, in F. F. Rosenbaum and E. L. Belknap (eds.), *Work and the Heart* (New York: Paul B. Hoeber, 1959); H. J. Montoye, Summary of research on the relationship of exercise to heart disease, *Journal of Sports Medicine and Physical Fitness,* 1962, *2,* 35.

6. S. Askanas et al., *Investigation into the effect of Medical Rehabilitation and of Therapeutic Procedure on Vocational Rehabilitation of Patients with Recent Myocardial Infarction* (Washington, D.C.: U.S. Department of Health, Education and Welfare, 1969); M. Cooper and K. H. Cooper, *Aerobics for Women* (New York: Bantam Books, 1972); D. C. Durbeck et al., The National Aeronautics and Space Administration–U.S. Public Health Service Evaluation and Enchancement Program, *American Journal of Cardiology,* 1972, *30,* 785; F. Heinzelmann, Social and psychological factors that influence the effectiveness of exercise programs, in J. R. Naughton and H. K. Hellerstein (eds.), *Exercise Testing and Exercise Training in Coronary Heart Disease* (New York: Academic Press, 1973); F. Heinzelmann and R. W. Bagley, Response to physical activity programs and the effects of health programs, *Public Health Reports,* 1970, *85,* 905; J. J. Kellerman et al., *Rehabilitation of Coronary Patients* (Washington, D.C.: U.S. Department of Health, Education and Welfare, 1969); R. B. Stuart, Exercise prescription in weight management: Advantages, techniques and obstacles, *Obesity and Bariatric Medicine,* 1975, *4,* 16.

7. Jean Mayer, *Overweight* (Englewood Cliffs, N.J.: Prentice-Hall, 1968).

8. H. K. Hellerstein et al., Principles of exercise prescription, in J. Naughton and H. K. Hellerstein (eds.), *Exercise Testing;* J. Naughton and R. Haider, Methods of exercise testing, in J. Naughton and H. K. Hellerstein (eds.), *Exercise Testing;* S. M. Fox, J. P. Naughton, and W. L. Haskell, Physical activity and the prevention of coronary heart disease, *Annals of Clinical Research,* 1971, *3,* 404; S. M. Fox, J. P. Naughton, and P. A. Gorman, Physical activity and

cardiovascular health: III. The exercise prescription: Frequencies and type of activity, *Modern Concepts of Cardiovascular Disease,* 1972, *41,* 25.

9. B. J. Sharkey, *Physiology and Physical Activity* (New York: Harper & Row, 1975).

10. R. Passmore and J. V. G. A. Durnin, Human energy expenditure, *Physiology Review,* 1955, *35,* 801.

Chapter 15

1. J. Grinker, J. Hirsch, and D. V. Smith, Taste sensitivity and susceptibility to external influence in obese and normal weight subjects, *Journal of Personality and Social Psychology,* 1972, *22,* 320; J. A. Grinker, Obesity and taste: Sensory and cognitive factors in food intake, in G. Bray (ed.), *Obesity in Perspective* (Washington, D.C.: U.S. Government Printing Office, 1975), p. 73.

2. R. E. Nisbett, Taste, deprivation and weight determinants of eating behavior, *Journal of Personality and Social Psychology,* 1968, *10,* 107; J. M. Price and M. Grinker, The effects of degrees of obesity, food deprivation, and palatability on eating behavior of humans, *Journal of Comparative and Physiological Psychology,* 1973, *85,* 265; J. Rodin, Effects of obesity and set point on taste responsiveness and ingestion in humans. *Journal of Comparative and Physiological Psychology,* 1975, *89,* 1003.

3. C. P. Herman and D. Mack, Restrained and unrestrained eating, *Journal of Personality,* 1975, *4,* 647.

Chapter 16

1. J. C. Gates, R. L. Hunenmann, and J. Brand, Food choices of obese and non-obese persons, *Journal of the American Dietetic Association,* 1975, *57,* 339.

2. B. A. Bullen, R. B. Reid, and J. Mayer, Physical activity of obese and nonobese adolescent girls appraised by motion picture sampling, *American Journal of Clinical Nutrition,* 1964, *14,* 211; R. B. Brandfield and J. Jordan, Energy expenditure of obese women during weight loss, *American Journal of Clinical Nutrition,* 1972, *25,* 971; R. J. Dorris and A. J. Stunkard Physical activity: Performance

and attitudes of a group of obese women, *American Journal of Medical Science*, 1967, *233*, 622; A. M. Chirico and A. J. Stunkard, Physical activity and human obesity, *New England Journal of Medicine*, 1960, *263*, 935.

3. Walter M. Bortz, Predictability of weight loss, *Journal of the American Medical Association*, 1968, *204*, 99.

4. U.S. Public Health Service, *Obesity and Health* (Washington, D.C.: National Center for Chronic Disease Control, 1966).

5. J. F. Munro, Endocrine and metabolic disease: Obesity, *British Medical Journal*, 1976, *1*, 388.

6. W. H. Sebrell, *The Nutritional Adequacy of Reducing Diets* (New York: Weight Watchers International, 1977).

7. J. D. Kirschman, *Nutrition Alamanac* (Minneapolis: Nutrition Search, 1973).

8. A. S. Bellack, R. Rozencsky, and J. Schwartz, A comparison of two forms of self-monitoring in a behavioral weight reduction program, *Behavior Therapy*, 1974, *5*, 523.

Chapter 17

1. A. Keys, F. Fidanza, M. J. Jarvonen, N. Kimura, and H. L. Taylor, Indices of relative weight and obesity, *Journal of Chronic Disease*, 1972, *25*, 329; R. T. Benn, Some mathematical properties of weight-for-height indices used as measures of adiposity, *British Journal of Preventive Social Medicine*, 1971, *25*, 42; W. Z. Billewicz, W. F. F. Kensley, and A. M. Thomson, Indices of adiposity, *British Journal of Preventive Social Medicine*, 1967, *21*, 122; G. A. Bray, Types of human obesity, *Obesity and Bariatric Medicine*, 1973, *2*, 146; C. Seltzer and J. Mayer, A simple criterion of obesity, *Postgraduate Medicine*, 1965, A101; U.S. Department of Health, Education and Welfare, *Skinfolds body girths, biacromial diameter and selected anthropometric indices of adults* Washington, D.C.: U.S. Government Printing Office, 1970; S. M. Garn, The measurement of obesity, *Ecology of Food and Nutrition*, 1972, *1*, 333.

2. T. Gordon and Y. W. B. Kannel, The effects of overweight on cardiovascular diseases, *Geriatrics*, 1973, *28*, 80.

3. W. M. Bortz, A. Wroldson, P. Morris, and B. Issekutz, Fat, carbohydrate, salt, and weight loss, *American Journal of Clinical Nutrition*, 1967, *20*, 1104; T. R. E. H. Pilkington, V. M. Gainsborough, and M. Carey, Diet and weight reduction in the obese, *Lancet*, 1960,

1, 856; T. Silverstone and T. Solomon, Long-term management of obesity in general practice, *British Journal of Clincal Practice*, 1965, *19*, 395; C. M. Young, N. S. Moore, K. Berresford, B. McK. Einset, and B. G. Waldner, The problem of the obese patient, *Journal of the American Dietetic Association*, 1966, *3*, IIII.

4. D. S. Janowsky, S. C. Berens, and J. M. Davis, Correlations between mood, weight, and electrolytes during the menstrual cycle: A reinantiotensin Aldosterone hypothesis of premenstrual tension, *Psychosomatic Medicine*, 1973, *35*, 143.

5. E. A. H. Sims, R. F. Goldman, C. M. Sluch, E. S. Horton, P. C. Kelleher, and D. W. Rowe, Experimental obesity in man, *Transactions of the Association of American Physicians*, 1968, *81*, 153.

Chapter 18

1. Surgeon General, *Obesity and Health* (Washington, D.C.: Department of Health, Education and Welfare, 1966).

2. D. Berkowitz, Obesity: Biological mechanisms, in L. Lasagna (ed.), *Obesity: Causes, Consequences and Treatment* (New York: Medcom Press, 1972).

3. G. V. Mann, The influence of obesity on health, Parts I and II, *New England Journal of Medicine*, 1974, *291*, 178, 226.

4. J. J. Alexander and K. L. Peterson, Cardiovascular effects of weight reduction, *Circulation*, 1972, *45*, 310; W. K. Kannel, N. Brand, and J. J. Skinner, Relation of adiposity to blood pressure and development of hypertension: Framingham study, *Annals of Internal Medicine*, 1967, *67*, 48.

5. J. H. Medalie, C. M. Papier, U. Goldbourt, and J. B. Herman, Major factors in the development of diabetes mellitus in 10,000 men, *Archives of Internal Medicine*, 1975, *135*, 811; T. D. R. Hockaday, Diabetes mellitus, *The Practitioner*, 1974, *213*, 535.

6. J. K. Alexander and K. L. Peterson, Cardiovascular effects of weight reduction, *Circulation*, 1972, *45*, 210; E. Fisher, R. Gregorio, T. Stephan, S. Nolan, and T. S. Danowski, Ovarian changes in women with morbid obesity, *Obstetrics and Gynecology*, 1974, *44*, 839; W. B. Kannel, N. Brand, and J. J. Skinner, Relation of adiposity to blood pressure and development of hypertension: Framingham study, *Annals of Internal Medicine*, 1967, *67*, 48; Massive obesity and nephrosis, *Nutrition Reviews*, 1975, *33*, 40; Respiratory complications of obesity, *British Medical Journal*, 1974, *2*, 519; A.

Rimm, L. Werner, R. Bernstein, and B. Van Yserloo, Disease and obesity in 73,532 women, *Obesity and Bariatric Medicine*, 1972, *1*, 77; G. Tibblin, L. Wilhelmsen, and L. Werko, Risk factors in myocardial infarction and death due to ischemic heart disease and other causes, *American Journal of Cardiology*, 1973, *35*, 514.

7. H. I. Kaplan and H. S. Kaplan, The psychosomatic concept of obesity, *Journal of Nervous and Mental Disease*, 1957, *125*, 181.

8. L. Luborsky, J. P. Docherty, and S. Penick, Onset conditions of psychosomatic symptoms: A comparative review of immediate observation with retrospective research, *Psychosomatic Medicine*, 1973, *35*, 187.

9. K. Abraham, The influence of oral erotism on character formation, in K. Abraham, *Selected Papers* (London: Hogarth Press, 1927); P. Burdon and L. Paul, Obesity: A review of the literature stressing the psychosomatic approach, *Psychiatric Quarterly*, 1951, *25*, 568; H. Bruch, *Eating Disorders: Obesity, Anorexia Nervosa and the Person Within* (New York: Basic Books, 1973); W. Hamburger, Emotional aspects of obesity, *Medical Clinics of North America*, March 1951, 483.

10. R. R. Keith and S. G. Vanderberg, Relation between orality and weight, *Psychological Reports*, 1974, *35*, 1205; R. A. Stewart, G. E. Powell, and S. J. Tutton, The oral character: Personality type stereotype, *Perceptual and Motor Skills*, 1973, *37*, 948.

11. L. P. Bronstein, S. Wexler, A. W. Brown, and L. J. Halpern, Obesity in childhood: Psychological studies *American Journal of Diseases of Children*, 1942, *63*, 238 (obese tended to be more intelligent); G. K. Gormanous and W. C. Lowe, Locus of control and obesity, *Psychological Reports*, 1975, *37*, 30 (I–E Scale did not differentiate); P. Balch and A. W. Ross, Predicting success in weight reduction as a function of locus of control: An unidimensional and ultidimensional approach, *Journal of Consulting and Clinical Psychology*, 1975, *43*, 119 (I–E Scale did differentiate); M. L. Held and D. L. Snow, MMPI, Internal-External Control, and problem check list scores of obese adolescent females, *Journal of Clinical Psychology*, 1973, *29*, 523 (MMPI did, but I–E did not differentiate); A. Kreze, M. Zelina, J. Juhas, and M. Garbara, Relationship between intelligence and relative prevalence of obesity, *Human Biology*, 1974, *46*, 109 (obese tended to have lower intelligence); R. Reivich, E. Ruiz, and R. Lapi, Extreme obesity, in N. Kiell (ed.), *The Psychology of Obesity* (Springfield, Ill. : Charles C Thumas, 1975; no known MMPI profile for obesity); M. Rotmann and D. Becker,

Traumatic situations in obesity, *Psychotherapy and Psychosomatics,* 1970, *18,* 372 (obese not more neurotic); J. Sallade, A comparison of the psychological adjustment of obese vs. non-obese children. *Journal of Psychosomatic Research,* 1973, *17,* 89 (obese children neither emotionally nor socially less well adjusted than nonobese); R. A. Wunderlich, Personality characteristics of super-obese persons as measured by the California Psychological Inventory, *Psychological Reports,* 1974, *35,* 1029 (C.P.I. did not differentiate); J. T. Silverstone, Psychosocial aspects of obesity, *Proceedings of the Royal Society of Medicine,* 1968, *61,* 371 (Cornell Medical Index showed obese not more neurotic than the lean).

12. N. Goodman, S. A. Richardson, S. M. Cornbusch, and A. H. Hastorf, Variant reactions to physical disabilities, *American Sociological Review,* 1963, *28,* 429; G. L. Maddox, K. Black, and V. Liederman, Overweight as social defiance and disability, *Journal of Health and Social Behavior,* 1968, *9,* 287; H. Canning and J. Mayer, Obesity: Its possible effect on college acceptance, *New England Journal of Medicine,* 1966, *275,* 1172; H. Canning and J. Mayer, Obesity: An influence of high school performance, *American Journal of Clinical Nutrition,* 1967, *40,* 352; D. Pargman, The incidence of obesity among college students, *Journal of School Health,* 1969, *29,* 621; K. T. Strongman and C. J. Hart, Stereotyped reactions to body build, *Psychological Reports, 1968, 23,* 1175; G. H. Elder, Appearance and education in marriage mobility, *American Sociological Review,* 1969, *34,* 19; R. Straus, Public attitudes regarding problem drinking and problem eating, *Annals of the New York Academy of Science,* 1966, *133,* 792; G. L. Maddox and V. Liederman, Overweight as a social disability with medical implications, *Journal of Medical Education,* 1969, *44,* 214; J. Rodin and J. Slochower, Fat chance for a favor: Obese-normal differences in compliance and incidental learning, *Journal of Personality and Social Psychology,* 1974, *29,* 557; W. J. Cahnman, The stigma of obesity, *Sociological Quarterly,* 1968, *9,* 283; E. Goffman, *Stigma: Notes on the Management of Spoiled Identity* (Englewood Cliffs, N.J.: Prentice-Hall, 1963).

Chapter 19

1. H. Bruch, Psychological aspects of overeating and obesity, *Psychosomatics,* 1964, *5,* 269; C. V. Rowland, Psychotherapy of six

hyperobese adults during total starvation, *Archives of General Psychiatry,* 1968, *18,* 541; A. J. Stunkard and J. Rush, Dieting and depression re-examined, *Annals of Internal Medicine,* 1974, *81,* 526; T. Robinson and H. Z. Winnik, Severe psychotic disturbances following crash diet weight loss, *Archives of General Psychiatry,* 1973, *29,* 559; A. J. Stunkard, The dieting depression, *American Journal of Medicine,* 1957, *23,* 77; D. W. Swanson and F. A. Dinello, Follow-up of patients treated for obesity, *Psychosomatic Medicine,* 1970, *32,* 209.

2. W. H. Biggers, Obesity, affective changes in the fasting patient, *Archives of General Psychiatry,* 1966, *14,* 218–221; E. Crumpton, D. B. Wine, and E. J. Drueick, Starvation: Stress or satisfaction? *Journal of the American Medical Association,* 1966, *196,* 394; W. G. Shipman and M. R. Plesset, Anxiety and depression in obese dieters, *Archives of General Psychiatry,* 1963, *8,* 26; R. I. F. Brown, The psychology of obesity, *Physiotherapy,* 1973, *59,* 216; G. G. Duncan, Correction and control of intractible obesity, *Journal of the American Medical Association,* 1962, *181,* 309; N. Fisher, Obesity, affect and therapeutic starvation, *Archives of General Psychiatry,* 1967, *17,* 227; J. T. Silverstone and B. D. Lascelles, Dieting and depression, *British Journal of Psychiatry,* 1966, *112,* 513; R. B. Stuart, The self-help approach to weight loss, in R. B. Stuart (ed.), *Behavioral Self-Management: Strategies and Outcomes* (New York: Brunner/Mazel, 1977); J. Grinker, J. Hirsch, and B. Levin, The affective responses of obese patients to weight reduction, *Psychosomatic Medicine,* 1973, *35,* 57.

3. R. B. Stuart, Sex differences in obesity, in E. Gomberg and V. Franks (eds.), *Gender & Psycho Pathology* (New York: Brunner/Mazel, in press).

4. E. V. Leckie and R. F. J. Withers, Obesity and depression, *Journal of Psychosomatic Research,* 1967, *11,* 107; W. G. Shipman and M. R. Plessett, Anxiety and depression in obese dieters, *Archives of General Psychiatry,* 1963, *8,* 530; J. T. Silverstone and T. Solomon, Psychiatric and somatic factors in the treatment of obesity, *Journal of Psychosomatic Research,* 1965, *9,* 249.

Index

The Chisholm Trail

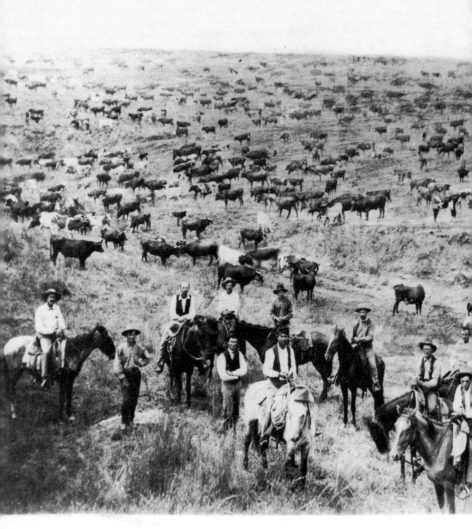

Cattle drive in Indian Territory. Herds were bedded on high ground to take advantage of the breeze. Courtesy of the Oklahoma Historical Society

The Chisholm Trail

High Road of the Cattle Kingdom

Don Worcester

Published for
Amon Carter Museum of Western Art: Fort Worth
by University of Nebraska Press
Lincoln and London

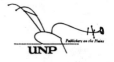

Publishers on the Plains

UNP

Second Printing: 1981

The Amon Carter Museum was established in 1961 under the will of the late Amon G. Carter for the study and documentation of westering North America. The program of the museum, expressed in permanent collections, exhibitions, publications, and special events, reflects many aspects of American culture, both historic and contemporary.

Copyright © 1980 by the University of Nebraska Press

Library of Congress Cataloging in Publication Data

Worcester, Donald Emmet, 1915–
  The Chisholm Trail : high road of the cattle kingdom.

  Bibliography: p. 189
  Includes index.
  1. Chisholm Trail. 2. Cattle trade—The West.
I. Title.
F596.W67   978'.02   80–12412
ISBN 0–8032–4710–9

Manufactured in the United States of America

To my son Harris

Contents

Illustrations

Preface

ALTHOUGH THE CHISHOLM TRAIL was open for less than two decades, millions of cattle traveled north over it. More than any of the other trails from Texas, it was the major route of cattle and horses, cowboys and cowmen, to Kansas railheads as well as the new ranches springing up all over the former ranges of the buffalo and the Plains Indians between 1867 and the Big Die-up of 1886–87. In fact, the name *Chisholm Trail* came to be applied indiscriminately to all of the cattle trails north out of Texas. This book is an attempt to portray, in text and photographs, the way of life created by the Chisholm Trail during the period of the great drives.

Although photography was in its early stages of development, some graphic photographs were made of ranch life and the trail before the end of the open-range, free grass era. Cowboy photographers have provided a valuable supplement to the memoirs of cowmen and cowboys. Using simple, often home-made cameras, the complicated wet plate process, and the collodion bottle and bath, they captured cowboys in action as well as at rest.

One of the most successful of the frontier photographers was L. A. Huffman, who arrived in Montana in 1878. A part-time rancher, Huffman was at home in cow camps and on roundups; many of his best photographs were taken from horseback. Two photographer-collectors who preserved valuable collections of old photographs in addition to the ones they took were Fred Mazzulla of Denver, Colorado, and N. H. Rose of Menardville, Texas.

I am grateful to Marni Sandweiss and Dr. Ronnie C. Tyler of the Amon Carter Museum of Western Art, Fort Worth, for their assistance in obtaining and selecting appropriate photographs. My thanks go also to my daughter and son-in-law, Barby

xi

and Michael J. Stephen of Helena, Montana, for their help in acquiring photographic and other materials, and to Keith Anderson, also of Helena, for sharing his father's old photographs with me.

Introduction

THE great cattle drives from Texas northward across the plains produced one of the nation's most enduring folk heroes. The cowboy, with his sombrero and lariat, mounted on a half-broken mustang, displaced the forest frontiersman with coonskin cap, squirrel rifle, and faithful hound in the pantheon of American folk heroes. Paradoxically, while the old-time frontiersman had been a free man, his own master, the cowboy was, as W. H. Hutchinson has noted, ever a "hired man on horseback" in the employ of cowman or syndicate. But, Hutchinson adds, "If you think all men are equal, you ain't never been afoot and met a man ridin' a good horse."[1] In the era of the long drives, from the 1860s to the 1890s, the cowboy became a legendary figure.

Trailing cattle was not new; Americans had "walked" cattle to market for more than two centuries, although the herds were small and easily handled by men on foot. A boy led a belled ox down the road and the cattle followed; a few men on foot brought up the rear to keep any from straying. They traveled through farming country and placed the cattle in fenced pastures each night. There was no need for night herding, no danger of stampedes. Fat cattle had been walked from Springfield, Massachusetts, to Boston as early as the 1650s. By the early nineteenth century, cattle were regularly driven from the Ohio valley to markets as distant as New York City.

There was nothing glamorous or captivating about these early cattle drives or the men who made them. While the term *cowboy* was used even before the American Revolution, it conveyed more contempt than respect. If there had been no Longhorns, mustangs, open range, or long drives it is unlikely that cowboys would ever have caught the public's fancy.

When the Civil War ended, an enormous tract of rich grassland in the central and northern plains remained the undisputed domain of warlike nomads whose way of life depended on the buffalo, or American bison. Cattlemen had not yet invaded this vast hunting ground, but as hide hunters decimated the buffalo herds in the next decade, millions of Longhorns from South Texas would take their places. Other cattle entered the northern plains from Oregon and Utah, and "Pilgrim," or farm, cattle were shipped from states east of the Mississippi River. The brief era of open range and free grass generated the greatest cattle boom in world history.

The age of the great cattle drives was one of rapid changes in American life both east and west, many of them stimulated by technological inventions. Eastern factories, developed or enlarged during the Civil War, supported a growing population and contributed to the increasing demand for beef. Railroads, pushing westward across the plains, provided transportation for live cattle to the packing plants of Chicago and St. Louis. Refrigerated railroad cars and ships introduced the dressed-beef trade to eastern and trans-Atlantic markets in the 1870s.[2]

The invention that had the most revolutionary impact on the cattle kingdom was barbed wire, invented by Isaac Ellwood, Joseph Farwell Glidden, and Jacob Haish of De Kalb County, Illinois, in the 1870s. In 1876 John W. ("Bet a Million") Gates demonstrated to skeptical Texas cowmen in San Antonio that the wire would hold Longhorns.[3]

This was one of those moments that bridge a chasm between two vastly different ages. Before Gates's demonstration, the era of open range and free grass was supreme. After it that age of pioneer cowmen was doomed, simply because a bunch of Longhorns had backed away from eight slender strands armed with tiny barbs. No one present foresaw how drastically "bob waire" would transform his way of life within a dozen years. Only gradually did the open-range cowmen realize that they, their Longhorns, and their mustang cow ponies no longer had a place in a land of privately owned and securely fenced pastures.

Wise cowmen began buying land by the section and enclosing it with barbed wire. The severe drouth of 1883 forced many cowmen to seek other grass and water; when they found fences in their way, they reacted angrily. The "Fence War" raged

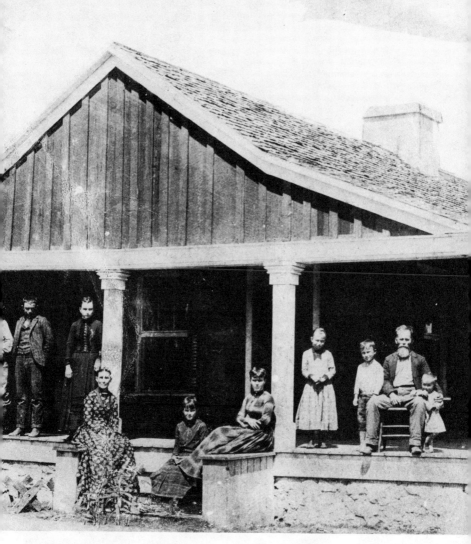

Rancho Perdido, Jim Wells County, Texas, in 1890. Built in 1871 by Martin Culver. Western History Collections, University of Oklahoma Library

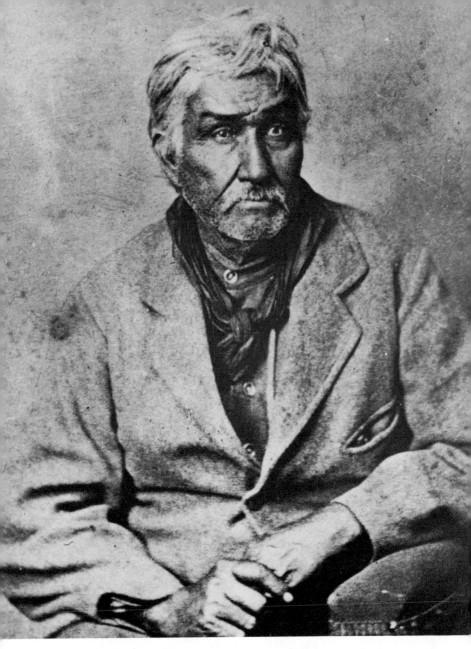

Jesse Chisholm, Cherokee-Scot trader, whose wagon tracks across Indian Territory became known as Chisholm's Trail. Texas cowmen gave his name to the entire trail from San Antonio to Kansas. Courtesy of the Oklahoma Historical Society sporadically for several years before the Texas Rangers put an end to fence cutting.

In 1879 fencing became a problem in Wyoming, for big outfits like the Anglo-American Cattle Company and Swan Land and Cattle Company enclosed whole sections of public land. In 1883 the secretary of the interior authorized settlers to destroy fences that were in their way to land they wished to homestead. Two years later Congress outlawed fences on federal lands, and President Grover Cleveland ordered them removed.[4] Northern ranchers gradually purchased and fenced their ranges, although the free grass era lasted longer in parts of Montana.

The six-shooter and repeating rifle were inventions that helped convert the central and northern grasslands from the buffalo range of the plains Indians to a major part of the cattle kingdom. By facilitating the extermination of the buffalo herds, these guns helped destroy the basis for the plains nomads' way of life, reducing them to the status of wards of the government. With the removal of these two obstacles to Anglo occupation of the plains, the cattle kingdom spread from South Texas to Montana and the Dakotas in less than a decade. "For every single buffalo that roamed the Plains in 1871," Richard Irving Dodge wrote, "there are in 1881 not less than two, and more probably four or five, of the descendants of the long-horned cattle of Texas. The destroyers of the buffalo are followed by the preservers of the cattle."[5]

The rapid spread of the cattle ranges occurred as millions of surplus animals were herded north from Texas. The oldest of the northern routes was the Shawnee Trail from San Antonio past Austin, Waco, and Dallas, fording the Red River at Rock Bluff near Preston. It passed through the Indian Nations, the lands of the Five Civilized Tribes, to Baxter Springs, Kansas, or Sedalia, Missouri. Most of the cattle driven up the Shawnee Trail were destined for feed lot or market rather than for stocking new ranches.

The routes by which most of the stock cattle reached the northern ranges were the Chisholm Trail to central Kansas and the later Western Trail to Dodge City. Of all the Texas cattle routes, the Chisholm Trail was the most used and by far the best known. Its name came from Scot-Cherokee Indian trader Jesse Chisholm, who in 1865 began hauling trade goods in wagons from his post near the future site of Wichita, Kansas, to Indian camps on the North Canadian River, about 220 miles to the south. Other parts of the trail were at first called by various names, but Texas trail men soon applied Chisholm's name to the entire route from San Antonio to Abilene and later Kansas shipping points. The "Chisholm Trail" was mentioned in Kansas newspapers in the spring of 1870, and in Texas papers by 1874.[6]

From South Texas, herds heading for the Shawnee and Chisholm trails followed the same landmarks toward San Antonio, San Marcos, or Austin. Near Waco the Shawnee Trail swung toward Dallas, while the Chisholm Trail continued north to Cleburne and Fort Worth. Beyond Fort Worth it followed along near the route of modern Highway 81, past Decatur to Red River Station, and over the sites of the future Oklahoma towns of Duncan, Chickasha, El Reno, and Enid. It crossed into Kansas where Caldwell was built as a trading post for trail crews in 1871. The trail swerved east of Jesse Chisholm's trading post, past the future site of Newton, and on to Abilene. Although Abilene was the first terminus of the Chisholm Trail, after 1871 the end of the trail might be any of several Kansas cowtowns, among them Ellsworth, Junction City, Newton, Wichita, and Caldwell. Even though most of the cattle were trailed on to the north or west of these towns, none of the northern routes was named after Jesse Chisholm.

All of the major trails were broad and general, not narrow lanes, and many minor trails joined them along the way. Cowmen using these feeder trails often gave them the name of the major trail they joined, adding to the confusion. Wayne Gard compared the Chisholm Trail to a tree: the roots were the feeder trails, the trunk was the main route from San Antonio across Indian Territory, and the branches were the extensions to the various railheads in Kansas.[7] When only a few herds were following a trail, they usually found adequate forage close by. But when many herds were on the move during any season, the later ones had to travel parallel to the tracks of the earlier ones to find

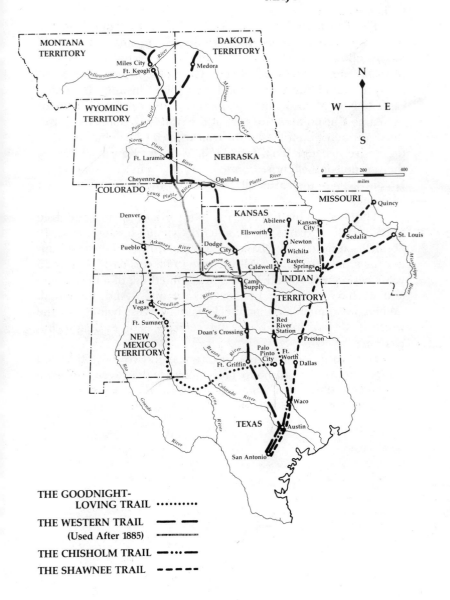

MAJOR CATTLE TRAILS

MONTANA
TERRITORY

DAKOTA
TERRITORY

Miles City
Ft. Keogh

Medora

WYOMING
TERRITORY

Ft. Laramie

NEBRASKA

Cheyenne

Ogallala

COLORADO

MISSOURI

Quincy

Denver

KANSAS

Abilene

Kansas
City

Ellsworth

Sedalia

St. Louis

Pueblo

Dodge
City

Newton

Wichita

Caldwell

Baxter
Springs

Camp
Supply

INDIAN

TERRITORY

Las
Vegas

Ft. Sumner

Doan's Crossing

Red
River
Station

Preston

NEW
MEXICO
TERRITORY

Palo
Pinto
City

Ft.
Worth

Ft. Griffin

Dallas

Waco

Austin

TEXAS

San Antonio

N
W   **E**
S

0   200   400
miles

Yellowstone River, *Powder River*, *North Platte River*, *South Platte River*, *Missouri River*, *Platte River*, *Arkansas River*, *Cimarron River*, *Canadian River*, *Red River*, *Brazos River*, *Colorado River*, *Pecos River*, *Rio Grande*, *Mississippi River*

THE GOODNIGHT-
   LOVING TRAIL ··········

THE WESTERN TRAIL — — —
   (Used After 1885) ▬▬▬▬

THE CHISHOLM TRAIL —··—

THE SHAWNEE TRAIL — — — —

grass. The drying up of streams and waterholes also caused variations in the route.

The Chisholm Trail was widely known by name, and the name was often applied indiscriminately to any route cattle might follow out of Texas.[8] Most of the men who used the trail probably had never heard of Jesse Chisholm or his wagon road; many thought it was named for Texan John Chisum, who trailed cattle to New Mexico. Some people even today restrict the use of the name Chisholm to the part of the trail he actually used. But since cowmen who followed the trail applied Chisholm's name to the entire distance from San Antonio to the Kansas railheads, there is no compelling reason to overrule them a century later.[9] No one even knows, after all, how or why the Shawnee Trail got its name.

The western myth that arose in the era of open range, free grass, and long drives has retained its vitality because, as C. L. Sonnichsen noted, our "basic need is a natural and normal hunger for a heroic past. . . . All we have to fill this basic need is 25 years between 1865 and 1890. It was something of a heroic age, and we have done our best to make it one." And, he added, "When we remember that the legendary West belongs to the world and not just to us, the subject assumes major importance."[10]

For two decades trail bosses, cooks, and cowboys followed Longhorns up the Chisholm Trail, unaware they were creating a "legendary West" that would long outlive the open range and the cattle kingdom. Their story is told in the following pages.

The Chisholm Trail

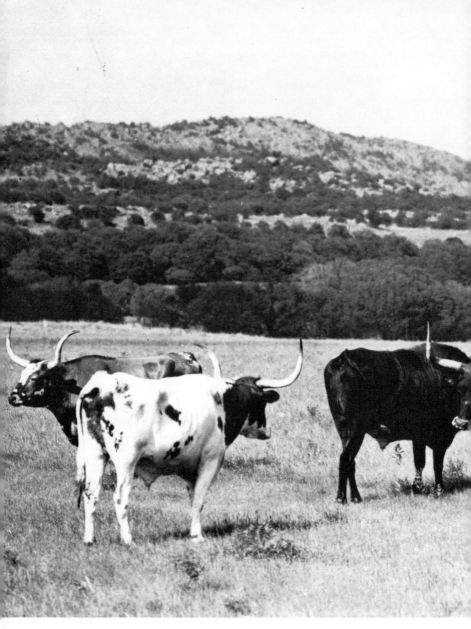

Modern Longhorn steers on the Wichita Wildlife Refuge, Oklahoma.
Photo by E. P. Haddon for the Bureau of Sport Fisheries and Wildlife.
Western History Collections, University of Oklahoma Library

CHAPTER 1

Cow Poor

Other states were carved or born
Texas grew from hide and horn.
Breta Hart Nance, "Cattle"

TEXAS had been a land of cattle and horses ever since the Spaniards introduced them in the seventeenth century. Anglo-Americans arriving in Texas after 1800 found thousands of Spanish cattle and countless wild horses, or mustangs (from *mesteño,* meaning a stray or ownerless animal). Anglos also brought livestock, which mixed with the native stock to produce the longhorns of South Texas. A German who traveled widely in Texas in 1849 differentiated between American and Mexican cattle, saying, "The former is tamer, the latter tends to become wild."[1] Other visitors, both earlier and later, commented on the long horns of the cattle they saw.

Longhorns were a robust breed of many colors—black, red, roan, white, brindled, yellow, and various combinations. They were long of leg and hard of hoof, perfectly adapted to the region, able to travel for grass and water and defend themselves against predators. They had developed an immunity to the tick fever that proved fatal to other cattle, but unfortunately they carried the ticks wherever they went. The Longhorns of the brush country were as wild and wary as any living creature, more difficult to stalk and kill than deer or buffalo. They roamed in scattered bands of perhaps half a dozen, hiding in the brush by day, coming out to graze at night.

Not all Texas cattle were Longhorns, nor were all immune to tick fever. The cattle of central and North Texas, which were a mixture of Shorthorns brought from the East or South and native or Spanish stock, were susceptible to the disease. Charles Goodnight described them as dark, line-backed, mealy-nosed, round-barreled, and well formed. Like the Longhorns, they easily became wild and difficult to handle, even dangerous.[2]

Anglos also brought Thoroughbreds and Quarter Horses, which they raised at first for racing. Eventually both were crossed with little mustang mares to produce larger and swifter cow horses. For many years, however, the mustang cow pony and the Longhorn were inseparable elements of the Texas cattle industry. Together they made the era of the long drives possible.

Although after the Civil War Texas was the unrivaled source of cattle, before the war the Five Civilized Tribes of Indian Territory raised and exported thousands of cattle to states to the north and east. The Cherokees, Choctaws, Chickasaws, Creeks, and Seminoles had learned open range cattle raising and trailing livestock to market on the southern frontier. Their trade with Missouri and Illinois antedated that of Texans by only a few years at most. The cattle the tribes brought to Indian Territory were apparently of good quality and, according to observers, "attained great size." By 1847 a regular trade had developed with buyers from Missouri, Illinois, and Indiana.[3]

During the Civil War both the Union and Confederate armies as well as other whites looted the herds of Indian Territory. The depleted herds were gradually rebuilt after the war to an estimated 700,000 by 1884. Trade with the states to the north was resumed, but, since these cattle were not carriers of tick fever, the traffic received little notice.[4]

Spaniards had trailed Texas cattle to Louisiana and northern Mexico in the eighteenth century. In the 1830s, Anglo cowmen drove small herds to New Orleans, and in the following decade they trailed cattle to Missouri, Ohio, and California.[5] By 1842 many men drove herds across Indian Territory for sale to army contractors who supplied Forts Smith, Gibson, Scott, and other military posts. These were fairly profitable years for some Texas cowmen.

By the early 1850s, Texans trailed cattle to Arkansas, Illinois, Kansas, Nebraska, Missouri, and Iowa. Illinois feeders regularly fattened Texas cattle during the decade, and hundreds of Longhorn steers were sold to freighters and farmers to be worked as oxen. Kansas City became a market for Texas beef, and some Texas cattle were trailed on to Chicago.

In 1853 Tom Candy Ponting and a partner came from Illinois to buy Texas cattle. In preparation for the drive they purchased a wagon, a canvas cover that also served as a tent, and a yoke of oxen. They bought six hundred steers and drove them across the Red River; the steers followed a belled ox that was tied to the back of the wagon. In Indian Territory they bought eighty more prime steers weighing about twelve hundred pounds for nine dollars a head. It took four months to reach Illinois.

After wintering the cattle they trailed 150 of them to Muncie, Indiana, then shipped them by rail to New York City, where beeves brought high prices. It had cost two dollars a head to trail the cattle fifteen hundred miles from Texas; it cost seventeen dollars a head to ship them six hundred miles to New York City. In the spring of 1855 Ponting and his partner sold some of their cattle in Chicago, too. In 1854 George Jackson Squires also went from Illinois to Texas for cattle. He bought five hundred Longhorns near Houston, drove them to Illinois, and later sold them in Chicago.[6]

Texans also trailed cattle to the California mining regions. In 1856 Frederick Law Olmsted saw near San Antonio a herd of four hundred steers heading west under a crew of twenty-five men, all mounted on mules. Most of the riders were working for their keep and transportation to the gold fields. They were five or six months on the trail, but a steer costing fourteen dollars in Texas brought one hundred dollars in California.

In the early days of cattle trailing, oxen hauled carts or wagons that carried bedding and supplies, mainly cornmeal and bacon. If an ox went lame, the men roped a steer and yoked it to the wagon. The food supply was never adequate, and the men usually had nothing to eat but beef before they reached their destination. Fortunately, the herds usually picked up strays along the way, for, as every Texas cowman knew, eating your own beef would make you sick.

Before the Civil War most trail herds numbered only a few hundred head, with four riders for each one hundred cattle.

The men usually had only two or three horses apiece, and these were often thin and sore-backed before the drive ended. Without tents or raincoats, the cowboys were at the mercy of the elements day and night. A man who was separated from the wagon overnight slept on a "Tucson bed"—stomach for a mattress and back for a cover.

The Shawnee Trail became hazardous for trail men and their herds even before the Civil War, for in 1855 an outbreak of "Texas fever" in Missouri killed thousands of cattle. The disease was correctly attributed to the arrival of Longhorns from Texas, but the trouble was blamed on the Longhorns' breath rather than on the ticks that carried the disease. The Missouri legislature banned Texas cattle, and irate Missouri farmers turned back Texas herds the next year. Some cattle crossed eastern Kansas to Kansas City and St. Joseph, and some reached Illinois, but similar epidemics of tick fever in Kansas also led to a quarantine against Texas Longhorns. In 1857, nevertheless, Jesse Day and Willis McCutcheon both trailed herds to Quincy, Illinois, where they sold them profitably. In 1858 Oliver Loving reached Illinois with a herd from his ranch in Palo Pinto County. The following year he wintered a herd in southern Kansas; in the spring of 1860 he drove it up the Arkansas River to Pueblo, Colorado.[7]

During the Civil War the populations of frontier areas in Texas, such as Parker, Palo Pinto, Denton, Wise, and San Saba counties, declined drastically, so that by 1866 no more than one-fifth of the old ranches were still occupied. When both state and Confederate forces were withdrawn after the war, frontier families were left defenseless against Comanche and Kiowa raiders, who ran off thousands of Texas cattle to trade to the Comancheros of New Mexico. Many men gave up the struggle and abandoned their ranches, but others, like the Lovings and Slaughters, moved their families to safety and remained with their cattle.[8]

When trailing cattle resumed, some Anglo cattlemen were not particular about whose animals were in their herds, and rustlers became active as the value of cattle rose. On one occa-

sion some northwest Texas cowmen caught up with a thief who
was driving off their cattle. They ate supper with him, then announced that they intended to hang him.

"Boys," he said, "I'll not argue with you, I'll not deny my
guilt or ask for mercy. You know me and I know you. I want at
least one honest man to have a part in my hanging. Now I want
the one of you who never stole a cow to step forward and put the
noose around my head." A moment of shocked silence followed,
then laughter. They let him go with a warning.[9] Other cow
thieves did not get off so lightly when caught, but most were
never apprehended.

Many Texans served in the Confederate Army, leaving
ranchers short-handed, unable to brand all of their calves or to
prevent their cattle from straying. It became customary at this
time to look out for others' cattle at branding time; when cows
from distant ranges were found, their calves received the mothers' brands. When the branding was finished, these strays were
pushed as far as possible toward their own ranges. As long as
only honest cattlemen were involved, such customs worked fairly
well, but many a Confederate veteran or his widow discovered
that his cattle had disappeared. There were, nevertheless,
thousands of unbranded cattle; by custom these belonged to the
man who burned his brand in their hides and notched his mark
in their ears.

In 1865 returning cowmen organized wild cow hunts to
replenish their herds, and the great era of "mavericking" began.
The term *maverick* came to mean an unmarked stray that was
presumed to be ownerless. The name, which spread over the
West, arose after Samuel A. Maverick received a herd of stock
cattle as a debt settlement and had them driven to a range on the
San Antonio River. The man in charge of the cattle neglected to
brand the calves. In 1855 Maverick sold the brand and his rights
to Toutant de Beauregard, who agreed to hunt and brand the
strays. Like later maverickers, Beauregard made the most of the
opportunity, rounding up and branding as "Maverick's" all the
unbranded cattle he found in a number of surrounding counties.[10]

W. S. James, an old-time Texas cowboy-turned-preacher who had "seen the elephant and heard the owl," wrote a book about life on the range to correct the errors in many books about the West. He thoroughly disapproved of mavericking and the scramble for unbranded cattle that it encouraged. The consequence was, he said, that the more successful men persuaded the legislature to enact laws that made it illegal to brand a calf one did not own. "There began the battle that for years waged unceasingly until the big fish swallowed up the little ones. We had as a result the cattle king and the common cow-puncher. The real difference being that the king no longer had to do his own stealing, for he was able to hire the cow-puncher to do it for him, and if the poor cow-puncher presumed to steal a little scrub for himself once in a while the king wouldn't kick unless someone tried to raise a fuss about it. If he could settle it without too much noise he would do it, and thus add one more link to the poor boy's chains with which to hold him in line. If there was too much noise about it, the king turned honest and sent him down East to work for Texas."

There were, James admitted, honest exceptions, but this is what mavericking generally produced. "When the business first began there were men with cattle who had never stolen, that really believed they were forced to do as other men in self-defense, who began taking lessons in stealing and wound up in the penitentiary. Some became wealthy and, thanks to true manhood, we are able to record that some men preferred to let poverty enter their home than that truth and honesty of purpose be dispossessed of their legitimate throne."[11]

The successful cattlemen, James added, perhaps in bitterness because he had not been one of them, were usually the ones who tended to the business of branding mavericks and looking after the ones they had already branded. "Show me a man who began in the cattle business as early as '68 or '70 who did not go busted, who can truthfully say that he never ate stray beef, never branded cattle whose ownership was questionable, and I will show you a man too good for Texas or Chicago."[12]

To James, "of all the contemptible cow thieves on earth it is the old donker who has stolen himself into respectability and then with his thieving old carcass togged up in a $50 suit of clothes bought with his ill-gotten gains to see him stacked up on a jury to try some boy for stealing a $5 yearling."[13]

Problems other than mavericking troubled Texas ranchers, for even though by 1866 many men had cattle to sell, all the markets were doubtful at best. During the war a few cowmen like Oliver Loving, Dan Waggoner, and Jesse L. Driskill had trailed herds east to supply the Confederate Army, while others had driven cattle to New Orleans. In the early years of the war Confederate money was accepted all over Texas. Later the only ones to profit were those who sold beeves to Union forces in New Orleans after the city fell, for they were paid in gold. The others still received Confederate currency, which soon went out of style.

One of the pioneer long drives was that of Nelson Story, a former overland freighter who followed gold seekers to Virginia City, Montana. Beef was scarce in Montana; in 1866 Story rode to Texas and bought a herd of mixed cattle for ten dollars a head and started them north. He and his men and the cattle survived a multitude of obstacles and hazards, man-made as well as natural. Story sold some of his cattle for a handsome profit and started a ranch with the rest.[14]

In 1866, Oliver Loving and Charles Goodnight pioneered a trail to New Mexico from northwest Texas by way of the future site of San Angelo to the Horsehead Crossing of the Pecos. The scarcity of water as well as Mescalero and Comanche attacks made the route hazardous. Goodnight returned to Texas for more cattle, while Loving drove the herd on to Colorado. Before Loving died of wounds inflicted by the Comanches, the two men had driven a number of herds to Fort Sumner, New Mexico, as well as to Colorado. They were the first Texans to establish a ranch in eastern New Mexico, in the Bosque Grande south of Fort Sumner.

In 1866 Texans drove upwards of two hundred thousand cattle to the north, east, or west, but few of them made profitable sales. Armed men met herds on the Shawnee Trail at the Kansas and Missouri borders and stopped them. Although a few men managed to evade the blockades and find buyers in Iowa and

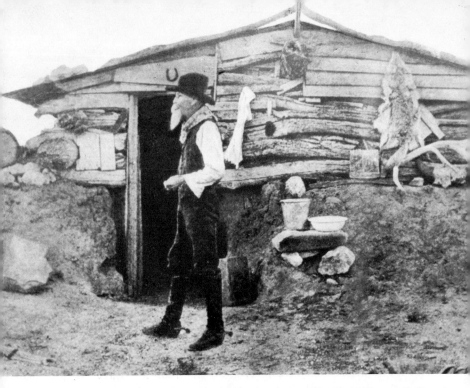

Early-day Kansas rancher and dugout cabin. Western History Collections, University of Oklahoma Library

elsewhere, others lost most of their cattle. Dan Waggoner sold twenty-five hundred steers in Sedalia, but his was one of the last herds to get through.[15] One trail boss who was forced to turn his herd west at the Kansas line succinctly expressed the feelings of many Texans. In Kansas, he said, there was nothing but "sunshine, sunflowers, and sons-of-bitches."

Among the few successful drovers were two young men who, with the help of twenty cowboys, started a herd from central Texas to their home state of Iowa in April. In crossing the Brazos they lost most of their cooking equipment. At that "all hands gave the Brazos one good harty dam" and continued on their way. They went by way of Baxter Springs and Council Grove, reaching Nebraska City in September. From Ottumwa, Iowa, they shipped the cattle to Chicago.[16]

Captain E. B. Millett turned east at Baxter Springs, but by the time he reached the Mississippi his cattle were in poor condition and virtually unsalable. Millett drove them on to central Illinois, where he wintered them. He sold the herd in the spring, but not profitably. He concluded that there was no money to be made by trailing Texas cattle, but after the Chisholm Trail was opened he changed his mind and drove many herds north. Men who found no other outlet for their cattle sold them to the coastal slaughterhouses to be killed for hides and tallow. Cattle disposed of in this way brought their owners about three dollars a head at best. Texas cowmen, up to their briskets in cattle for which there was no profitable or stable market, faced ruin.

At this critical moment a young cattle dealer of Springfield, Illinois, Joseph G. McCoy, purchased some cattle that W. W. Sugg had brought from Texas in 1866. McCoy shipped his cattle to eastern markets, where they sold readily for high prices. The American population was rising, and the growing demand for beef exceeded the supply. McCoy was one of several men who were determined to meet that demand, but first he had to locate a dependable supply of cattle at reasonable prices.

Charles F. Gross, who in 1865 had surveyed a route for a military telegraph line from Shreveport, Louisiana, to Brownsville, told McCoy where he could find the cattle. He had, Gross said, seen thousands of cattle along the Texas coast "running wild and waiting for someone to gather them and drive them to the northern market."

Sugg confirmed the great numbers of cattle in South Texas and the low prices they brought. He also warned McCoy about the difficulties that drovers encountered on the old Shawnee Trail into eastern Kansas and Missouri. McCoy immediately sensed that a bonanza awaited the man who could find a way to deliver low-cost Texas cattle to eastern markets. The main problem was getting cattle safely to some railhead not under quarantine. At first he considered receiving cattle on the Arkansas River near Fort Smith, where they could be shipped by river or by rail. Other men had similar ideas, but none that proved effective.

In Kansas City, McCoy talked to Marsh and Coffey, who traded for cattle in Indian Territory and along the Red River. They suggested central Kansas as a possible shipping point, for the Eastern Division of the Union Pacific Railroad (later the Kansas and Pacific) had laid tracks westward as far as Salina, Kansas. The Kansas quarantine law applied only to the settled area, leaving the lands to the west open to Texas cattle. Marsh and Coffey warned McCoy, however, that shipping costs from central or western Kansas might leave no profit margin on the cattle. Much depended on railroad freight rates.

When McCoy approached the Union Pacific freight agent at Wyandotte, Kansas, he found the man interested and cooperative. The agent gave him a railroad pass to Salina. On the return trip McCoy had the train stop in Abilene, a hamlet of one-room cabins, two saloons, a post office, a blacksmith shop, a six-room hotel, and a sawhorse beside the railroad track that served as a platform on the rare occasions when the train stopped to discharge passengers.

Because it was unusual for a train to stop in Abilene, almost everyone in town came to see who had arrived. McCoy found them more receptive to his project than anyone elsewhere. He learned that there was plenty of low-priced land available for corrals and shipping pens.

The train also stopped at Junction City, east of Abilene, but although its location was satisfactory, the price of land was too high. While dining there at the Hale House, McCoy discussed his project with Colonel J. J. Myers, a well-known cattleman from Lockhart, Texas, who urged him to put his plans into operation as quickly as possible.

Remembering the warning of Marsh and Coffey, McCoy went to St. Louis to discuss freight rates with officials of several railroad companies, but met mild interest, indifference, or hostility. Union Pacific officials doubted the feasibility of his program, but agreed to let him proceed at his own expense, promising to pay him one-eighth of the freight charges on each carload of cattle shipped, about five dollars. The president of the Missouri Pacific replied to McCoy's question about freight rates by ordering him out of the office. The freight agent of the Hannibal and St. Louis Railroad promised reasonable rates to Chicago, where the Union Stockyards had been built in 1865. As a result of these meetings, Chicago rather than St. Louis became the primary market for Texas cattle.

Kansas quarantine law banned Texas cattle east of a line approximately sixty miles west of Abilene. Fortunately for McCoy, the governor of Kansas was convinced of the benefits the cattle trade would bring and was willing to overlook a minor violation of the quarantine law. "I regard the opening of that cattle trail into and across Western Kansas," Governor Crawford announced, "of as much value to the state as is the Missouri River."[17] McCoy immediately set about making his shipping pens a reality.

There was need for haste, for it was already June, midway through the season for trailing cattle. McCoy bought 250 acres northeast of Abilene and persuaded the railroad to build a siding that would hold one hundred cattle cars. Aware that only the strongest fences would stop Longhorns, he built his shipping pens and corrals of railroad ties. Work on the pens began on July 1, and in two months they were ready for one thousand cattle, with facilities for weighing and for loading forty cattle cars in two hours. Construction of the three-story Drover's Cottage and a bank also got under way.

Farmers east of Abilene protested McCoy's cattle business until they learned that trail bosses were willing to pay high prices for eggs, potatoes, onions, corn, and hay. "If I can make money out of the Texas trade," said the leader of the opposition, "I'm not afraid of Texas fever but if I can't, I'm damned afraid of it."

Although the trailing season was well advanced, McCoy sent handbills to Texas towns and advertisements to newspapers, informing cattlemen of the new market at Abilene. He also sent riders to tell trail bosses who were holding herds in Indian Territory because they knew of no place to sell them. By mid-August a herd that northern cattlemen had bought in Indian Territory was grazing near Abilene, waiting for the pens to be completed.

The first herd that came directly from Texas to Abilene was owned and managed by Colonel O. O. Wheeler and two partners. Wheeler had been driving cattle from southern California to San Francisco, but a drouth had greatly reduced herds. He went to San Antonio, and with his partners purchased twenty-four hundred Longhorn steers and one hundred cow ponies. They hired fifty-four cowboys, arming them with Colt revolvers and Henry repeating rifles, for there was great danger of Indian attacks on the southern plains.

Wheeler and his partners drove their herd along the old Shawnee Trail, leaving it when it swung east toward Dallas. They continued on past Fort Worth and across the Red River. In Indian Territory they came upon Jesse Chisholm's wagon tracks and followed them. Wheeler planned to winter the cattle in Kansas and then drive them through South Pass to San Francisco.

Abilene proved to be the last stop for Wheeler's herd, for his partners, fearing cholera as well as Indian attack, refused to continue. To Wheeler's disgust they shipped the cattle to Chicago from McCoy's pens. Because there had been frequent rains the grass was poor and the lean cattle did not bring a satisfactory price.

Dan Waggoner was one of the North Texas cowmen who learned of the Abilene market in time to trail a herd there in 1867. Other herds headed up the same route from Jack County.[18] Ultimately thirty-five thousand cattle were shipped from Abilene that first season, but because of widespread fears of tick fever, there was little profit to be made in shipping Texas cattle to market until 1868, when they had become popular with meat packers.

News of the cattle market at Abilene spread over the Texas ranges in the fall of 1867, as ranchers prepared herds for the trail in 1868. McCoy sent men to survey the route across Kansas, to shorten it where possible, and to mark it with mounds of earth.

By the spring of 1868 Abilene had been transformed from a sleepy hamlet to a boom town, as men and women flocked there for the pleasure and profit of relieving Texas trail hands of their hard-earned pay. But competitors were already after the Texans' money. Junction City ran ads in Texas newspapers and sent riders to warn trail bosses to avoid sinful Abilene. McCoy countered by sending W. W. Sugg to urge them to take advantage of the facilities and buyers at Abilene. Sugg, who knew many Texas cowmen, was successful, and by mid-April, as several herds approached Abilene, some buyers were already waiting for them.

Cattle continued to arrive, but the buyers had satisfied their needs, and sales ceased. Resourceful as ever, McCoy hired two Spanish California ropers and four Texas cowboys, Mark A. Withers, Jake Carroll, Tom Johnson, and Billy Campbell, and took them and their horses west to the buffalo range. He had cattle cars reinforced and adapted to hold buffalo bulls, wild horses, and elk. Signs on the sides of the cars advertised McCoy's Abilene cattle sales.

McCoy sent the cars to St. Louis, where the cowboys staged roping and riding exhibitions that attracted huge crowds. The cars went next to Chicago, where the performances were equally well attended. While this was going on, McCoy invited Illinois cattle dealers and feeders to accompany him to western Kansas on a buffalo hunt. As a result of these efforts, which cost McCoy six thousand dollars, many more cattle buyers came to Abilene, and all of the cattle were sold, more than seventy-five thousand head for the season. Packers had discovered that the meat of Longhorns was better for packing than that of other breeds, for there was less waste.

Because of widespread losses of cattle in Illinois after Long-horns were brought there for fattening, the state legislature considered a bill prohibiting the importation of Texas cattle. McCoy attended the sessions to lobby against the bill, and finally secured an amendment permitting the entry of stock that had been held over on the plains for the winter. "Wintered" cattle were free of the ticks and no longer spread the deadly fever. It was astonishing, McCoy noted, how many cattle certified as having been wintered appeared at Abilene in the summer of 1869.[19]

In Texas, cattle were always sold by class rather than by weight, and all animals of any class brought the same price regardless of size or condition. A man buying cattle anywhere in Texas paid a fixed price for each yearling, two-year-old, and so forth. But at the railheads buyers bought steers for shipping to market by the pound. Texas cowmen quickly recognized the opportunity to increase their profits by getting their steers to market as fat as possible.

In 1870 more than 300,000 head of Texas cattle were driven to Kansas. Because the railroads east of the Missouri were waging a rate war by lowering shipping charges, some cowmen made profits of between fifteen and twenty-five dollars a head. The result was that in 1871 Kansas was deluged with Texas cattle, for upwards of 600,000 head were trailed north. Heavy rains made the grass poor and the cattle weak. In the meantime the railroads had agreed on high rates for shipping cattle. About half of the cattle were not sold and had to be wintered on the plains. Severe weather, including ice storms, killed an estimated 250,000 head, and many cowmen, including Dan Waggoner, suffered heavy losses.

Although Texas cattlemen had trailed herds to distant markets before the Civil War, the herds were small, and it was only after the Chisholm Trail was opened and traveled by dozens of herds that trail bosses became proficient in handling large numbers of cattle with few men. The first herd up the Chisholm Trail had employed fifty-four cowboys for twenty-four hundred steers, but the large number was partly for protection against plains Indians. Expert trail bosses found that with ten or twelve riders and a cook they could manage a herd of twenty-five hundred head, the optimum size for successful trailing. Under an experienced trail boss and favorable conditions the steers gained weight along the way.

The opening of the Chisholm Trail gave Texas ranchers a large and stable market for their cattle. In the first few years the trail herds were composed largely of "mossy horns" up to ten or twelve years old. As the number of older steers was reduced, trail herds bound for market were mainly beeves, steers that presumably were four years old. Many stock cattle—cows and bulls—were trailed north to the new ranches that spread rapidly as the plains Indians retreated and the buffalo disappeared.

As the plains tribes were gradually confined to reservations, the new Indian agencies added considerably to the demand for Texas cattle, for all of the tribes that had depended on the buffalo had to be fed beef. No state was better prepared to meet this demand than Texas. And when new army posts were garrisoned, the army's requirements also rose. Government contracts provided an important stimulus to cattle raising and the trailing business as long as it lasted.

CHAPTER 2

From Wild Cow Hunts
to Roundups

"The trail life as a whole is easy compared to
ranch life."

Duke and Frantz

PUTTING together a herd of ten- or twelve-year-old steers for the
trail was difficult and often frustrating work, for mossy horns
were hard to catch and troublesome to control. It took expert
cowhands, especially Mexican vaqueros, to separate Longhorns
from their refuges in the Brasada, or brush country between the
Nueces River and the Rio Grande. "Brush popping" was the
hardest kind of cow work.

The only horses suitable for brush popping were the little
mustangs, or Spanish Texas cow ponies, which enjoyed the
chase and were as fearless as the wild cattle. These ponies were
cheap, and cowmen considered them expendable; they were
often gored and nearly always crippled before their work in the
brush was done. Brush popping was a much tougher test of man
and horse than handling cattle on the open range. There were,
in fact, few similarities between the two types of cow work.

Lee Moore, who in the 1880s was a ranch foreman in Wyoming, recalled conditions in Texas immediately after the Civil
War, when recently discharged Confederate soldiers came home
to their ranches. Most immediately banded together in small
groups to recover lost herds. "We didn't call it roundup in those
days," he said. "We called it cow-hunts and every man on this
cow-hunt was a cattle owner just home from the war and went
out to see what they had left to brand up." Moore, a boy at this
time, was looking for his father's cattle.

"We had no wagon," he continued. "Every man carried his
grub in a wallet on or behind his saddle and his bed under his
saddle." Moore was put on day herding the cattle gathered. "We

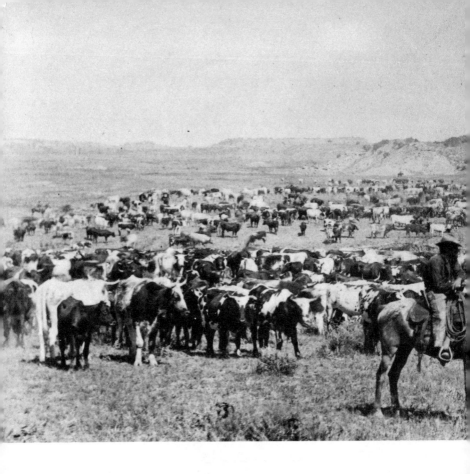

Roundup crew and herd in Colorado. Note four-mule chuck wagon, and brand on cow pony on right. The remuda is behind the chuck wagon. Courtesy of the Amon Carter Museum of Western Art, Fort Worth

would corral the cattle every night at some one of the owners' homes and stand guard around the corral."

The men played poker every night for stakes of unbranded cattle. Yearlings were valued at fifty cents a head, and so on up to five dollars for the best beeves. If a man ran out of cattle to wager, he could get back in the game easily; for ten dollars he could buy a stack of twenty yearlings. The cow hunt continued all summer. Every few days each man drove his cattle to his own range, the process later called a throwback.[1]

When a crew was getting ready for a cow hunt in the

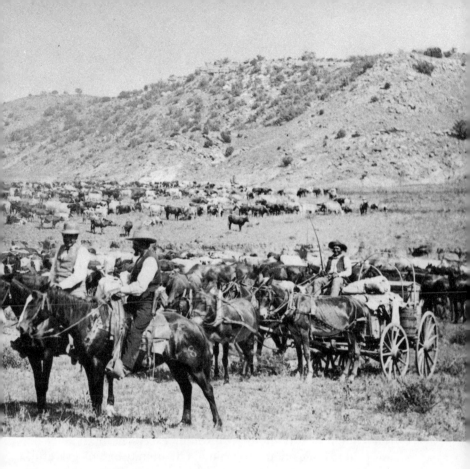

Brasada, each man made himself a supply of rawhide hobbles for his cowponies, braided extra rawhide reatas, and repaired any of his equipment in need of it. Every man wore heavy bull-hide leggins, or chaps, a thick brush jacket of leather or Mexican cloth that thorns could not penetrate, a tough hat, and heavy leather gauntlets to protect hands and forearms. The saddles had tapaderos, or leather stirrup coverings, to protect the rider's feet.

When all was ready, they loaded cornmeal and bacon on a pack horse or two, and turned out the decoy herd of tame cattle to use in controlling the wild ones. The only difference between tame and wild cattle was that the tame ones did not high-tail it for distant parts the moment they saw a man on horseback.

Because the range cattle had been neglected during the war years, there was an unusually large number of ten- or twelve-year-old mossy horns among the brush cattle. These were out-laws when it came to being herded by men on horses, and it was necessary to clear them out as quickly as possible, for they made younger cattle more difficult to handle. Mossy horns were as wild as mustangs, and they preserved their freedom with determination. The brush in which they hid was composed of mesquite trees, prickly pears, and a rich variety of other thorny shrubs.

The brush poppers set up camp near a strong corral made by digging a trench about three feet deep and setting up a palisade of ten-foot posts bound at about eye level with strips of rawhide. The corral had wings extending out from both sides of the gate to help keep the cattle from turning back or breaking out.

The cow hunt began when the riders placed the decoy herd in the brush. The moment they entered the brush a mile or two from the decoys, the ponies became especially alert and ready to run, for they could detect the presence of wild cattle before their riders could. When they heard cattle crashing through the brush the eager ponies dashed after them, their riders hanging on and dodging tree limbs and prickly pears as best they could. Some of the ponies threw themselves sideways through the thickets. A rider might be anywhere on his pony except in the saddle; he was paid to hang on, not to maintain his dignity or look graceful, and brush ponies would not stop for anything once the chase began.

Trusting to their ponies' sense of direction, the brush pop-pers tried to run the wild cattle toward the decoys. If all went well, wild and tame cattle were mixed, and the hands quickly surrounded them, loudly singing unmelodious tunes as they rode, presumably to calm the nervous cattle. Slowly and care-fully they eased the herd out of the brush toward the corral near camp. The farther they traveled from the brush the more des-perate the mossy horns were to break away.

Mishaps were frequent, for sometimes wild cattle dashed into the decoy herd so fast there was no stopping them, and the whole bunch left that part of the country. Often, too, on the way to the corral they might lose half of the morning's catch. If a steer broke out and a man went after it, other cattle would race through the gap thus created in the line of riders. Once wild cattle had escaped from a herd they were harder than ever to pen and control. On bad days brush poppers found that by the time they had the herd in the corral there were fewer cattle than they had started with in the morning.

After some brush cattle had been gathered, part of the decoy herd was left with them, and they were closely herded when turned out to graze during the days. In the afternoon the day's catch was brought up and the two herds were thrown together and eased toward the corral. Often they began milling outside the gate, and at such times a few usually escaped. As soon as the gate was closed on the herd, the riders galloped off to rope and tie those that had escaped.

Roping mossy horn outlaws in the brush was the most dangerous part of brush popping, for the ropes had to be tied to saddle horns. A roped bull or steer might dash around one side of a mesquite tree, while the cow pony went the other way. Bull and pony met, often with disastrous results, for a cornered Longhorn was as dangerous as a bear with a sore paw. A powerful mossy horn might break rope or cinch, or turn and charge pony and rider. At such times a rider saved himself by cutting the rope or shooting the Longhorn.

When a cowboy roped a steer in the brush, he tied its head up against a tree. If the decoy herd was near, it was brought up and the steer released into it; usually it went to the center of the herd and stayed there. If the decoy herd was too far, it meant bringing an ox and necking the two together. By passive resistance the ox eventually took the fight out of the steer, and showed up with it hours later at the corral.

Another method of catching outlaw steers was hunting and roping them on moonlight nights when they came out of the brush to graze. At times it was possible to get between the wild cattle and the brush before daybreak, but roping wild cattle was a painfully slow way to build up a herd. Often, however, it was the only way to catch the old mossy horns.

After a small herd had been gathered it was moved to ranch headquarters while the cowboys returned to the brush for more.

Even when moving such herds there was always the likelihood that one of the old outlaws would make a break for freedom. The nearest rider raced after it, and, while riding at full speed, "tailed" or "busted" the steer. Tailing required a fast pony that knew its work, and a skillful, daring rider. As the pony drew alongside the racing steer, the cowboy grabbed its tail and wound it around his saddle horn. The pony put on a burst of speed and turned slightly away, sending the steer flying end over end, perhaps breaking its horns or even its neck. Dazed, it usually trotted meekly back to the herd and gave no more trouble, at least for the rest of the day. As cattle increased in value, such destructive methods were abandoned.

Although Anglo cowmen brought with them from the southern frontier many of the techniques of handling range cattle, tailing was one of the skills they learned from Mexican vaqueros, for whom it was a Sunday sport and popular diversion. A number of vaqueros would round up and pen a bunch of wild bulls. Then amid shouts one bull was let out through the gate, to race over the prairie with a shrieking vaquero in pursuit. He tailed the bull and then rode back to the pen while another took his turn. Injuries occurred, for the swift bulls occasionally turned and charged pony and rider.

Another method of taking the fight out of an outlaw bull or steer was to shoot it through the thick part of its horn. If the bullet struck dead center the shock and pain usually made the animal less pugnacious and more cooperative thereafter. Since such shots were usually made while pony and steer were running at full speed, it was not always possible to hit a horn dead center. If the shot went a bit low and killed the steer no one complained, for cattle were cheap and outlaws were more trouble than they were worth. Cowmen were determined to rid their ranges of troublesome mossy horns, and no one cared if a few were killed in the process.

Brush popping was a special type of cow work for both men and ponies, and its story has never been fully told. Because it was brutally hard on the ponies, three times as many were needed by brush poppers as were required for regular range work. After a day's run the brush ponies were usually full of thorns; many were stiff and lame before they warmed up. The work was equally hard on riders, but brush poppers boasted that they could go anywhere a cow could and stand anything a horse could.

At the end of a day's riding the men pulled thorns from themselves and their ponies. For painful wounds and bruises the remedies were poultices of prickly pear leaves and applications of coal oil or kerosene for both men and horses.

The mossy horns were well known in their own and nearby areas; to "run like a Nueces steer" was a common expression for the most abandoned type of running through or over obstacles. Wild brush cattle had at least one name that was printable—"cactus bloomers."[2]

Cow hunts in the Brasada were dangerous at all times, and not only because of the wild cattle or occasional Comanche raiding parties. The brush country was also the refuge of outlaws, for sheriffs, unless careless of their lives, rarely entered the area in search of wanted men. The Nueces River was the "deadline for sheriffs." Ranchers found it wiser to help fugitives than to arrest them, for it was unhealthful to earn the enmity of men who lived outside the law. As a result of these perils every brush rider was armed, in the early days with cap and ball revolvers known as "outlaws" because when a man pulled the trigger he never knew how many chambers would fire.

Less spectacular denizens of the brush were the lice that swarmed over the men and their clothing. The vaqueros learned from the plains Indians to place their clothes on ant hills until the ants had carried off all of the lice. Then they washed themselves and their clothes with suds made from yucca roots, allowing the suds to dry in order to kill the nits.

Brush poppers lived in isolation from the rest of the world for months at a time, gathering wild cattle for others to drive to the main ranch and put in trail herds. There was no mail, no regular payday. When a man needed clothing or gear or tobacco, it was brought from the main ranch with provisions and charged against his pay. Some vaqueros worked for years without settling their wages, but no wise rancher tried to cheat them. For one thing, it was customary to take a man at his word; for another, cheating a vaquero was a risky way to save a few dollars. Vaqueros were artists with rawhide reatas, and on occasion two mounted men dueled with their reatas until one was caught and dragged to his death.

Brush poppers occasionally got well acquainted with outlaw steers that would not stay captured. In the spring of 1872, for example, a herd of twelve hundred mossy horns was gathered and delivered to a buyer who had come from Kansas with a crew of "shorthorns"—men from farming country. Unaccustomed to handling wild cattle, they reached Kansas with only their saddle horses and work oxen. Some of the wild steers were back in the brush before the next year's cow hunt.

Texans who were accustomed to working in the Brasada often were as reluctant as the cactus bloomers to leave the brush country. One little Texas brush popper tried year after year to accompany a herd up the trail, but each time when they left the wooded regions he fled back to the brush, for the treeless prairies made him nervous.

One spring when he started up the trail as usual, the cowboys hog-tied him and put him in the wagon. They kept him there until he was too far out on the plains to turn back; he stayed with the herd out of fear of leaving it and crossing the plains alone. "You know," he confessed, "when I get out on that big prairie I feel kind of naked."[3]

Mossy horn steers that refused to be driven away from the brush country with trail herds were treated somewhat in the same fashion as the brush popper. After collecting them a second time, when they started up the trail the cowboys necked them to tamer animals. After a few weeks they were herd broken, and had forgotten about turning back.

At first all of the big ranches were near the coast, but bold men began pushing north and west, coming into conflict with the Kiowas and Comanches. One of these was John Simpson Chisum, who in 1854 began ranching in Denton County. He moved his operations in 1862 to the area around the junction of the Colorado and Concho rivers, then in the 1870s moved his cattle to the Bosque Grande on the Pecos in New Mexico.

In 1856 the Reverend George W. Slaughter and his son C.

C. Slaughter settled with their cattle in Palo Pinto County, along with other pioneer families. In times of serious troubles with the Indians, some ranchers sold their cattle for anything they could get and pulled up stakes for safer country. C. C. Slaughter, by buying cattle at such times, became the biggest cowman in this region.

During and after the Civil War, Comanches and Kiowas ran off thousands of Texas cattle to trade to Comancheros from New Mexico. In 1864, for example, they escaped with ten thousand head from Young County, and in the following year drove away two thousand of Charles Goodnight's cattle from the Young-Throckmorton country. These costly raids continued until the mid-1870s, when troops finally defeated the Kiowas and Comanches at Palo Duro Canyon and confined them to their reservations in Indian Territory.

Not all losses were to Indian raiders, for there were also unscrupulous Anglos who stole their neighbors' cattle. Before ranches were fenced, cattle often strayed a hundred miles or more from their home ranges. It was customary, therefore, when a rancher gathered a herd for market, to include all suitable animals regardless of brands. Honest men kept records of these strays and notified their owners. Once a year ranchers held "stock meetings" to settle accounts with the owners of branded strays they had sold, charging only one dollar a head for selling them, a fee owners were quite willing to pay. In 1866 this practice was legalized by the "tallying law" providing for inspectors to make counts of all brands and classes of cattle in trail herds and to record the tallies with county clerks. As long as only honest men were involved, the system was satisfactory, but some men defrauded the owners of cattle they had sold.[4]

There were also cow thieves at work. Many ranchers suffered heavy losses when neighbors sold herds or whole brands. Men buying cattle on range delivery often rounded up all of the cattle regardless of brands and drove them away. Ranchers whose cattle were in such drives, if they learned of it in time, had to follow the herds and cut out the brands that had not been sold, but often they were unaware of their losses until the next roundup. Because of the growing demand for cattle, the Big

Steal persisted. It was not even partially checked until cattlemen formed associations such as the one organized at Graham in 1877.[5] These associations hired inspectors to pursue rustlers and recover stolen cattle, but by that time some cowmen had lost every animal they owned and given up ranching. By the late 1870s cattle were scarce on some Texas ranges.

The old-timers who had clawed out their ranches in the face of Indian raids and cow thieves were convinced that they should enjoy exclusive use of the ranges even if they owned little land. They considered it an infringement of their rights when nesters began plowing up small plots; cowmen looked on the land as having been made for pasture only.

Texas cowmen, according to Joseph McCoy, were prodigal, selfish, and suspicious of "Northern men." They would, he said, stand by their contracts, but not always by their oral agreements, and in his view they were no more courageous than men in general.[6]

"Sanguine and speculative in temperament," McCoy continued, "impulsively generous in free sentiment; warm and cordial in their friendships; hot and hasty in anger; with a strong inate [sic] sense of right and wrong; with a keen sense for the ridiculous and a general intention to do that that is right and honorable in their dealings; they are, as would naturally be supposed, when the manner of their life is considered, a hardy, self-reliant, free and independent class acknowledging no superior or master in the wide universe."[7]

In Texas, despite what McCoy thought, there were few written contracts among old-time cowmen. As one remarked, "I'd rather argue with you a week before a trade than a minute afterwards." Binding contracts were sealed by "It's a trade" and a handshake.[8]

Not all successful Texas cowmen were of masculine gender, for there were also "cattle queens" such as Lizzie Johnson and Mabel Day, who through wisdom and determination made their way on a man's range. Lizzie Johnson earned money to enter the cattle business by teaching in her father's school—the Johnson Institute—near Austin, and by writing and selling articles under a pen name. In 1871 she registered her own brand in Travis

County and expanded her herd in the conventional fashion by having her cowboys mark mavericks with her brand.

When she was thirty-six, Lizzie married Hezekiah Williams, a widowed preacher whose lack of business acumen was undermined further by his fondness for hard liquor. A shrewd businesswoman, Lizzie had no intention of allowing Hezekiah to squander her wealth, so she insisted that their marriage agreement include a contract allowing her to retain both her property and future profits. She and Hezekiah used the same foreman on their ranches, and according to legend she ordered him to put her brand on Hezekiah's unbranded calves. Whether apocryphal or not, this story simply reflects Lizzie's ability to match wits with men and come out a winner.

Lizzie accompanied her own herds up the trail; Hezekiah took his herds at the same time, but these were two independent operations. Lizzie's only concession was to let him share her buggy. She was completely at home with cowmen and, though ever a lady, talked their language. On a number of occasions she saved Hezekiah with substantial loans, but they were dutifully repaid. When he died she bought him an expensive coffin, scrawling across the bill, "I loved this old buzzard this much."[9]

Mabel Day, another Texas cattle queen, inherited her husband's ranch of 77,550 acres in Coleman County, along with upwards of $100,000 in debts. She had to contend with a number of predatory cattlemen, including her late husband's brother and former business associates, who wanted her land and cattle. Hers was a discouraging struggle, but she refused to accept defeat. The courts ignored her protests when the administrator of her husband's estate tried to sell her brother-in-law eighteen hundred yearlings at more than $9,000 below market value. Only after she had posted a bond of $150,000 did the court appoint her executor of the estate. Even then her situation remained precarious.

By negotiating a loan in New York City and a contract with Kentucky bankers and distillers who wanted to buy into the cattle business, she managed to retain her land. At that time the "Fence War" broke out, and miles of her fences were destroyed, an expression of resentment against outsiders investing in Texas cattle ranches. Although she never was able to liquidate all of her debts, her long battle to retain possession of the ranch was successful.[10]

These were but two of the women who were active in the cattle business. There were others, and many ranchers' wives accompanied their husbands up the trail to Kansas. In chapters entitled "Hairpins on the Trail," "Amazons of the Range: The Lady Ranchers," and others, Joyce Gibson Roach has described many women involved in ranching, trailing, and other activities related to the cattle ranges.[11]

As ranching spread out of the brush country to the open plains, the wild cow hunts of the early days became large-scale, cooperative roundups. Each spring the ranchers of a section of the range would agree on a date and a roundup boss. Each of the big outfits sent its crew, remuda, and chuck wagon to the meeting place; small ranchers sent only a man or two. Distant ranchers sent representatives ("reps") to gather their strays. Reps were top hands who knew every brand and earmark of the whole region; they often represented a number of distant ranchers.

While the roundup was on the range of one of the big outfits, the foreman of that ranch was the one who decided where the circle riders would go and where the cattle were to be gathered. He also sent some of his own men, who knew the country, to accompany the circle riders. These men rode their "long horses,"—frequently outlaws with great endurance that couldn't be used for cow work. They swept a large area on the run, driving all of the cattle toward the gathering ground at the center of the circle. Riding hard, the circle riders might cover forty miles before all of the cattle were on the gathering ground.

After lunch and a change of horses, the men sorted, or cut, the cattle, separating them by brands. The local rancher was the first to cut out his cattle from the herd, which might number five thousand head. It was here that the top riders on cutting horses moved quietly into the herd and separated the cows and calves according to brands.

When this was finished, the branding began. The best ropers skillfully tossed loops on the calves and dragged them to the

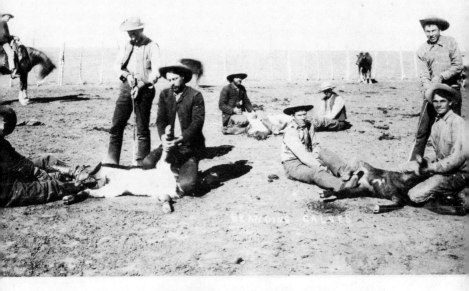

Branding calves on an Oklahoma ranch in 1888. Not shown are the ropers and fires for heating branding irons. Wrestling calves at branding time was hard work. Courtesy of the Oklahoma Historical Society

fire, calling out the brands of the cows so the calves could be correctly marked. Flankers grabbed the calves and held them down; one man did the branding while another cut the owner's earmark and castrated the bull calves. Every tenth bull calf was left intact to serve as a range bull; no effort was made to choose the best animals for herd sires.

At first the mavericks belonged to the ranch that claimed the range. Later the cattle raisers' associations sold the mavericks at auction, using the funds to aid cattlemen.

After the branding was completed, the herds from other ranges were moved along to the next gathering ground. Every few days men came to drive them back to their own ranges, the process called a "throwback." In the meantime, the herds had to be kept under control day and night to prevent them from straying or mixing with others. This meant that the cowboys rode hard all morning, wrestled calves in the heat and dust all

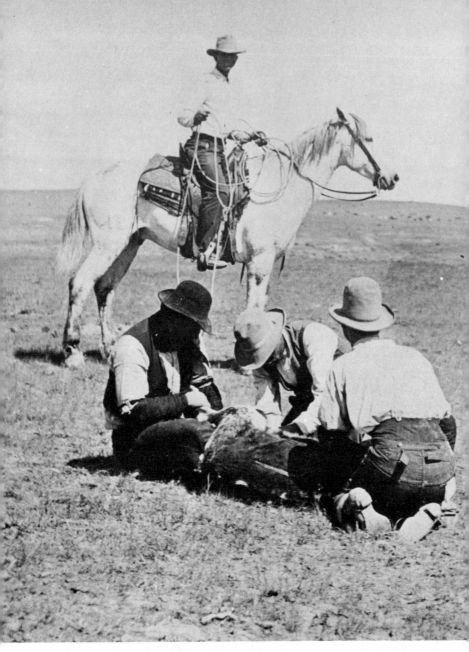

Cowboys castrating a bull calf, Judith River roundup, 1910. Courtesy of Keith Anderson, Helena, Montana afternoon, and then took a turn at night herding. Depending on how large an area the roundup covered, they might be out with a wagon for several months at a time.

The spring gathering was the calf roundup, for it was primarily to brand the new calves. The beef roundup in the fall was for the purpose of separating steers that were old enough to market, but it was also a time for branding late calves or any that had been missed in the spring.

When the big ranches were fenced with barbed wire in the late 1870s and 1880s, the old-time cooperative roundup was no longer necessary, for cattle could not stray from their own ranges. It was also possible, once pastures were securely fenced, to control breeding and begin upgrading herds. Many ranchers bought Shorthorn or Hereford bulls, for these cattle reached maximum weight much sooner than Longhorns.

The coming of barbed wire also meant that ranchers had to acquire title to rangeland, for it was no longer possible to own merely enough land for ranch house and corrals and to control strategic water sources. Old-timers who had grown up in the era of free grass and open range refused to accept this unwanted change without a struggle; one called barbed wire the curse of West Texas. Although the use of barbed wire in Texas began in 1876, most free grass men didn't feel the pinch until the summer drought of 1883. When they found access to grass and water elsewhere cut off, they realized for the first time the full impact that barbed wire was having on their way of life. The "Fence War" began as free grass men cut down mile after mile of barbed wire fences. As the conflict became more intense through central Texas, the governor called a special session of the legislature, which made fence-cutting a felony as of January 1884. In the meantime, cattle thieves had taken advantage of the opportunity to strip some ranches of cattle and horses.

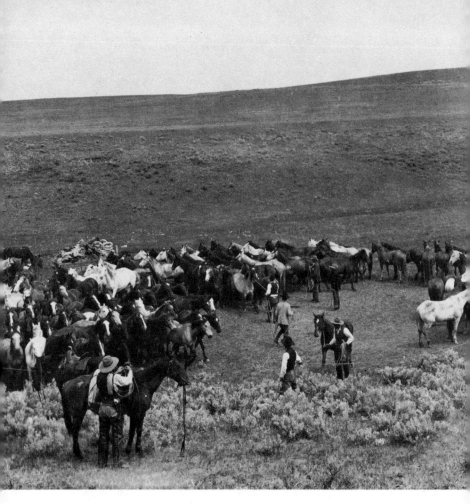

After the rain, in the rope corral. Horses were trained to respect the rope corral on the trail. In the background is the hoodlum wagon loaded with bedrolls; the team is harnessed, ready to be hitched. Photo by L. A. Huffman. Courtesy of the Amon Carter Museum of Western Art, Fort Worth

CHAPTER 3

Life on the Trail

"This procession of countless cattle on their slow march to the north was one of the most interesting and distinctive features of the West."

Richard Harding Davis

WHEN the Chisholm Trail opened the way to an expanding market, Texas cowmen welcomed the opportunity to sell their surplus cattle. Most of the men who took part in the early drives knew little about what to expect north of the Red River. For trail bosses and cowboys alike, the only place to learn trailing techniques was on the trail.

A man who planned to put together a herd in the spring began his preparations in the fall by visiting ranchers and arranging with each for the delivery of a certain number of beeves to a fenced pasture at a specified date. The drover acquired a chuck wagon, engaged a cook, bought horses for the remuda, then hired the experienced cowboys who were available and enough youths to make up a crew.

Cook and crew assembled before the ranchers began delivering their cattle. Some or most of the horses might be half-wild and unbroken, and the cowboys went to work on them. Each man, starting with the boss, chose his string of mounts; from it he selected the most reliable animal for his night horse. The remuda had to be trained to stay in the rope corral used on the trail as a catch pen. It was simply several lariats tied together and attached to trees or chuck wagon wheels, and was only the symbol of a corral. But when a horse broke out, a cowboy roped and "busted" him hard. By the time the herd was ready, every horse in the remuda respected the rope corral.

As each rancher brought in his beeves the boss cut out and rejected any considered unsatisfactory. He counted the others

33

into the pasture, making a tally of the various brands, so owners of strays could be reimbursed after the cattle were sold. When the herd had been gathered, the trail crew spent the next few days putting a road brand on them, to identify any that might stray. The road brand also enabled inspectors to check trail herds for cattle being moved illegally. Road branding was a Spanish practice adopted unofficially at first; in 1871 a law required that all cattle being moved out of the state must bear road brands that were large and easily identified. In the early days the cattle had to be roped and thrown; later long chutes were built so that fifteen or twenty could be branded at one time, speeding up the process and reducing the danger of injuries to men and animals.

When all was ready, they shaped up the herd, opened the pasture gate, and headed north, accompanied at first by extra hands. For several days they pushed the cattle fairly hard to get them away from their customary ranges and to make them too tired to run at night. After about a week the cattle usually settled down and were considered trail broken. Then the extra hands took their bedrolls and headed home.

Once across the Red River the herd was in Indian Territory, and in the late 1860s and early 1870s the danger of Indian attack made all hands apprehensive. In 1867 the Kiowas, Comanches, Southern Cheyennes, and Arapahoes had been persuaded to accept the Treaty of Medicine Lodge Creek, in which they gave up the right to roam and presumably accepted the concept of confinement on reservations. Some of the warriors of these tribes, however, preferred to die fighting instead of starving to death on the reservations. When they came upon a herd they might simply demand a few cattle, or they might attack the cowboys and stampede the cattle and horses.

Indians weren't the only hazard to early trail herds, for buffaloes and mustangs might charge through the line of cattle, scattering them beyond recovery. Trail bosses hired "buffalo whoopers" to ride ahead of the cattle each day and frighten away any herds of buffalo or mustangs that were close enough to the trail to cause trouble.

By the time a herd reached Indian Territory its travel was

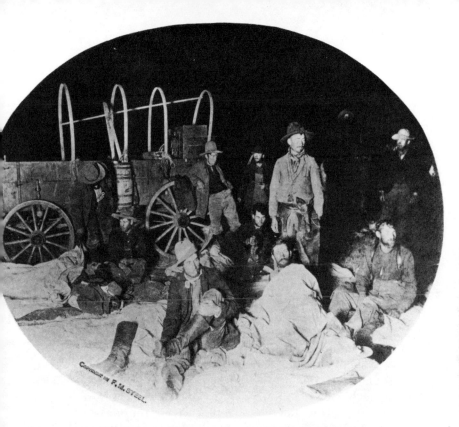

Crew bedding down for the night by the hoodlum wagon. Cowboy removing boots still has hat on. The hat was the first item of clothing put on in the morning and the last to be removed at night. Photo by F. M. Steel. Courtesy of the Amon Carter Museum of Western Art, Fort Worth

usually routine, and the cattle moved along by habit. The strongest steers had taken their place as leaders; others had positioned themselves somewhere in the long column, and they took approximately the same place each day. At the rear were the drags, the weak and sore-footed cattle whose protection and safe delivery were vital to the success of the drive.

The greenest men were assigned to the drags, for good hands wouldn't accept the distasteful, dirty, menial task because of the constant dust. Drag riders came away from the herd each evening with a heavy coating of dust on their hats and dust as "thick as fur" on their eyebrows and mustaches. Flankers and swing men on the side away from the wind were not much better off. The thousands of cattle pulverized the ground into fine dust, "and looking at a herd being driven at a distance one could only see a great cloud of dust rising to the heavens."[1]

A typical day began with the last change of guards before breakfast at three-thirty or four o'clock in the morning. Those heading for their blankets for half an hour more of precious sleep awakened the cook, who stirred up his fire and started breakfast. The rattle of pots and pans told the wrangler it was time to ride out and look for the remuda. When breakfast was nearly ready, the boss and the pointers arose so they could eat and be with the herd when it drifted from the bed ground. The cook called the men, who arose, put on their hats, then struggled to get their feet into damp, tight-fitting boots, hopping around on one foot and filling the air with profanity. Next they tied up their bedrolls and threw them beside the wagon. By the time the men had finished breakfast the wrangler was ready to push the horses into the rope corral.

There were no pets among the horses, and not one of them would allow a man to walk up and tie a rope around its neck; range horses that were easy to catch were easily stolen. On roundup or the trail the usual practice was for one or two of the best ropers to do all of the corral roping. Since not all cowboys were expert ropers it saved time and was easier on the horses for cowboys to hand their lariats to the roper and call out the names of the horses they wanted.

By the time the boss and pointers reached the herd the cattle were beginning to leave the bed ground and graze, always toward the north. The pointers positioned themselves well back from the lead steers so the cattle could spread out and graze along at their own pace. The boss loped ahead to decide on watering places for the day and a suitable place to rest the herd at noon.

As the herd moved slowly away from the bed ground the riders eased into position around it. Pointers and drag riders resumed the same place each day, but swing and flank men rotated. As the herd grazed along for several hours all the men had to contend with was boredom, for usually there was little to occupy them unless the boss signaled a change of direction.

When the cattle had eaten their fill they began walking steadily along the trail, stretching out into a long line.

At noon the boss signaled to push the herd off the trail; no other order was necessary, for the men knew exactly what to do. Half of the crew—left point man, right swing, left flanker, and right drag rider—headed for the wagon. They ate quickly, saddled fresh horses from the remuda, and loped back to the herd. To a hungry man with the herd there was no more welcome sight than his relief coming at a good clip.[2]

At supper time the riders again came in shifts to eat. If there was no nighthawk to herd the remuda, every man hobbled his own string except for his night horse, which he saddled and picketed near where he threw his bedroll. Because of the widespread belief that white horses attracted lightning in the dark, they were shunned as night horses. At least one episode suggests that there may have been some foundation for this belief about white animals and lightning. In 1854 a herd bound for California was struck by a violent thunderstorm in southwestern New Mexico. A bolt of lightning struck a white steer, then leaped to another white one fifty yards away, killing both.[3]

When the herd was bedded down for the night, about nine o'clock, all but the first or cocktail guard headed for the wagon. At times the men sat around the wagon for a time talking or listening to some cowboy fiddler playing "Billy in the Low Ground," "Dinah Had a Wooden Leg," "Hell among the Yearlin's," or other favorites of the day. Much of the talk was about the stars.[4]

Cowboys knew the major stars and planets from nights on guard around a herd, and had their own names for them. They learned to tell time by the rising or setting of certain stars or constellations with surprising accuracy. The Big Dipper, which Mexicans called *el reloj de los Yaquis*—the Yaquis' watch—was the principal cowboy timepiece. The men of the last guard agreed, however, that the Morning Star was the most beautiful sight in the sky, for its rising meant that the cook was starting breakfast and the wrangler was riding out after the remuda.[5]

Night herding was one of the daily trials of the cattle drive, although when the weather was pleasant and the cattle were quiet, it meant only the loss of two hours of sleep. Lack of sleep was, in fact, the most persistent complaint on the trail, for even under the most favorable conditions there was never time for a full night's sleep for any man. When conditions were bad, the men might go without sleep for forty-eight hours. At such times some kept themselves awake by rubbing tobacco juice in their eyes. As one trail boss said, "If you expect to follow the trail, son, you must learn to do your sleeping in the winter."[6]

The men who had to night herd from midnight to two in the morning had about three hours' sleep, then about an hour and a half more when they came off guard. But if the crew got one hour of sleep or none it made no difference, for in the morning the wagon and the herd moved on. If all hands were in the saddle all night following a stampeding herd or one drifting before a norther, at daybreak they ate breakfast, saddled fresh horses, and went back to the cattle to start another day's work.

Night herding got to be as much a part of a cowboy's life as anything else on the trail. The men had the same hours every night and by habit awakened when their turn came. Usually a sleeping man could hear the hoofbeats of the night guard's horse trotting toward the wagon. He would climb out of his blankets, pull on hat and boots, gulp down a cup of coffee, and untie his night horse. After one herd had reached the Mussel-shell River in Montana, the boss decided night herding was un-necessary. Every man woke up when it was his turn to go on guard, wondering what was wrong.[7]

It was at night that electrical storms caused much trouble. Anything, on occasion, could set off a stampede, but thunder and lightning started more runs from bed grounds than any-thing else. Signs that trouble was coming were often detected in the nervousness of the cattle, but many a rider's first warning came from the actions of his night horse, which always alerted him to any dangers it sensed.

Far in the distance a line of dark clouds might appear near the horizon, clouds that were eerily lighted by flashes of light-ning so far away the men could barely hear the thunder. The air would turn deathly still and humid; sweat poured down the riders' faces and stung their eyes. Gradually the flashes became brighter and the rolls of thunder grew louder. A heavy mist rose from the ground, so that the riders strained their eyes to see their ponies' ears, for these relayed warning signals.

Balls of electricity—Saint Elmo's fire—played around the tips of the horses' ears and the steers' horns, leaping snakelike from tip to tip around the herd, while the riders held their breath and hoped they had left everything metallic in the wagon. Deliberately, as if controlled by malevolent spirits, the blackest clouds poised menacingly over the herd.

A blinding flash of lightning lighted up the countryside; then all was plunged into total blackness. By the time the deafening thunderclap had ended, the rumble of hoofs and clatter of horns rose above the roar of the storm. Longhorns did not rise to their feet and then stampede—it was "one jump to their feet and running and the next jump to hell." As Charlie Russell said, "The confidence a steer's got in the dark is mighty frail."[8]

Blinded by the lightning, the cowboys could only loosen their reins, strangle their saddle horns, and hope their ponies did not fall over a bluff. Running cattle invariably turned gradually to the right. The night ponies, wise to the way of Longhorns, edged forward on the dead run along the left side of the herd to press the leaders into turning, to make a mill or pinwheel. If the cattle were spread out on a wide front there was no hope of starting them milling, but if they were strung out in a line the leaders could be turned and the others would follow. Once the cattle were milling they stopped running; when they were quiet the cowboys unpeeled the mill much as they had started it, and again tried to settle the cattle down for the night. They never returned to the original bed ground, for that would invite another stampede.

Some storms moved off quickly, before the cattle had run far or scattered badly. Others seemed strangely attached to the cattle, and herd and storm roared along together for miles. On such occasions the weary riders and their ponies simply hung on. Every time there was a flash of lightning over the herd a

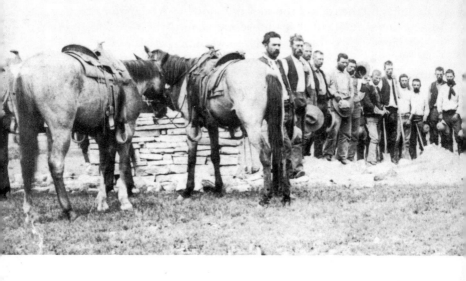

A cowboy's funeral, one of the few times cowboys were bareheaded. The Montana Historical Society

momentary silence followed as all the cattle leaped into the air at the same time. When they hit the ground together the earth trembled.

Under these circumstances all the riders could do was to follow bunches of cattle that turned off to one side or the other and hold them together till morning. When the sun finally rose, the men with small bunches of cattle drove them toward the wagon, or in what they thought was the right direction. They pushed the cattle onto the highest ground so they could look for other riders.

Gradually the herd was reassembled and strung out to be counted. When they knew how many were missing, riders combed the country for miles around looking for strays. If fortunate, they might recover all but a few that were killed or maimed in the flight. But if the cattle had run all night, several hundred might never be found.

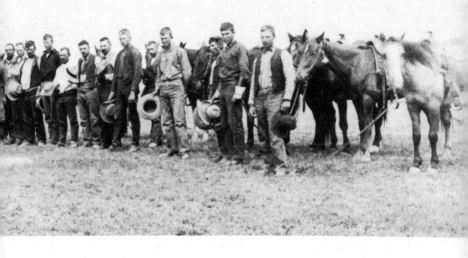

After one stampede Teddy Blue Abbott helped bury a cowboy whose horse had fallen in front of the cattle. Not knowing that a man had fallen, the other cowboys had milled the cattle at that place until morning. After that episode the men were ordered to sing or yell when running with a stampede, so others could tell where they were. But cattle would not run over a man if they could avoid it; more men were killed by lightning than by stampeding cattle.[9]

At a particular time when the cattle were ready to run, almost anything could start a stampede. One was caused by a steer getting his hoof caught in an empty tomato can. Another time a night guard's horse got his hoof caught in the tree of a McClellan saddle. One herd was passing Camp Verde when the remuda, frightened by the army's camels, stampeded and scattered the cattle so badly that it took days to find them. On another occasion Jim M. Dobie had made the first day's drive with a herd and penned it in a pasture so the trail crew could have a good night's sleep. Before anyone got to sleep a peacock screeched and the cattle were gone. As a result no one slept.[10]

As Charlie Russell noted, stampedes were noisy, but any harm they caused was usually to the cattle. The losses might range from a few steers crippled to the loss of the entire herd. The extreme disaster occurred to a herd of two thousand steers belonging to Wilson Brothers. When the steers were west of the Brazos, an electrical storm started them running, and the whole herd plunged into "Stampede Gully." Every animal was lost.

Rainstorms might blanket the trail for days, turning the prairie into a miserable bog and making the grass poor so the ponies grew weak and the cattle lost weight. Cooks were hard pressed to prepare hot food, and the men were soaked to the skin and cold for days at a time. No one slept in a dry bed. When relieved from duty with the herd, three exhausted men would lie down in a triangle, each resting his head on another's ankles to keep his face out of the water.

One trail crew driving a herd of yearlings north was struck at night by a blue norther near a dry lake bed that was covered with large tumbleweeds. Soon the tumbleweeds were flying among the bleating yearlings, which scattered in all directions. In the dark it was impossible to tell yearlings from tumbleweeds, and one cowboy chased a bunch of weeds for half a mile trying to force the leaders to turn.[11]

At times storms struck when several herds were in the same area, perhaps waiting for a swollen river to subside. When that happened ten thousand cattle from four or five herds might be so badly mixed it took a week to separate them. Usually there was not enough time to complete the job down to the last steer, and each boss had to rely on the others to keep track of the cattle they sold and reimburse the owners.

Even when the cattle did not stampede, electrical storms could be terrifying, and they sometimes killed men and animals. In 1885 young John Conner was nighthawk of a remuda on the Salt Fork of the Red River when a severe thunderstorm struck. As the air became charged with electricity the horses crowded around him, heads between their front legs and moaning loudly. More terrified than the horses, Conner slid to the ground and lay flat until the storm passed.

During thunderstorms cowboys often prayed loudly, making all sorts of promises, then laughed about them in the morning. In one violent hailstorm on the North Platte, however, old Matt Winter lost his temper. Shaking his fist skyward, he shouted, "All right, you old bald-headed bastard son of a bitch up there, if you want to kill me come on and do it!" The other cowboys fearfully begged him to stop.[12]

After a brutal thunderstorm near the Platte the men with an Olive herd were in the saddle several days rounding up the scattered cattle, stopping only long enough to eat and saddle fresh horses. When the herd was finally gathered, one weary cowboy said to Teddy Blue Abbott, "Teddy I am going to Greenland where the nights are six months long, and I ain't going to get up until ten o'clock the next day." "What the hell are you kicking about?" the boss asked. "You can sleep all winter when we get to Montana."[13]

After trailing became fairly routine, trail bosses or cowboys often put a fast horse in the remuda, not for use on the trail but for racing against others when a number of herds were close together or at some trail town. Cowboys bet heavily on their favorites. In the spring of 1877 young Jesse James Benton joined Tobe Odem's big herd of beeves from Goliad. Benton, whose family had recently moved from Kentucky, took along the small Thoroughbred mare, Gray Eagle, that his father had given him when he thought she wouldn't amount to much because of her size. But Gray Eagle proved to be exceptionally fast for short races, defeating many larger Quarter Horses.

There were other herds on the trail, and Odem, after satisfying himself as to the mare's speed, matched her against a big buckskin from another remuda, a horse that had won many races. The bet was for half interest in a bunch of "pick up" steers, or strays. Cowboys from all of the herds in the vicinity came to watch and wager; Odem confidently bet five hundred dollars in cash as well as the cattle. Because the buckskin was large and well known, most of the cowboys bet on him, but they were disappointed, for Gray Eagle easily beat him. Odem, who won nearly four hundred steers as well as considerable cash, gave Benton fifty dollars of his winnings.[14]

Horse racing was not the only excitement for Odem's men that trip. Near Dodge City six well-dressed women came out to the herd in a coach to visit Odem. The cowboys gave them all nicknames; one who was over six feet tall they called "Latigo Liz." The women stayed several days, insisting that they must see a stampede.

On the second afternoon Odem told them, "There's a bad storm coming and they will sure run tonight." He assigned each lady a dependable night horse and a cowboy for a partner, to keep her out of danger. The storm struck and the steers ran; drenched and with hair flying, the ladies had a great time.

In the morning "an old mutton-head cowboy" told Latigo Liz that she didn't need to be afraid of cattle or buffalo running over her.

"Why?" she asked.

"Because you could just jerk up your dress and stand on one leg and they would think you had clumb a tree, and pass you by."

Latigo Liz laughed. "I do not doubt it at all," she said. Jeff, the Negro cook, was horrified at the old cowboy's remarks, and chided him for his bad manners.[15]

Before the stocking of the northern ranges generated a steady demand for Texas horses as well as cattle, after a herd was sold in Kansas the cowboys, accompanied by the cook and chuck wagon, drove the remuda and perhaps a lead steer back to the home range. On these trips they amused themselves by roping buffalo, hunting, or fishing.

Later, remudas were sold along with the cattle heading for Wyoming or Montana, except for one horse apiece for the men. Eventually all of the horses were sold, and the men were given "cowboy tickets" to Texas on one of the railroads. The first trips by rail were usually entertaining for the passengers, for the cowboys ducked whenever the train went across a bridge or under a trestle. One night some cowboys were asleep on a train that had stopped on a siding to let another pass. When the other train came roaring and whistling past it frightened the cowboys out of their wits. They ran down the aisle, with "Dog Face" Smith in the lead. "Stampede!" one shouted. "Circle your leaders and keep up the drags!"[16]

Conditions on the trail were much improved in the 1880s over those of the previous decade. The chuck wagon was fully developed, and since it was drawn by a four-mule team it was able to carry a wider variety of foods. Saddles, too, were greatly improved, so that sore-backed horses, common on earlier drives, were now rare.[17]

At the outset of the trailing era, the men had used any type of saddle available and wore whatever clothing they might possess, often remnants of Confederate uniforms. They looked, Jesse Benton noted, "like a bunch of cotton-pickers." New styles gradually developed as certain items of clothing or equipment proved their durability and usefulness on the long drive. In 1867 the prevailing saddle style had narrow stirrups and long tapaderos. Riders rested their weight on their toes when they stood in their stirrups. Saddle trees varied widely, but the favorite had a broad horn pointing upward at a forty-five-degree angle. Bridles were functional rather than ornamental, made from rawhide rubbed and grained until reasonably soft and pliable. A few men wove horsehair bridles or bought them from vaqueros. There were also bridles of braided rawhide, and the best lariats were of the same material.

Homespun clothing was protected against hard and constant usage by adding leather caps at the knees and leather seats. Some men made leggins (chaps) of calfskin, hair side out, or of tanned buckskin fringed down the outsides.[18]

By 1872 everything had changed to some degree, especially styles of equipment. Broad stirrups, invented by an old fellow who ranched along the Llano River, had become popular because they were easier on the feet. Riders now shortened their stirrup leathers so that their knees were bent when their feet were in the stirrups. Saddles had broad, flat horns and were higher in front than in the back; most of them also had saddle pockets of goat or bear skin. Spurs with long shanks had replaced those with little straight shanks and sharp rowels. Cowboys now also wore buckskin gloves.[19]

One of the earliest saddles made in Anglo Texas was the little apple horn from Corpus Christi, which was widely used in the 1870s and 1880s even though its tree often caused sores on the horses' backs. Another saddle soon available was made in Fort Worth by Padgett. It was an improvement over the apple horn, but it also contained flaws in design. Still others were

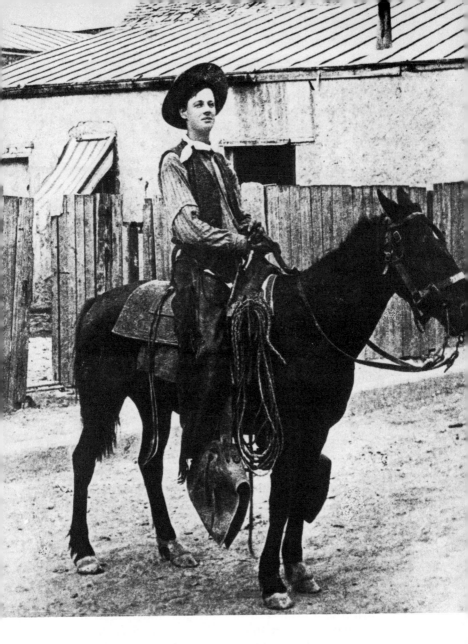

An old-time Texas cowboy on a twenty-dollar pony and forty-dollar saddle, San Antonio, 1880. He has tapaderos on his stirrups and rawhide lariat on his saddle. Western History Collections, University of Oklahoma Library.

produced by Frazier and by Dunn Brothers, Andrews, and Alexander of San Angelo, Texas, and by Gallup in Pueblo, Colorado. For a time one of the most famous saddles was made by H. H. Heiser of Denver.[20]

The California saddle, long used by Mexicans of that region, became popular among cowboys all over the West, for it was comfortable for both horse and rider. The merits of the California saddle, according to Randolph Marcy,

> consist in its being light, strong, and compact, and conforming well to the shape of the horse. When strapped on, it rests so firmly in position that the strongest pull of a horse upon a lariat attached to the pommel can not displace it. Its shape is such that the rider is compelled to sit nearly erect, with his legs on the continuation of the line of the body, which makes his seat more secure. . . . His position is attained by setting the stirrup-leathers farther back than on the old-fashioned saddle. The pommel is high, like the Mexican saddle. . . . The tree is covered with raw hide, put on green and sewed; when this dries it contracts and gives it great strength. It has no iron in its composition, but is kept together by buckskin strings, and can easily be taken to pieces for mending or cleaning. It has a hair girth about five inches wide.
>
> The whole saddle is covered with a large and thick sheet of sole leather, having a hole to lay over the pommel; it extends back over the horse's hips, and protects them from rain, and when taken off in camp furnishes a good security against dampness when placed under the traveler's bed.
>
> The California saddle-tree is regarded by many as the best of all others for the horse's back, and as having an easier seat than the Mexican.[21]

Texans always used double-rigged or rim-fire saddles because they tied their lariats to the saddle horns, and the extra cinch was needed when they roped bulls or heavy steers. Dally ropers, who wound the lariat around the saddle horn and could let out slack if necessary, preferred the single-rigged or center-fire California saddles. The saddle came to be a cowboy's most prized possession. "He sold his saddle" meant that a man was down and out, finished, disgraced. He "hung up his saddle" when he was too old to ride; when he "sacked his saddle," it was time for his funeral.[22]

The old saddles had long seats and no swell, which made it difficult for riders to stay on bucking horses. Cowboys often rolled up their slickers or blankets and tied them across the front of the saddle, thereby creating a swell, or "buckin' roll," that aided them in staying on bucking horses. In the 1890s some saddle makers introduced swelled forks like those of modern bronc saddles. The first one, called the "Ellensburg," was made in 1892 by the T. M. Farrell shop in Ellensburg, Washington. Cowboys everywhere at first made fun of the swell-fork saddles, but men who rode the "rough strings" soon appreciated the advantages.[23]

At first saddles were purchased from local shops, but soon they were available from mail-order houses. Catalogs and order blanks from the Garcia Saddle Company of Elko, Nevada, or the Visalia Saddle Company of Visalia, California, or similar ones in Denver and elsewhere were placed in bunkhouses all over the cattle kingdom. The Justin Boot Company, at the suggestion of rancher O. C. Cato, designed a self-measuring method of determining boot sizes. Thereafter boots could also be ordered ready-made.[24]

Before good manila hemp ropes were available, braided rawhide lariats were most widely used, though some men used cotton, sea grass, or Mexican maguey ropes. None was serviceable under all conditions. After sea grass ropes became plentiful, they replaced both rawhide hobbles and reatas.

Except for Bull Durham roll-your-own cigarettes and high-heeled boots, which remained virtually unchanged for more than half a century, most clothing and equipment changed from time to time. Slickers and tarpaulins came into use and were of great service in keeping the men and their bedding dry. Both were made of strong cotton cloth so thoroughly saturated with linseed oil that they readily turned water. Tanned leather replaced rawhide in bridles, and instead of simple split-ear headstalls they had brow and nose bands, throat latches, chin straps, and roller bits.

In the early 1870s wide-brimmed black or brown low-crowned beaver hats were popular, replacing sombreros for a time before they were also superseded by Stetson hats, introduced in the 1870s. In the 1870s, too, the heavy denim riveted pants made by the Levi Strauss Company of San Francisco, and Justin boots made in Texas, both began playing their key role in cowboy clothing. Before the coming of Levis the striped or checkered woolen "California" pants made in Oregon City had been considered the best for riding. "Justins," "Levis," and "Stetsons" became synonymous with boots, pants, and hats in much of the West.

By the 1880s regional styles had developed in clothing, riding gear, and ways of handling horses and cattle. A glance at a strange rider was usually enough to determine where he was from. Montana cowboys, for example, wore narrow-brimmed, low-crowned Stetsons creased with four dents, never with a leather or horsehair hat band. They also customarily wore vests. In the winter Montana cowboys wore the heavy wool California pants with buckskin sewed over the seat and down the insides of the legs. They also wore heavy Angora chaps of white, black, burnt orange, or red colors.[25]

Texans, whether on their home ranges or on those the Matador and other big outfits leased in Montana, wore high-crowned, wide-brimmed hats with creases down the middle and no dents. Most still tucked their pants in their boots. They wore leather shotgun chaps with fringes, or bat-wing chaps.

The Texans also used their small mustang cow ponies or larger Quarter Horse and mustang crosses. The Montana cowpunchers (this term was rarely used in Texas) rode larger, longer-legged, and heavier horses that were strong enough to battle snowdrifts in the winter.[26]

Once the herd reached the end of the trail and the hands were paid and allowed to go into town, they were more eager to catch up on entertainment than on sleep. First they visited a barbershop and had their shaggy manes trimmed. Then they bought a new outfit of clothing from the skin out, bathed, dressed, and headed for the nearest saloon, dance hall, or gambling house.

In releasing their pent-up feelings young cowboys were

boisterous and noisy, and if they could not make loud enough sounds with their vocal cords they made up for it by firing their pistols. The dance halls in the cattle towns along or at the end of the trail were their favorite haunts. Men were obliged to buy drinks for their partners between dances, and one might surmise that the dancers became increasingly carefree as the night wore on. Joseph McCoy commented that "few more wild, reckless scenes of abandoned debauchery can be seen on the civilized earth, than a dance house in full blast in one of the many frontier towns. To say they dance wildly or in an abandoned manner is putting it mild."[27]

When new ranches were opened on the northern plains, many Texas cowboys stayed on with the cattle and remained thereafter in Wyoming or Montana. Others headed for Texas by horse or by train, vowing never again to take part in a long drive. But when spring came and trail bosses were signing up crews, the vows were often forgotten. As Ben Borroum of Del Rio expressed it, "Like many others, when I had work for the time being I did not think I would ever make another trip up the trail, but also like many others, when the next drive came I was 'rarin' to go."[28] There was a fascination about going up the trail that young cowboys found impossible to resist.

The Trail Boss

"The trail drives produced a man unlike any
other that had as yet appeared in the West."
Clifford Westermeier

THE trail boss was the key man in a successful cattle drive, for he
bore the whole responsibility for getting the herd safely to its
destination in good condition. Jim Flood, Andy Adams's semi-
fictional trail boss, explained their duties to his cowboys before
they started up the trail.

"Boys," he said,

> the secret of trailing cattle is never to let your herd know
> that they are under restraint. Let everything that is done be
> done voluntarily by the cattle. From the moment you let
> them off the bedground in the morning until they are bed-
> ded at night, never let a cow take a step, except in the
> direction of its destination. In this manner you can loaf
> away the day, and cover from fifteen to twenty miles, and
> the herd in the meantime will enjoy all the freedom of an
> open range. Of course, it's long, tiresome hours to the men;
> but the condition of the herd and saddle stock demands
> sacrifices on our part, if any have to be made. And I want to
> caution you younger boys about your horses; there is such a
> thing as having ten horses in your string, and at the same
> time being afoot. You are all well mounted, and on the
> condition of the *remuda* depends the success and safety of
> the herd. Accidents will happen to horses, but don't let it be
> your fault; keep your saddle blankets dry and clean, for no
> better word can be spoken of a man than that he is careful
> of his horses. Ordinarily a man might get along with six or
> eight horses, but in such emergencies as we are all liable to
> meet, we have not a horse to spare, and a man afoot is
> useless.[1]

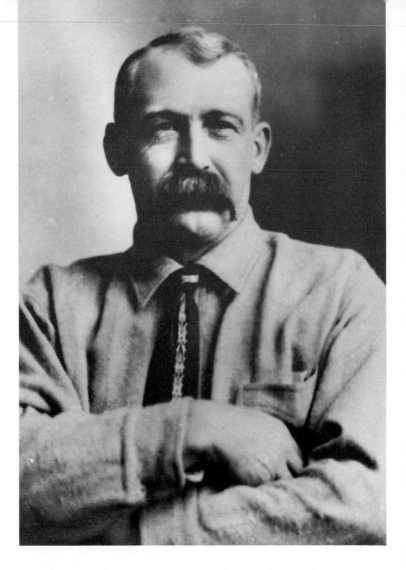

Andy Adams, whose books on trailing cattle were based on experience. *The Log of a Cowboy* and *The Outlet* are regarded as the most authentic accounts of life on the trail. Courtesy of the Amon Carter Museum of Western Art, Fort Worth

It is unlikely that any trail boss ever stated the requirements more clearly or succinctly than Flood. It often happened, before successful trailing practices became well known, that riders used up their horses and were practically afoot before the drive ended. "Watch out for the cows' hoofs and the horses' backs" was the first rule of trail bosses.

Managing a trail herd required knowledge gained only by experience with cattle, horses, and men as well as acquaintance with the country, the rivers, and the weather. The good trail boss was a man of stoic patience and endurance who was also cautious, alert, and fearless. He might drive himself and his men, but he pushed the cattle only on the rare occasions when it was necessary to cover long distances between watering places.

At the outset the trail boss had to select his crew for the drive, and this required the ability to size up men so as to pass over any of doubtful quality. On the trail tension was often high for days, and men who were likely to break down, become quarrelsome, or panic in emergencies were poor risks. Since only about one-third of the trail hands made the trip more than once, most crews included men who were inexperienced in trailing cattle. At times when dozens of herds were going up the trail, bosses often had to search widely to find enough men.

When young cowboy James Henry Cook asked trail boss Joel Roberts for a job with his herd, Roberts looked him over and said, "Now if you can ride the next four months without a whole night's sleep, and turn your gun loose on any damned Injun that tries to get our horses, well get ready."[2]

On the trail the boss and point riders ate before the others, while the herd began drifting from the bed ground. The boss rode ahead to check on grass and water and to choose the bed ground for the night. He was in the saddle as long as any man with the drive, and might ride thirty or forty miles each day while the herd traveled twelve or fifteen. Because of the need to find good grass and water, herds seldom traveled in a straight line to the north.

After he had scouted ahead, the trail boss might appear on a hill a mile from the herd, where he employed signaling techniques similar to those of the plains Indians. A motion of his hat meant for the men to move the herd out. The pointers repeated it to the swing men, who passed it along to the flankers, who relayed it to the drag riders bringing up the rear.

If the streams ahead had dried up and water was scarce, the boss returned to the herd and told the men to move the cattle faster. This meant that flank and swing and drag riders rode closer to the cattle, causing them to walk faster and graze less. The boss saddled a fresh horse from his string and galloped off to search for water. When he had found an adequate stream, directly ahead or to either side, he rode back to a hill from which he could see the herd, then signaled to the pointers which direction to take.

To signal a change of direction the trail boss galloped his horse in the direction to follow, then signaled with his hat to come along. Again the point men relayed the signal down the line to the drags. If the turn was to the right, the point, flankers, and swing men on that side dropped back and away from the cattle. The men on the left pressed the steers, forcing them to turn, with the result that the whole herd swung in the desired direction at the same time. If the swing men and flankers performed their job skillfully, the sore-footed drag cattle were spared about three hundred yards of walking. Making it easier on the weaker cattle was one of the signs of good trail management. The drags determined the speed of the herd; the stronger cattle often had to be held back so that gaps did not occur in the line. Whenever there were gaps the cattle trotted to catch up with those ahead, and running cattle lost weight. One of the drag riders' jobs was "keeping up the corners" to prevent the rear cattle from spreading out more widely than the swing cattle in front of them, to avoid danger of losses from overheating. The heat generated by a herd was surprising even when it moved slowly, but especially during stampedes.

The trail boss also checked on the horses frequently, to see if any were missing. Experienced men could glance at a remuda of a hundred horses and know when two or three were not there. Most could also name the ones that were absent.

Grazing and watering were daily necessities that must be

accomplished perfectly if the herd was to arrive in good condition. When there were many herds on the trail, finding good
grass became critical for the trail boss. Cattle bedded down at
night without having had their fill of grass and water were likely
to stampede, and running cattle might be lost or crippled. At
intervals along the way the cattle were strung out and counted.
This was, of course, always done after a stampede or any
difficulty in which some cattle might have been separated from
the herd.

Veteran trail bosses like Jim Dobie and Ab Blocker learned
that the most effective way to control a stampede was to leave all
of the men but one or two experienced cowboys at the wagon.
Two or three men were usually able to calm the cattle more
quickly than a lot of yelling cowboys.

Watering a trail herd was an orderly process. First the cook
watered his team and filled the barrel, then the remuda was
watered. Next came the cattle; when they had finished drinking,
the trail crew had its turn. "I ain't kickin'," one remarked, "but I
had to chew that water before I could swaller it." One of the
highest compliments that could be paid a trail boss was that he
was skillful in watering a herd. J. A. Smiley commented that
Henry Eubanks of the XIT was "a real cowman and the best trail
man I ever saw. He could water more cattle in a small lake of
water and never get it muddy than any man I ever saw."[3]

Burgess and Harry Rutter watered two thousand head at a
spring that was about as big as a wagon box, according to Teddy
Blue Abbott. If the big beeves had been allowed to crowd in,
they would have made a mud hole out of it. The two men
brought them up in little bunches and watered a few at a time.
"It was," Abbott concluded, "the slickest piece of cow work I ever
saw in my life."[4]

Crossing rivers was another test of skill, for if the water was
high, or "swimming," it was difficult as well as dangerous. If a
river was low, there was danger of cattle being caught in quicksand. Ordinarily, if the lead steers were strung out and allowed
to approach the water slowly, they would plunge in and head for
the opposite bank. The herd willingly followed the leaders. Trail

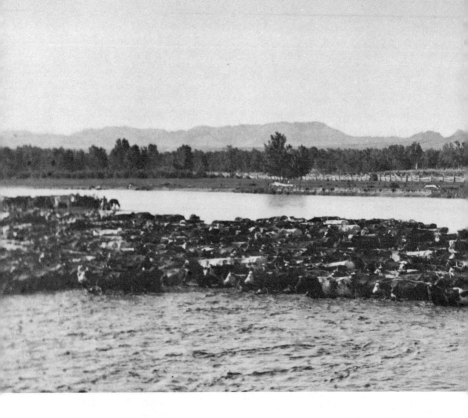

N Bar herd crossing the Powder River in Montana, 1886. The N Bar was owned by E. S. (Zeke) Newman of El Paso, Texas. Photo by L. A. Huffman. Courtesy of the Amon Carter Museum of Western Art, Fort Worth

bosses learned not to push cattle into a river when the sun was low and facing them, for they would start milling halfway across, and many might drown.

The Red River was especially treacherous, for storms upstream often made it rise suddenly, even while a herd was crossing. More trail hands were drowned in the Red than any other river. The Cimarron was also difficult to cross, for it had a bottom of quicksand in which cattle bogged down if they stopped to drink. Pulling cattle out of quicksand was hard, time-consuming work. Some streams contained poisonous gypsum deposits that killed many cattle.

Often when a river was flooded over its banks a number of herds had to wait for it to subside. This happened at the Red

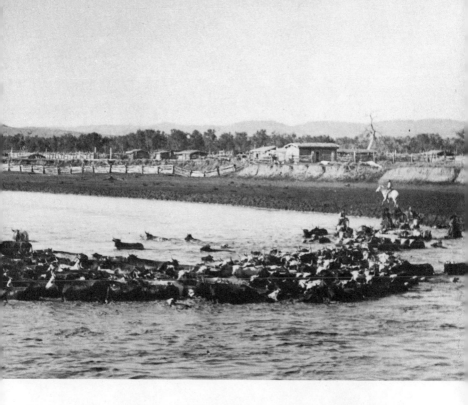

River Station crossing in the spring of 1871, when heavy rains raised the river over its banks until it was a mile wide. Mark Withers, who had earlier taken part in Joseph McCoy's wild west show, started from Caldwell County with twenty-two hundred head of mixed cattle. It rained every day, and the Colorado and Brazos rivers, which were usually easy for cattle to wade across, were both swimming when his herd reached them. When he was still three days' travel from Red River Station, Withers heard thousands of cattle bellowing. The sound grew louder the next day, and it never ceased.

Withers left his herd and rode ahead, to find the Red River a foaming torrent full of uprooted brush and trees. He saw a number of trail bosses and cowmen gathered there, including Shanghai Pierce. Pierce, whose voice could be heard farther than that of any other Texan, was doing the talking. There were sixty thousand cattle waiting to cross; Pierce urged everyone present to move his herd back ten or twelve miles. With so many outfits so close together, he said, if any herd started to run there

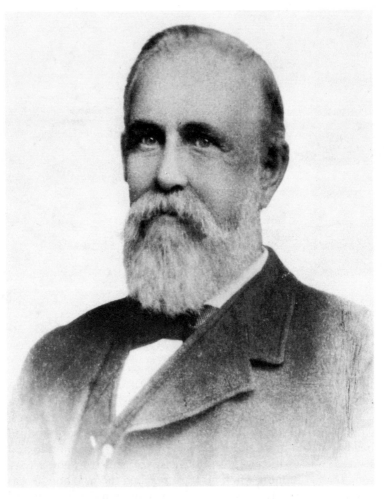

Abel H. ("Shanghai") Pierce, Texas rancher and trail driver. Western History Collections, University of Oklahoma Library

would be hell to pay, and all would lose money. It was clear that it would be days before any herd could cross, but none of the bosses was willing to drop back and risk losing his turn at crossing.

The first outfit that had reached the river was an all-Mexican crew with a small herd from Refugio County. After a few days the rain stopped and the sky cleared. Late in the afternoon the vaqueros drove a small bunch of steers down the cut and into the water, with one rider accompanying them. The powerful current swept them downstream; a submerged log shot to the surface, striking the vaquero's horse and unseating the rider. He tried desperately to grab a steer's tail but failed to reach it. Another vaquero spurred his horse into the current in a vain effort to save him; both men and the cattle were swept under.

A few nights later one of the waiting herds stampeded, and soon all of the cattle for miles around were milling. As Shanghai Pierce had predicted, everyone lost money, for cattle were crippled and killed, and it took ten days to separate the herds.

Dick Withers, like his brother Mark, was an experienced trail boss. In 1879, with ten cowboys, a cook, and a wrangler, he drove fifty-five hundred mixed cattle to Ogallala for J. F. Ellison. At the Red River one man was too sick to continue, and two quit. Although it was an unusually large herd, Withers eased it along with only a skeleton crew. At Dodge City he hired more cowboys and continued.

At Ogallala, Nebraska, Ellison instructed Withers to cut out one thousand cows, one thousand yearlings, and seven hundred two-year-old steers. When Ellison rode out to the herd, he found the cowboys cutting out some "long yearlings" as two-year-olds. "Dick," he warned Withers, "a Texan is going to receive those cattle and he knows ones from twos." But when Withers and the Texan classed the cattle, they agreed on eight hundred yearlings and nine hundred two-year-olds, which meant unexpected profits for Ellison. He was so pleased he bought supper for the whole crew and gave Withers train fare back to Texas.[5] Contracts calling for cattle of a certain age were filled by substituting younger ones when older cattle were scarce. It was surprising, cowboys wryly noted, how much cattle aged on the trail.

A trail boss always had to be prepared for the unexpected. In April 1879 a herd of Tom Snyder's steers started up the trail a short distance south of Victoria, with Dick Arnett as boss. As usual, early in the drive the cattle were nervous and easily stampeded, and on the second day the herd passed through the main street of Victoria. A woman saw them coming and was afraid that the steers would break down her fence and destroy her roses. She ran out to the fence, waving bonnet or apron at the cattle. It was said that cowboys feared nothing more than a good woman, and clearly the steers shared this feeling, for the leaders turned back and the rush was on. Only the quick thinking of trail boss Arnett saved Victoria from a Longhorn tornado. "Give way at all street crossings and let the cattle have room," he shouted. Dashing about and giving orders, he prevented the steers from taking short cuts through the houses. Several blocks of homes were surrounded by wild-eyed Longhorns, but they soon became quiet and were easily driven on through the town.[6]

The next night the cattle were bedded in a wide lane east of Gonzalez. The lane had high rail fences on either side, so night guards were stationed only at each end. During the night the herd stampeded and could not be checked. When the cattle were rounded up and counted the next day one hundred steers were missing. Four seedy-looking characters rode up and offered to bring in strays for one dollar a head, but accepted fifty cents instead. They brought in sixty, and it seemed likely that they had stampeded the cattle. The trail crew brought in twenty more, so they were only twenty short.

When the herd reached Fort Worth, Arnett held it over for a day while he and the cook bought everything needed for the five-hundred-mile trek to Dodge City. Several representatives of Fort Worth business houses rode up with whiskey, cigars, and similar gifts for the trail boss. All trail hands loved practical jokes, and on this occasion Arnett stayed with the herd while the cowboys indicated that gray-haired "Shug" Pointer was trail boss. Pointer had solemnly accepted the proffered gifts when one of the cowboys rode up and said, "Shug, the boss says come on, you lazy cuss, and get to work, or he'll turn you off at Fort Worth." All of the hands had a good laugh over the expressions of shock when the Fort Worth solicitors realized they had been taken in.

Tom Snyder rode the train to Dodge City ahead of the herd. Learning that many cattle in other herds had died from drinking gypsum water at several crossings, he sent a man to guide Arnett and the herd through the danger areas. At one of the bad crossings the cattle were thirsty, but the sight of dead cattle all around was proof that the water was poisonous. The men bunched the cattle near the crossing, then rushed at them shouting and waving slickers, to stampede them across the shallow stream. Even though some of the cattle tried to turn back to drink, the cowboys got the herd safely out of danger.

When they crossed the Cimarron near the Kansas line, Arnett learned that there was no more water for the cattle until they reached the Arkansas River at Dodge City, nearly one hundred miles away. The herd had been grazing along, making about twelve miles a day. Now it had to be pushed so as to cover the one hundred miles in four days. By the fourth day the cattle were staggering from thirst, and the herd stretched out five miles or more. Fortunately, it rained and small pools of water formed, which helped save them.

North of Dodge City there were daily rumors of Indian war parties in the area. Finally Arnett met some Texas cowboys with a herd of eight hundred horses they were taking to Ogallala, Nebraska, to sell to ranchers. The boss of the horse herd asked Arnett if he had seen any Indians. Arnett replied that he had not seen any, but had heard something about them every day. The boss of the horse herd admitted that he and his men had had so much trouble with sod-busters that they began spreading reports about Cheyenne war parties and then making night drives, knowing that men who feared an Indian attack would not interfere with the horse herd.[7]

Relations between trail bosses and Kansas sod-busters ranged from hostile to cordial, for although there was mutual resentment, each also had something the other needed. The settlers plowed furrows around their fields in place of fences, but Longhorns were not kept out of cornfields by scratches in the earth. When cattle crossed the furrows, the trail boss was fined for trespass.

But when night approached it was a different situation, for farmers offered fresh eggs, vegetables, and other inducements to trail bosses to bed their cattle on the farmers' land in order to obtain a supply of fuel for the coming winter. When the herds left the next morning the farmers guarded their donations "like a Texas man does a watermelon patch" until the cow chips were dry enough to gather and store.[8]

Before their trailing business became so large that they had to hire a number of crews, the Snyder brothers were their own trail bosses. They began by buying cattle on credit and trailing them to Abilene. Over the years Snyder herds were driven to New Mexico, Colorado, Nebraska, Wyoming, and Montana, where they helped stock new ranches.

The Snyders were pious folk, and they enforced strict rules of conduct for their cowboys. "First, you can't drink whiskey and work for us. Second, you can't play cards and gamble and work for us. Third, you can't curse or swear in our camps or in our presence and work for us." Once when Tom Snyder and his crew were riding south to pick up a herd at Victoria, a young man joined them. Soon he was cursing everything in sight, and for one so young his vocabulary was rich and varied and reasonably colorful.

Finally Tom Snyder stopped him. "Young man," he said, "we will be pleased to have your company if you will not swear so much, but if you cannot quit cursing, please fall behind or ride ahead of us. We propose to be gentlemen."

"Mister, is you a Christian?" the startled youth asked.

"I hope so."

"And a cow driver?"

"Yes. Why not?"

"That's awful damn strange," the boy shouted as he galloped away.[9]

Like the Snyder brothers, "Uncle Henry" Clare of Bee County was another trail boss who could not stand profanity. Whenever things went wrong his strongest expression was "O my stars, boys, don't let 'em run!"[10]

One of the best-known trail bosses was Albert Pickens ("Ab") Blocker, who trailed cattle year after year in the employ of his brother John. He had gone up the trail as a youth but reluctantly abandoned it one season to help his mother on her farm. After all the hard work involved in raising a crop of cotton, it sold for only four cents a pound. Ab gave up farming in

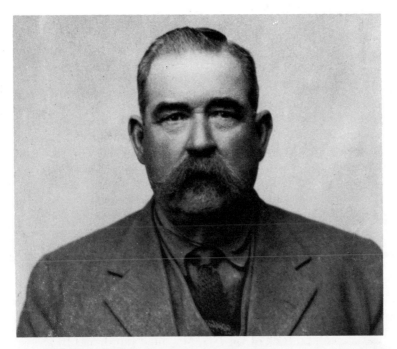

John R. Blocker, head of Blocker Brothers, trailing contractors. Western History Collections, University of Oklahoma Library

disgust and returned to the only life that suited him, and to his preferred diet of beef, potatoes, and whiskey.

The Blockers had the reputation of being hard taskmasters. One cowboy said that when working for the Blockers he could always count on "two suppers ever' night . . . one after dark and the second befo' sunup next mornin'." John Blocker possessed, nevertheless, an element of chivalry. When a widow tried to sell him one hundred steers for ten dollars a head he refused, but threw the steers in with his herd. After the cattle were sold he brought the widow fifteen hundred dollars. She tried to pay him the customary one dollar per steer, but he shook his head. "The boys didn't know they were in the herd," he told her.

During the few years he was married, Ab's wife shocked him by giving birth to a daughter. When a neighbor's wife asked Ab how she was doing, he replied, "Oh, she's just as porely as she can be. She's had everything from hollerhorn to a baby."

"Hollerhorn" (hollowhorn) was his term for any bovine ail-
ment.[11]

The kinds of harassment trail bosses might face on the way
north were experienced by Doc Manahan of Fairfield, Texas,
when he delivered a herd of wild two- and three-year-olds to
Fort Reno and other posts in 1873. Since the herd had been
purchased by the government, Manahan had an escort of twelve
troopers. In Llano County eight mean-looking armed men rode
into camp; the leader claimed that the herd was on his land, and
demanded fifty cents a day for horses and twenty-five cents for
cattle. Doc Manahan pulled him off his horse and thrashed him,
which was all the payment he got.

When Manahan's herd reached the Red River, it was rising,
and he had to wait five days for it to subside. In Indian Territory, U.S. marshals told him that two weeks earlier rustlers had
killed most of the men with a herd of fifteen hundred cattle and
had stolen the entire herd. Across the Washita armed men demanded the right to cut the herd for strays. Well aware that this
was a common trick of rustlers, Manahan ran them off.

After the herd had crossed the Cimarron a thunderstorm
started a stampede that lasted three hours. In the morning
Manahan counted his crew and the herd and found two men
and thirty head of cattle missing. An Indian rode up and informed them that he had seen dead cattle at the foot of a cliff.
With the dead cattle, Manahan discovered the bodies of his
missing men, one a sergeant of the escort.

At the Kansas line more armed men rode up, claiming the
right to inspect the herd for ticks, and demanding payment of
twenty-five cents a head for the service. When Manahan threatened to have them arrested, they withdrew. Fake inspectors
were common, not only at the Kansas border, but even at the
Red River crossing. In 1873 two "inspectors" ordered a trail boss
to pay fifty dollars apiece for two strays in his herd. He had his
cowboys tie the men and throw them in the wagon, setting them
afoot somewhere in Indian Territory.[12]

On the trail, strays, either from the range the cattle were
passing through or from earlier herds, often joined the drive.
After inspectors were placed at the Texas border, these animals

were cut out. But trail bosses never objected to having strays accompany their cattle, for they could provide beef for the crew or for Indians who demanded a "wohaw" or two, or they could be sold in place of cattle lost on the trail. ("Wohaw" was what Indians thought ox drivers called their cattle). As one man remarked about unbranded cattle that joined his herd and refused to be turned away, "But it is remarkable the way these cattle persisted in following the herd. Naturally our sympathy was with them."[13]

William Jackson was bossing his own herd and crew when a stray with Ike Pryor's road brand joined his cattle. Jackson planned to turn the stray over to Pryor at Dodge City, but near Fort Sill a band of Kiowas or Comanches stopped him. The leader handed Jackson a slip of paper. It said to treat this Indian well and give him a beef, and there would be no trouble. Pryor had signed the note.

Chuckling to himself, Jackson called one of his men and told him to cut out Pryor's steer and give it to the Indians. It might seem that when a herd of two thousand steers was stretched out half a mile or more, finding any particular animal would be hopeless. But since trail cattle took approximately the same places every day, it required only a few minutes to locate the steer and cut him out.

After water holes or streams along the trail were fenced, cowmen were forced to pay for each head watered; in some cases they were refused water. In the early 1880s Shanghai Pierce accompanied one of his herds north, and found water scarce. When the thirsty cattle finally reached a water hole, local ranchers armed with Winchesters denied him water, even after he grudgingly offered to pay. He drove his cattle up the trail that night and bedded them down without water.

With a few reliable men Pierce rode back and drove off a herd of steers that belonged to the men who had refused him water. He ordered his men to push them hard toward Kansas, "till their tongues dragged the ground."

Several times the next day the ranchers rode up and asked to cut Pierce's herd for their lost cattle. It was customary, when a herd crossed another man's range, to let him inspect it for his strays. On this occasion Pierce was more obliging than usual, allowing them to take all the time they wanted, in order to give his own men more time to get the lost steers beyond reach. This continued for several days; each time Pierce was polite and agreeable. But on the fourth day, knowing that his men were safely away, he armed the rest of his cowboys. When the ranchers came again to cut his herd he said, "No damn grease sack outfit can trail cut my herd four successive days. Get goin'." Although it was dry, he solemnly remarked later, considering the "natural increase" of his cattle on the road, it turned out to be a profitable drive.[14]

One man started up the trail with his own herd from his ranch near Decatur in the spring of 1868. They camped a few nights later near Victoria Peak, northwest of where Bowie is now located. That night Comanches drove off the entire remuda except the night horses, which were tied near the wagon. The two men on the first guard saw the Comanche raiding party; knowing that in those days when a man lost his hair it was not all he lost, they preserved theirs by dashing all the way back to Decatur, where they breathlessly announced that Indians had killed everyone with the herd. The owner rode thirty-five miles back to his ranch, bought horses, hired two men, and was back with the herd by the next day.

When a trail boss allowed himself to be pushed into doing something against his better judgment, the results were likely to be disastrous. One held up his herd at the Canadian River when it was at flood stage. Because his men poked fun at him for being so cautious, he ordered the herd moved into the river, leading the way himself.

The river was not to be crossed that day, and the boss and his horse were swept under. When the men finally recovered his body, they found a letter from his wife in his coat pocket. In it she begged him not to try to cross rivers when they were flooding.

In 1874, Sol West was given charge of a herd belonging to his brother. They agreed on the selling price, and would split profits between them. Sol was one of the youngest men who ever bossed a herd up the trail, and no man with him was over twenty. Eager to be the first to reach market, he set out from Lavaca County on February 27 and had a difficult time because of blizzards which scattered the cattle. Worse than that, every horse froze to death and he had to replace the entire remuda. On his return his brother went over the expenses carefully and figured the profits to be a dollar and a half. He handed Sol seventy-five cents, asking if he planned to buy another herd or start a bank.[15]

Controlling men was occasionally a problem for trail bosses, especially when they had to hire strangers after a drive had started. In 1888, S. D. Houston was driving twenty-five hundred steers north from the Pecos River region, when he was obliged to hire four men. After visiting Fort Sumner he returned to the herd and saw only one man with it. The new hands were at the wagon, all of them armed. Houston got his own gun and ordered them to drop theirs. They obeyed. Houston immediately moved camp, leaving the four men behind with nothing but their saddles.

Short-handed, Houston had to leave the Pecos and cross the Staked Plain, a ninety-mile drive without water. He had the wrangler turn the remuda in with the herd and help with the drive. They reached the Canadian without losing any cattle. At Clayton, New Mexico, he hired a youth named Willie Matthews, who stayed with the herd until it was near the Colorado-Wyoming border and then quit because of homesickness. A short time later a lady visited the herd—it was the same Willie Matthews. She was the daughter of an old-time trail driver from South Texas who was determined to see for herself what "going up the trail" was really like.[16]

Among the best-known trail bosses was Dick Head, "one of the best cattlemen that ever came from Texas." He was a large, good-looking man with a black beard and "eyes that seemed to penetrate you."[17] He had trailed cattle to California, and he bossed dozens of herds to Kansas and beyond.

When Millett and Mabry contracted to deliver fifty-two thousand cattle at Ogallala and elsewhere in 1875, they hired Dick Head to serve as general manager for the drive. Head successfully supervised the seventeen herds on the trail, bringing them to Ogallala in good condition and earning his employers substantial profits.

Till Driscoll, another experienced trail boss, was in the employ of Schreiner and Lytle. When he trailed herds in the early 1880s he refused to allow his cowboys to carry guns. There was no longer danger of Indian attack, but when hungry Kiowas and Comanches demanded a "wohaw" or two for allowing cattle to cross their lands, it would have been easy for a trigger-happy cowboy to start a disastrous clash.

Driscoll never let his men crowd the cattle off the bed ground, but allowed them to remain until they were ready to graze off of their own accord. As a result there were few sore-footed cattle, and his herds arrived in good condition.

At the height of the trailing era, when a number of contractors sent up from five to fifteen herds each season, experienced trail bosses were in great demand. The techniques of trailing large herds were well known by this time, but there were still unforeseen dangers. Many drives were unsuccessful, and some were disasters, but that was in the nature of the business. The vast majority of herds made the journey in relative safety and without major calamities, some traveling all the way from the Rio Grande to the Dakotas.

The trail boss belonged to the era of the great cattle drives, and when it ended there was no longer any need for the type of field officer he represented. Like the mustang and the Longhorn, the trail boss vanished soon after barbed-wire fences began cutting up the Chisholm Trail.

CHAPTER 5

The Cook and His Castle

"Only a fool argues with a skunk, a mule, or a
cook."

NEXT in rank and pay to the trail boss was the cook, lord of the
chuck wagon, headquarters and home for trail hands. Trail
bosses were only occasionally tyrannical toward the crew; chuck
wagon cooks competed for the distinction of being known as the
"techiest" one on the trail in any year. A widespread reputation
of unrivaled crankiness was a source of satisfaction. No cook
would admit, of course, that he was proud of the food he served,
or that he greatly valued the crew's appreciation of his efforts.

It is hardly surprising that chuck wagon cooks were easily
irritated much of the time. They had to feed eleven or twelve
hard-working men three times a day regardless of weather or
anything else; it was difficult enough when the weather was
pleasant. Sandstorms, hailstorms, and drenching rains that
soaked the fuel and left the ground under water often chal-
lenged the cooks' ingenuity. What they accomplished under the
most adverse conditions was astonishing. The trail boss worried
about the welfare of the cattle and horses—neither animals were
given to complaining—but the cook was responsible for keeping
the men well fed and reasonably contented. Nothing made tired
men forget their weariness faster than a hot, tasty meal ready to
eat the moment they slid from their saddles. Because of his
impact on the crew's morale, a capable cook was essential, a man
to be humored by all hands.

The chuck wagon was the cook's castle, and no man dis-
puted this with impunity. "The space for fifty feet around the
cook is holy ground," Bruce Siberts wrote, "and the cook is the
Almighty. If things go wrong, he will raise hell. Maybe he will
anyway. He is the only one who can cuss not only the hands but
the boss too."[1]

From the two-wheeled ox carts that carried provisions and

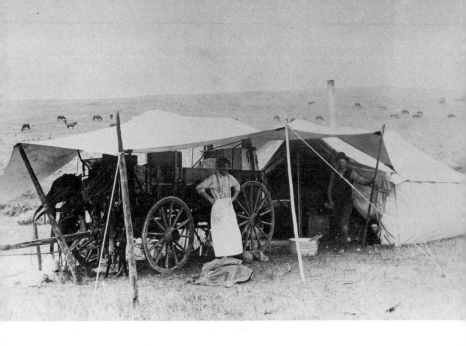

Oscar Anderson's cook, Judith River roundup, 1910. Remuda is grazing in the background. Courtesy of Keith Anderson, Helena, Montana

served as mess wagons, the chuck wagon gradually evolved. Charles Goodnight is usually credited with inventing the chuck wagon, or at least with perfecting it. In the spring of 1866 he bought an army wagon with wide wheels and rebuilt it with the toughest wood he could find, such as thoroughly seasoned bois d'arc. The key element in Goodnight's design was the chuck box fitted across the rear of the wagon as a cupboard. The cover of the chuck box was hinged and had a dropleg, so that it served as the cook's work table.[2]

Each chuck wagon carried a water barrel strapped to one side, and a *cuna,* or cradle—"cooney," the cowboys called it, or "possum belly," or "the bitch"—slung under the wagon bed. The cooney was simply a cowhide suspended by the four corners to hold firewood or buffalo chips as an emergency fuel supply. It was the duty of the wrangler or the nighthawk to keep the cook supplied with firewood, but since the cowboys were also concerned they watched for dead branches they could rope and drag into camp.

Space for carrying food was extremely limited. Only easily

handled nonperishables such as cornmeal, beans, bacon or sow-belly, molasses, and coffee were the cook's regular supplies, while canned tomatoes and dried fruits were occasional luxuries. It required culinary artistry and imagination to concoct combinations of these limited ingredients that were not exactly like those of the day before or the day after. Whenever a beef was butchered the cook used only the choice cuts, for without refrigeration meat soon spoiled. In the early years buffalo, antelope, and wild turkeys enabled cooks to vary their menus. There were always lots of rabbits near the trail, but no cowboy would eat "nester food" unless he was starving, for "anybody that would eat rabbit would talk to hisself, and anybody who talks to hisself tells lies."[3]

Awakened usually by the last guard to go out to the herd, or by the built-in alarm clock in every trail cook's head, the cook arose before anyone else except the trail boss. When breakfast was nearly ready, he sent the wrangler out to bring in the remuda and called for the hands to "come and get it." The men ate, threw their dirty dishes and utensils into the "wreck pan" lying under the chuck box lid, turned their night horses loose, and saddled fresh ones from the remuda. Two men harnessed the chuck wagon mules and left them standing by the wagon. As they rode out to the herd, the last night guard headed for the wagon and a hasty breakfast. While the shifts of riders were eating, the cook prepared lunch to be served at noon when they threw the herd off the trail to rest.

After the last man had eaten, the cook washed dishes, pots, and pans while the wrangler loaded the Dutch ovens and the trail hands' bedrolls. Any cowboy who failed to tie up his bedroll and put it by the wagon might discover at night that his blankets still lay on his tarpaulin where he had left them that morning. The herd was already strung out grazing when the wagon and remuda left the camp ground and passed the slowly moving cattle. In five to seven miles they reached the place the boss had chosen for the noon stop. The cook unhitched his team, donned his flour sack apron, and began preparing the next meal.

At noon, while the cattle rested, the men rode to the wagon, half of them at a time, to eat a hurried meal and saddle a fresh horse. As soon as all had eaten and returned to the herd, the cook washed the dishes and then drove on to the place where the herd would be bedded down for the night.

At the night camp the wrangler dug a trench for the fire from six to ten inches deep and about two feet long. He placed the oven rack over the hole, and the cook suspended the Dutch ovens from it. Enough sourdough biscuits were made to last a day, so that they did not have to be baked at every meal. Some foods such as beans, which required four or five hours of cooking, were placed over the coals several times after meals had been served. Undercooked beans rattled noisily on the tin plates, a sound no cook wanted to hear. Chuck wagon cooks had much to remember and much planning for coming days if meals were to be ready on time. Since the herd wouldn't reach the bedding ground for several hours after the noon stop, the cook also had time to nap or hunt or fish.

At dark the cook pointed the wagon tongue toward the North Star. Before riding ahead each morning, the trail boss took note of the direction. This was usually the only "compass" available, and on cloudy nights it was undependable.

Few cooks were young, which may have accounted for some of their crankiness. Often they were crippled cowboys who could no longer do cow work. In the early years many were ex-slaves; others were Mexicans. Since the number of good trail cooks was never equal to the demand, good and bad they were humored and pampered regardless of color. One of the cardinal rules of the trail was that "only a fool argues with a skunk, a mule, or a cook."[4]

Cooks were usually paid more than cowhands, but no one complained, for there was no doubt that a good cook deserved all he was paid. His was a long, lonesome work day, and his hours of sleep were few. He had to drive an ox or mule team over rough ground and keep the wagon repaired until the herd was sold and delivered.

The cook also served as nurse and physician, handling all ailments from aches and pains to broken bones. Common complaints such as carbuncles, however, the cowboys treated themselves by placing a chew of tobacco on them. Among his limited

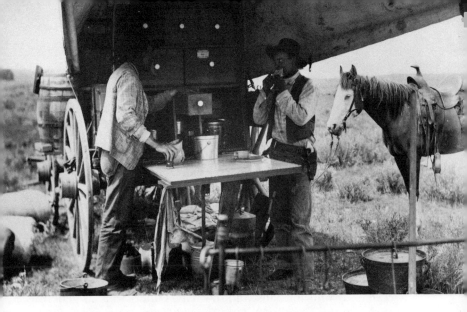

Roundup cook and pie biter—the wrangler—on a Montana range. Pot rack and hooks are in foreground, Dutch ovens on the right. Water barrel is on left side of wagon. Photo by L. A. Huffman. Courtesy of the Amon Carter Museum of Western Art, Fort Worth

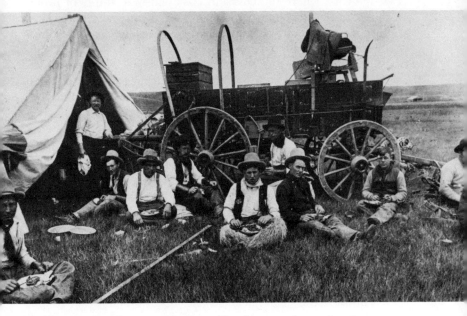

Mealtime on the 2D range, Montana. Man in center is wearing Angora chaps. Cook has removed flour sack apron for photographer. The Montana Historical Society

supply of condiments the cook stored a few simple multipurpose medicines such as turpentine, liniment, quinine, and calomel, as well as some reasonably clean rags that could serve as bandages. His remedies for various ailments were typical of the folk medicine of the frontier. When dealing with dysentery caused by drinking alkali water, he boiled bachelors' buttons if they were in bloom, or fed sauerkraut if available. He might also make fry cakes using a batter of flour and salty water, or concoct a brew from the inside bark of cottonwood trees.[5] On occasion he was also a barber.

The food supplies chuck wagons carried were often decided as much by herd owners as by available space. Some owners, especially contract drovers, were tight-fisted, supplying mainly coffee, cornmeal, beans, and sowbelly. Others were as generous as conditions permitted, but perishable foods were, of course, out of the question, except for a meal or two when laying over at Fort Worth or when grangers in Kansas had eggs and vegetables for sale. In 1879 a Snyder herd on its way to Wyoming passed by Dodge City, where the boss and cook laid in a supply of provisions. Among the items purchased was a rare keg of pickles. Once the keg was opened, the men ate nothing but pickles until they were all gone.[6]

A staple of the chuck wagon was Arbuckle coffee, which came roasted but unground from Arbuckle Brothers of Pittsburgh. Strong, black coffee was served at all meals, and the pot sat on the coals all night so night herders could gulp down a cup before riding out to the herd.

Dried frijoles, or beans—red, pinto, or navy—high in protein and easily carried, were an important element in chuck wagon cooking. They were also inexpensive and easily obtained in Texas, although the cook had to spend some time picking out pebbles and other inedibles before soaking them overnight and cooking them for half a day or more.

The cook also kept a keg of sourdough fermenting; sourdough biscuits baked in a Dutch oven were daily fare that men were always ready to eat. The dough was also used to make crusts for other dishes and desserts.

Besides the "eatin' irons" and cooking utensils like pot

hooks, Dutch ovens, and coffee mills, chuck wagons also carried the cowboys' "war bags" containing their extra clothing. In addition there were usually an ax, a shovel, chains, and guns and ammunition, especially during electric storms, when the riders hastily got rid of everything metallic. When danger from rustlers or Indians threatened, the cook handed out the guns as the riders dashed by the wagon. Once when Comanches approached a herd, the boss had every gun passed out to the riders, leaving the cook with nothing but his butcher knife for defense. "By Jacks," he protested, "when it begins to thunder and lightning you fill this wagon full of six-shooters, but when the Indians are around the guns are all gone and who is going to protect me?"[7]

Trail bosses chose their cooks carefully and held onto good ones year after year if possible. But since there were more jobs than dependable cooks, bosses and crews were sometimes deeply disappointed. During a storm Mark Withers and his crew were out with the herd all night and much of the next day without rest and with only a "Spanish supper"—tightening the belt a notch or two. When the cattle were finally under control, Withers and half of the men rode to the wagon for coffee and a hot meal. There was not even a fire going, for the cook was rolled up in his blankets asleep. Somehow the infuriated Withers and his men refrained from shooting the cook, but Withers fired him and sent him on his way on foot.

On a drive from the Mexican border to Montana in 1896, five different cooks served part of the way with the herd. The cattle were shipped by rail whenever grass was scarce, and there were far too many towns where whiskey was available. When one cook was too drunk to work, the trail boss sacked him and hired another.[8]

It happened occasionally that after the chuck wagon had been rafted across a river, the water rose suddenly and spilled over its banks before the cattle had been crossed. In the spring of 1874 this happened at the Salt Fork of the Canadian River near the Kansas line. There were two wagons and twenty-four riders under trail boss Asa Dawdy. The wagons crossed safely, when the river suddenly rose and flowed a mile over its banks. Separated from the wagons for seven days without even their

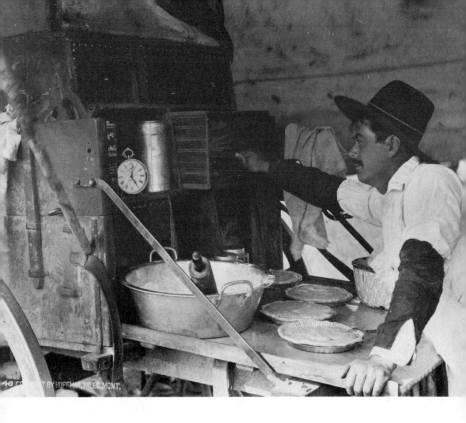

"Mexican John," well-known XIT ranch cook in Montana. Photo by L. A. Huffman. Courtesy of the Amon Carter Museum of Western Art, Fort Worth

bedding, the men had nothing to eat but meat without salt.[9]

Most cooks had nicknames, often two. One was the name the cook wished to be called; the other was the cowboys' graphic but secret name for him. Bilious Bill, who cooked for the LU outfit, was always taking "sody" to settle his stomach. Vinegar Joe was known for his mock lemon pies made with vinegar. Bilious Bill and Vinegar Joe were once camped near each other on a roundup and each tried to outdo the other in a display of talents. A war between them was barely averted when Bilious Bill's pet, a retired chuck wagon mule that followed him everywhere, discovered the pies that Vinegar Joe had put out to cool and ate them all.[10] Dirty Dave was a cook whose name reflected his mania for washing dishes. "He's so plumb soap-

and-water crazy, so damn clean," a cowboy said, "that he's dirty."[11]

One cranky cook called Gray Jack lost his pipe, which only increased his irritability. At last, when he emptied the coffee pot, he found the missing pipe. Naturally, the cowboys could only congratulate him on his good fortune, for if they antagonized him they might find that there were worse things than coffee flavored with tobacco ashes and nicotine. A rough form of trail justice caught up with Gray Jack, for which he could blame no one but himself. One morning after all of the men had eaten and ridden out to the herd he discovered blankets and a tarp that had not been rolled up and tied according to the rigid trail etiquette. With a wicked grin Gray Jack attached tarp and blankets to a wagon wheel, which reduced them to shreds. When he looked for his own bedroll that night, he discovered that it was his own he had tied to the wagon wheel.[12]

In 1877 a trail outfit hired an inexperienced young man as cook at Fort Worth. One afternoon the boss told him to cook some dried apples for supper. He heaped a pot with dried apples and added water. As the apples swelled they overflowed the pot. Some of the cowboys saw the cook's predicament, and watched him. He dug a hole, and as the apples fell from the pot, he buried them in it. He had a new nickname next day—Apple Jack.[13]

One cook served dried apples until the men stopped eating them. Then he used them to make fried pies. When he heard a cowboy say, "Tromp on my corns and tell me lies, but don't pass me no apple pies," the cook was miffed. There was no more stewed fruit of any kind the rest of the trip.[14]

The tastiest dish chuck wagon cooks prepared was "son-of-a-bitch stew." Moved by sensitiveness unknown to old-time trail hands, modern writers usually call this popular dish "son-of-a-gun stew" or, more daringly, "SOB stew."

Son-of-a-bitch stew could be made only when a yearling had been slaughtered. The ingredients were brains, tongue, liver, heart, sweetbreads, kidneys, lights (lungs), and marrow gut, all cut into small pieces. Cooked in a Dutch oven, it made a rich, savory meal, especially with the cook's secret flavoring added. As one cook described it, "you throw ever'thing in the pot but the hair, horns, and holler." The longer it cooked the better it tasted, and a cook was mightily offended if anyone could guess all of the ingredients.[15]

After the early years big outfits often included both a night-hawk and a wrangler in the crew. The nighthawk herded the remuda all night, so that it was not necessary to hobble the horses as before. Days he drove the extra "hoodlum," or bed wagon, and doubled as a cook's louse, helping with the dish washing and other chores. When the wagons reached the next stopping place at noon or night, the nighthawk crawled into or under the wagon to catch what sleep he could.

Although the nighthawk remained one step lower than the wrangler in the hierarchy of trail hands, both boys were sub-jected to constant teasing. Nevertheless, at every opportunity the cowboys taught them to rope and other skills, and after one drive as wrangler a youth might graduate to riding drag the next year, a short step up the ladder.

One of the most bizarre cases of recruiting cooks occurred, according to legend, in Cheyenne, Wyoming, in the fall of 1876. A herd of Longhorns from Texas was crossing Wyoming on its way to an Indian agency in the Dakotas, when the cook died. The trail boss sent two cowboys into Cheyenne with orders to find a replacement and get him out to the herd pronto, for the season was getting late.

A short time earlier Custer and the Seventh Cavalry had made history on the Little Big Horn, and three Japanese gener-als and their aides had come to study the American Indian fighting army in the field. General Phil Sheridan had them with him in Cheyenne; the next stop would be Deadwood, where they would confer with General George Crook when he came in from his Sioux campaign.

Two Japanese captains in civilian clothes were wandering around Cheyenne one afternoon looking for excitement. They saw two dusty Texas cowboys riding up the street. The cowboys stopped and seemed to be discussing the Orientals. What they said was probably to the effect that "yonder's a couple of Chinks, and I hear tell that all them Chinks is good cooks."

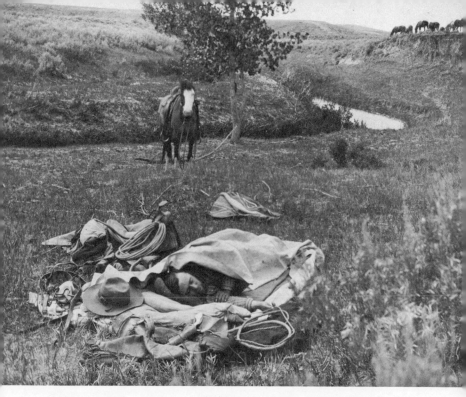

The nighthawk in his nest. After herding the remuda all night he drove the hoodlum wagon to the next stop, then caught what sleep he could. Photo by L. A. Huffman. Amon Carter Museum of Western Art, Fort Worth

The captains watched impassively as the cowboys untied their lariats and shook out loops. In a moment the loops sailed through the air and pinned the captains' arms to their sides. They protested vigorously in their native tongue as the cowboys hauled them up behind their saddles, wheeled their ponies, and galloped out of town. When they reached the herd they dumped the two officers unceremoniously on the ground and pointed to the chuck wagon.

Not knowing a word of English, the captains were unable to explain that they were neither cooks nor Chinese. As the herd moved toward the Black Hills, the captains struggled with the four-mule team the wrangler had hitched to the chuck wagon.

General Sheridan was irritated but apologetic when he learned from the generals that two of their aides had mysteriously vanished. He took his guests on to Deadwood with him, explaining that his men would find the missing aides and bring them to Deadwood.

The trail-broken Longhorns moved steadily toward the Black Hills without protest, but the crew was on the verge of mass desertion. Their "Chinese" cooks were a disaster—they couldn't cook beans or biscuits. Even worse, they couldn't even brew a decent pot of coffee.

As the herd approached Deadwood, the boss managed to hire a stove-up miner who could make sourdough biscuits and boil beans. The boss paid off the "Chinese" cooks along with some uncomplimentary remarks they fortunately couldn't understand. The two captains were so happy to escape alive they declined to press charges. The trail boss shook his head in bewilderment as he watched them hurry up the road. Good cooks were sure hard to find.[16]

CHAPTER 6

The Cowboys

"Ma, do cowboys eat grass?"
"No, dear, they're partly human."
Rawhide Rawlins (Charlie Russell)

COWBOYS, along with mustangs and Longhorns, were key but passive elements of the long drives and the cattle kingdom. Others made the financial arrangements; the cowboys simply did the work. They were, in fact, faceless youths on horseback, for most were known only by their first names even to their companions. Unless they wrote or dictated memoirs, today even their names are forgotten. As daring, graceful riders, nevertheless, they won a lofty place among American folk heroes, displacing the Daniel Boones and Kit Carsons of forest and mountain.

An estimated thirty-five thousand to fifty-five thousand men rode up the trails with cattle and horses. Perhaps one-fifth were black cowboys or Mexican vaqueros, and about one-third made the trip more than once. Nearly all were in their teens or early twenties when they first went up the trail; only cooks and bosses were likely to be over thirty.

Cowmen, as Lewis Atherton has pointed out, were as owners and managers considerably more important than the cowboys they employed. Despite this and the fact that ranching was the only American business that "evoked a literature, mythology, and graphic symbolism of its own," popular attention has always been focused on the cowboy rather than the cowman.[1]

Much has been written about these cowboys and the adventuresome, exciting lives they led. Most writers have viewed them favorably, whether accurately or imaginatively. A few, however, have taken a less flattering view of the hired men on horseback. Bruce Siberts felt that most of those in South Dakota were below average as humans.[2] Joseph G. McCoy, whose main

81

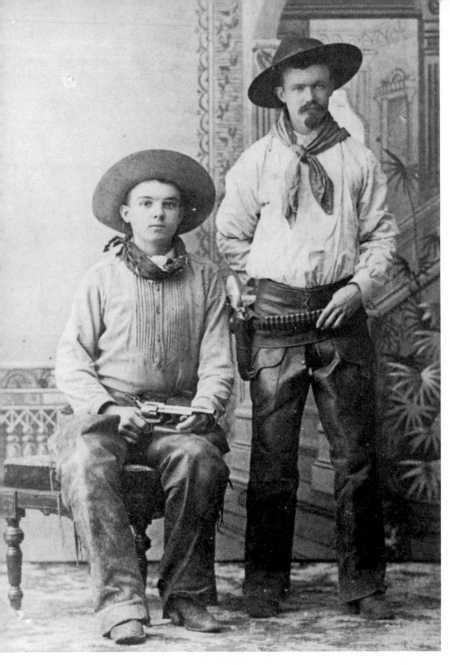

LU Ranch cowboys Thomas Aston and Dogie Taylor, 1889. Photo by L.
A. Huffman. The Montana Historical Society

contact with cowboys was when they hit town at the end of the drive, spoke of them without trying to conceal his contempt. John Clay and Theodore Roosevelt both praised and criticized the cowboys they knew in Wyoming and the Dakotas.

Clay's criticism concerned the men who worked for the Scottish syndicate he represented, mainly in the Sweetwater valley of Wyoming. As the cattle came up from Texas to stock the northern ranges, he wrote, many cowboys came with them. The majority were well trained and no worse morally than the ordinary run of young fellows. But the great movement of cattle gave criminals and the indifferently honest the chance to move into new surroundings where they were unknown. The crew of the 71 (71 quarter circle), he added, was as mean a lot as ever got together, for though able, they were undependable, inclined to gambling, and held human life as of little value. It was, nevertheless, a pleasure to watch them sweep around a herd with an easy grace and careless abandon, never missing a point. Riding and roping were second nature to them. But cowboys usually degenerated and disappeared, he noted; old cowboys were rarely seen.[3]

Clay was especially disgusted with the cowboys who struck for higher wages on the 1884 Sweetwater roundup. He pointed out, with evident satisfaction, that the ones who quit all dropped out of sight, while those who remained loyal all became successful ranchers.[4]

Midwestern newspapers as well as the people of the Kansas trail towns mercilessly caricatured the youthful and unschooled Texas cowboys. The attitude of the people who profited by cheating and swindling the cowboys is not surprising, for one may drink milk without admiring cows. But these people saw cowboys only after months on the trail, not at work. Others, who watched them in action, generally respected them for their hard work and loyalty, their universal generosity, and their unfailing good humor.

The editor of the *Topeka Commonwealth* wrote on August 15, 1871,

> The Texas cattle herder is a character, the like of which can be found nowhere else on earth. Of course he is unlearned

and illiterate, with but few wants and meager ambition. His diet is principally navy plug and whisky and the occupation dearest to his heart is gambling. His dress consists of a flannel shirt with a handkerchief encircling his neck, butternut pants and a pair of long boots, in which are always the legs of his pants. His head is covered by a sombrero, which is a Mexican hat with a high crown and a brim of enormous dimensions. He generally wears a revolver on each side of his person, which he will use with as little hesitation on a man as on a wild animal. Such a character is dangerous and desperate and each one has generally killed his man. . . . They drink, swear, and fight, and life with them is a round of boisterous gayety and indulgence in sensual pleasure.[5]

Another view of the cowboy was that of salesman John McCoy, who arrived in Fort Worth in 1876:

The life of the cowboy is one of considerable daily danger and excitement. It is hard and full of exposure, but it is wild and free, and the young man who has long been a cowboy has but little taste for any other occupation. He lives hard, works hard, has but few comforts and fewer necessities.

He has but little, if any, taste for reading. He enjoys a coarse, practical joke, or a smutty story; loves danger but abhors labor of the common kind; never tires of riding, never wants to walk. . . .

One thing is certain about the cowboy. He is undoubtedly the Good Samaritan in the parable which was designed to hold up for commendation the most noble attribute of human nature. A Pharisee the true cowboy never is.

But the cowboy is more than a Good Samaritan. We do not read in the Bible that, in relieving the sufferings of the man who had fallen among thieves, the Samaritan parted with anything in which he was actually in need. The cowboy is not only generous when generosity costs him nothing, but he is generous when generosity involves actual personal hardship.[6]

Cowboys fought with guns but disdained fighting with their fists. They were common men without education, but, said Teddy Blue Abbott, "They set themselves away up above other people who the chances are were no more common and uneducated than themselves." They were fiercely independent, a quality that easterners and Britons like John Clay failed to comprehend. In Texas a cowboy's string of horses was virtually his personal property, and not even the owner dared tamper with them. Montana rancher Granville Stuart, unaware of this rigid custom, once sold a horse out of a man's string without consulting him. The offended cowboy asked for his time. When others explained his error to Stuart he was able to persuade the man to stay.

"Cowboys are ultra sensitive, diffident, and superstitious about anything that they do not understand," cowman Frank Hastings noted. "They possess a quality that is not necessarily courage, but rather the absence of fear."[7]

Cowboys were proud and sensitive, Abbott admitted. "But that sensitiveness on their part and the belief that their outfit was the best on earth was all to the advantage of the owners, and that was why John Clay was such a fool when he made that speech . . . in 1914, attacking the old-time cowpunchers."

What Clay said that provoked the rebuke was that "the chief obstacle on the range at that time was the cowboys, who were mostly illiterate, uncivilized; who drank and thieved and misbranded cattle, and with a kind of rough loyalty, never told on one another in their crimes."

"John Clay was a hard-fisted, money-loving Scotchman," Abbott continued, "who had no understanding of the kind of men who worked on the range. . . . They were all like a bunch of brothers. And if they weren't, they were no use as an outfit and the boss would get rid of them."[8] It should be added, in at least partial justification of Clay, that many men for whom sheriffs were looking in Texas and elsewhere changed their names and headed for Wyoming and Montana. Also, Texans were unable to generate much loyalty for eastern or British syndicates like the ones Clay represented.

In *The Story of the Cowboy*, Emerson Hough described the

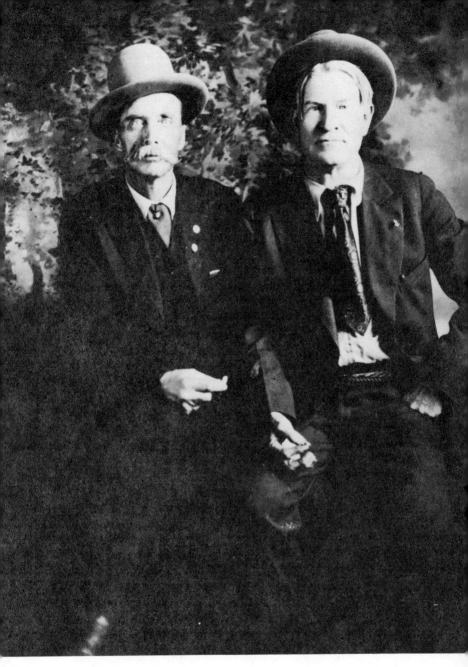

"Teddy Blue" Abbott and cowboy artist Charlie Russell. The Montana Historical Society

cowboy as simply a part of the West; anyone who did not understand the one could not possibly understand the other. "Never,"
he wrote, "was any character more misunderstood than he."
People remember the "wild momentary freaks of man" but not
the lifetime of hard work and loyalty. The cowboy should be
seen in connection with his surroundings to know him as he
actually was, "the product of primitive, chaotic, elemental forces,
rough, barbarous, and strong." Then, "because at heart each of
us is a barbarian," he will appeal to "something hid deep down in
our common nature. And this is the way we should look at the
cowboy of the passing West . . . as a man suited to his times."[9]

Cowboys were products of the great age of open range and
free grass, of freedom-loving Longhorns and wiry little mustangs, and of the cattle kingdom stretching from the Rio Grande
to the Mussellshell. As Don H. Biggers remarked about the cowboys of that era, "No class of men ever worked harder, endured
more exposure, encountered greater danger, had fewer of life's
common comforts or less time to devote to the cheerful side of
existence."[10] Richard Irving Dodge added, "I doubt if there be
in the world a class of men who lead lives so solitary, so exposed
to constant hardship and danger, as this. . . . For fidelity to duty,
for promptness and vigor of actions, for resources in difficulty,
unshaken courage in danger, the cow-boy has no superior
among men."[11]

The trailing of hundreds of cattle over trackless prairies,
coping with thousands of rampaging buffalo, bands of playful
mustangs that charged among the cattle, and resentful plains
warriors came immediately after the Civil War. "It was," says
western historian Clifford Westermeier, "the trail drives that
made him a type—gave him his personality and exalted his spe-
cialized form of work. The trail drives produced a man unlike
any other that had as yet appeared in the West."[12]

Because the increase in numbers of range cattle had been
unregulated during the Civil War, postwar cattle trailing expanded almost explosively after the Chisholm Trail opened the
way to profitable sales. Texans suddenly found themselves with
vast herds of cattle and a distant, expanding market. The cattle
had to be moved, but there was no comparable supply of experi-

enced cowboys to move them. Early trail crews, or "crowds,"
were, therefore, mixtures of skillful Mexican vaqueros and
equally adept ex-slave cowboys, on the one hand, and green boys
fresh from farm or city on the other. Many of these youths later
praised the Mexicans and black cowboys for their willingness to
teach them to rope and ride and other skills needed for survival
and success.[13] In a fairly short time, because of the many hours
they spent in the saddle day after day, the greenies were con-
verted into cowboys if they could stand the hard life as well as
being the butt of camp jokes. Experienced cowboys who could be
spared from ranch work for the trail were never numerous
enough to fill the trail crews, so trailing continued to be a training ground for cowboys.

Young men came from far and near—East, Midwest,
South—to work on Texas ranches and to "go up the trail." A
large number of them soon realized that ranch life was not as
pictured in dime novels, and quietly disappeared, but dozens of
others realized their dreams. Some, like Ad Spaugh, left one-
room sod-buster's cabins and wandered into cow camps, where
amiable Texans took an interest in them and gave them the
opportunity to begin doing a man's work at the age of fifteen.[14]

In the late 1860s most of the Anglo Texas cowboys were
former Confederate soldiers in fact or by association, and they
remained unreconstructed rebels at heart. Much of the end-
of-the-trail boisterousness of Texas cowboys had undertones of
Yankeephobia. The people of the Kansas cowtowns who eagerly
separated trail hands from their money were all "no'therners" or
"Yankees" to Texans. This same attitude carried over to eastern
and British cattlemen and syndicates who hired Texans for their
ranches in Wyoming, Montana, or the Dakotas. Texas cowboys,
accustomed to cowmen who worked alongside them and treated
them as equals, resented the absentee owners who regarded the
cowhands as servants and whose visits to the ranches were like
circuses. Only rarely could Texas cowboys develop a genuine
respect for and feeling of loyalty toward these men.

Cowboy W. S. James was born in Tarrant County, Texas, in
1856, "the ugliest little bundle of humanity that could have been
found in seventeen states and fourteen territories," he confes-

sed. His father moved his herd to one of the western counties, probably Palo Pinto, where James grew up in the saddle.

"In reality the cow-boys might properly be divided into three classes," James wrote. "First, No. 1, the genuine, because of his true manhood, not only in his relationship to those with whom he is daily associated in handling cattle, but with all the world. One who has as much respect for the rights of others, though he be miles away, as for his immediate neighbors. I mean by that, a man who is strictly honest, one whom it does not affect in his general health to eat a piece of an animal of his own mark and brand."[15]

The second was the true type of western hospitality, liberal to a fault, especially in his moral views, who had an elastic conscience ready to serve him. His education often assisted him in interpreting to his own advantage the brands of cattle from northerly ranges. Eating his own beef "shore makes him sick."

James described the third class of cowboys—the typical cowboy—as "a big-hearted, whole-souled bundle of humanity, kind-hearted, generous to a fault, possessed of all the frailties common to mankind, and not the biggest rascal on earth by a jug full."

After the Civil War, Texas became the refuge of renegades from North and South, who were a greater scourge than Indians had ever been. It was they who gave the state a reputation for lawlessness and violence. Before the war, stealing cattle and horses was virtually unknown; horsestealing was regarded as worse than murder. Cow stealing, or rustling, began during the last years of the war.

Despite the undercurrent of Yankeephobia, any man who proved himself and who could take a joke was accepted. A genial old gentleman from the East came to Texas and bought two thousand choice steers. When he and some cowboys drove them to his camp, he wore a silk hat. He lay down for a nap under an oak tree, placing the hat on the ground by his side. He was awakened by the tramp of horses' hoofs as the cowboys rode into camp, and he listened to their talk.

"What must we do?" one asked.

"What is it?"

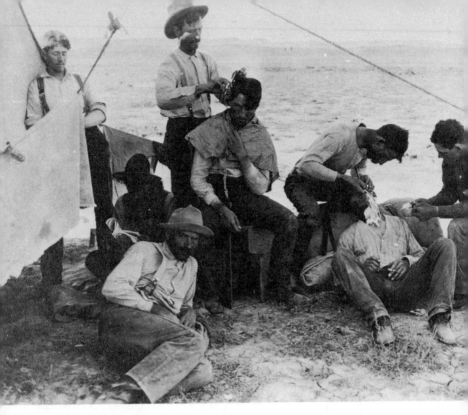

Circle Ranch roundup camp, 1906. Cutting hair was once one of the cook's skills. Here cook Ralph Waite is having his hair cut. The Montana Historical Society

"It's a bear."

"It's a venomous kypoote. It's one of those things that flew up and down the creek and hollowed 'wala wahoo' in the night time."

"Boys," one cowboy said, "it's a shame to stand peaceably by and see a good man devoured by that varmint." He called, "Look out there, mister, that thing will bite you," and drew his pistol. The old gentleman "got a ten cent move on him" and didn't stop to get his hat. By the time he was ten or fifteen feet away, every man had put a bullet or two through the hat, shooting the crown off.

Finally one of the cowboys dismounted and, with a stick, cautiously turned the hat over. "Boys, it's shore dead," he said. The old gentleman had a hearty laugh, called the cowboys to his

wagon, and took out a jug of "sixteen-shooting liquor." Together they celebrated the death of the terrible varmint. One of
the cowboys lent him a hat until they could chip in and buy him
one, the best to be had. After three days on his new ranch,
everyone, including the cook, was ready to fight his battles for
him. It would have been a far different story if he had been
angry over what they had done. They would simply have told
him that if he brought wild animals into camp he could expect
that they would be killed.

Before the Civil War, slaves were valued far more than cowboys, as one incident in Abel "Shanghai" Pierce's early ranch life
illustrated. One of the most powerful of Texas cowmen after the
war, Pierce recalled that as a young man working for W. B.
Grimes he and a slave cowboy named Jake drew straws to see
which of them got to ride an outlaw dun horse. Jake won, but the
outlaw fell on him, leaving him stretched out unconscious on the
ground. Grimes's aunt had been watching, and she concluded
that Jake was dead. "There's $1500 gone, Bradford!" she
shouted at Grimes. "Why didn't you let Abel Pierce ride that
horse instead of Jake?"[16]

Some youths who aspired to be cowboys came from as far
away as the British Isles, and a few of the successful ones wrote
or dictated memoirs, which help us visualize cowboy life as they
saw it. Among them was Frank Collinson, who came to San
Antonio from England in 1872. There he went to work on John
T. Lytle's ranch south of the city. Two ex-slave cowboys, both
top hands, taught him every step in the process of breaking
broncos and handling cattle. Collinson became a top hand and
spent the rest of his life on the plains.

In 1874, Collinson went up the trail with a herd of thirty-six
hundred of Lytle's steers to the Red Cloud Sioux Agency, then
at Fort Robinson, Nebraska. The herd was composed largely of
big brush steers that had been purchased in small bunches from
many ranchers. Collinson considered the trail drive as nothing
but hard work, though others like Teddy Blue Abbot viewed it
differently.

Abbott had accompanied his family from England to Nebraska in 1871, when he was eleven. His first trailing experience

was in 1873, when he accompanied his father to Texas to buy three hundred big steers from John R. Blocker. His father doubled his money on the cattle, breaking some to sell as oxen by yoking them and tying their tails together while they tore up the pasture for several days.

Although there were many Texas cattle and cowboys in Nebraska at that time, there was nothing north of Ogallala except Indians and buffalo. Texas cowboys were, according to Abbott, a wild, reckless breed, and he seems to have fitted in with them very well. His father was a tyrant, but the Texans were the most independent class of men on earth. They taught Abbott to ride and rope.

Abbott left home for good when he was eighteen, while his father and brothers continued the struggle to raise crops. Only one brother chose another career, said Abbott, "and he ended up the worst of the lot—a sheepman and a Republican."[17]

Because he arrived in Montana with a trail herd from Texas, Abbott was always regarded as a Texan. There was nothing about him to make him appear to be anything else, for like most Texas cowboys he was ready for any prank or other activity that tempted him. On one occasion he rode to New Mexico to help Bill Charlton receive a herd of seven hundred "wet" horses at the Rio Grande. Charlton paid the Mexican vaqueros three dollars a head for the stolen horses, then drove them to Nebraska and sold them to settlers for twenty-five to thirty dollars apiece.

Abbott's worst experience was helping the FUF crew gather wild brush cattle. Totally unprepared or equipped for brush popping, Abbott saw his clothes torn to shreds, and he picked thorns out of his knees all the way to Kansas. He swore never to go near brush country again.[18]

Unlike his countryman, Collinson, Abbott thoroughly enjoyed life on the trail. Some of the accounts of hardships were accurate, he admitted, "but they never put in any of the fun, and fun was at least half of it." In his later years he grumped that the famous collection *Trail Drivers of Texas* sounded like a bunch of preachers.

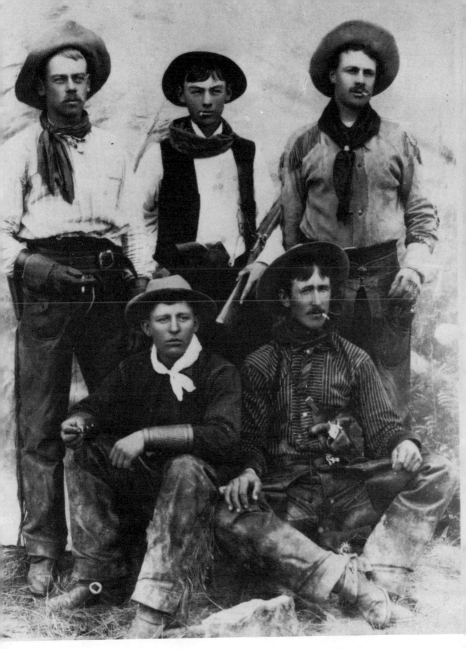

Montana cowboys at Big Sandy, around 1890, all looking like "strong, silent men." The Montana Historical Society

Another young man who headed west to become a cowboy was James Henry Cook, who in the early 1870s got his first job at Ellsworth, Kansas, working for a cowman holding a herd there. When the outfit returned to San Antonio, Cook went along. There he hired on with Ben Slaughter's foreman, John Longworth, to gather brush cattle. All of the other members of the crew were Mexican vaqueros; without them no cow hunt in the brush could succeed.

Even before they got into action Cook began learning some of the things a cowboy needed to know, such as providing beef when in camp. As they were preparing to head into the Brasada, Slaughter told Cook to kill a stray for beef. Cook leveled his rifle at a fat heifer.

"Hold on, young man, hold on," Slaughter said with some irritation. "Don't you see that's a T-Diamond?"

"Yes. Whose brand is that?"

"I reckon it's my brand. We don't kill that kind in this country. Kill an LO or a WFC (any brand but his own); they taste better."[19]

The vaqueros, who were paid only ten dollars a month while Cook received twelve dollars, generously taught him everything he needed to know, from making rawhide hobbles and braiding rawhide reatas to handling broncos and catching mossy horn outlaws in the brush. Under their tutelage Cook became a cowboy.

Like many young men, Cook was eager to go up the trail. When he learned that trail boss Joel Roberts was hiring, he asked for a job. Roberts knew of Cook's reputation as a marksman and hired him.

On his first trip up the trail Cook served as wrangler during the day. He also took his turn at night herding, and soon learned a lesson in the dangers of curiosity. Circling the herd he noticed an old black cow that continually grazed away from the others. Finally, after she had been turned back a number of times, she lay down, still away from the herd.

As he rode on his rounds Cook passed nearer and nearer to the black cow, wondering how close she would let him come. Finally he reached out and touched her neck with his boot. With a loud snort she bounded into the herd; the cattle were already on their feet and running, for the moment she snorted there was a roar and clash of horns and hocks and a trembling of the earth. Sleeping men knew instinctively what to do, for the roar of a stampede was like no other sound. Every man pulled on his boots and ran for his night horse; in moments the whole crew was racing through the night toward the sound of running cattle.

In the morning the cattle were strung out and counted; about five hundred were missing, causing a delay of several days while the strays were rounded up and more cattle were added from other Slaughter herds to replace the missing ones. Like many trail hands who caused stampedes through some act of foolishness or carelessness, Cook never admitted until years later that he had started the cattle running.[20]

Baylis John Fletcher was born in Williamson County at the edge of the Texas hill country; in 1879, at the age of nineteen, he rode up the trail with a herd belonging to his neighbor, Captain Tom Snyder.

In Indian Territory the trail boss, Dick Arnett, roped a wild mustang, which hit the end of the rope so hard it threw Arnett's horse. It fell hard on Arnett's right leg, reinjuring a wound he had received during the Civil War. Badly crippled, Arnett had to lie in the wagon for a week. It was then, when he was working with a crew of untrained trail hands, each acting as his own boss, that Fletcher became fully aware of the need for a competent trail boss in absolute control of herd and men. Fortunately, a man Tom Snyder sent to guide them through the saline and gypsum region took charge of the herd until Arnett recovered.

Another Texan who spent his life in the saddle was G. R. (Bob) Fudge, who was born in Lampasas County in 1862. When he was ten, his father, mother, sister, two brothers, and two aunts and uncles headed for California with one thousand steers and two hundred horses. In New Mexico, Comanches killed one uncle and ran off the cattle and all but four horses. Soon after that all but Fudge, his mother, and two brothers died of smallpox. The survivors returned to Texas.

At the age of twelve Fudge went to work for a rancher, and

was on his way to becoming a rarity in those days, a 250-pound cowboy. In 1881, at the age of nineteen, he helped trail a Higgins and Shankin herd to Colorado, and the following spring rode with a Blocker herd to the Little Big Horn country of Montana. Fudge made many trips up the trail, and worked eighteen years for the XIT ranch on its Montana range. The wildest trip he ever made was driving eight hundred horses to Wyoming, for they stampeded every night, making as much noise as a freight train.[21]

For several years during the height of the cattle kingdom, becoming a cowboy was almost a passion among eastern college men. Despite their genteel background some of them readily adapted to the hard life and became as skillful riders and ropers as their Texan instructors. A few young easterners like Edgar Beecher Bronson even won the respect of the Texas cowboys.

Unlike many aspiring cowboys who headed for Texas to learn the trade, Bronson went to Wyoming in June 1872. His friend Clarence King gave him a letter of introduction to his partner, N. R. Davis. Bronson arrived in Cheyenne with his cowboy outfit already purchased, his first mistake. Davis looked him over, barely concealing his contempt at the sight of laced boots, leggings, short hunting spurs, little round felt hat, and Colt .45. He steadied himself, drew his breath, and ordered Bronson to get rid of everything but the pistol. Starting Bronson almost in his underwear, Davis got him properly outfitted with a bridle, forty-pound saddle, rawhide lariat, California spurs with two-inch rowels, high-heeled boots, heavy leather chaps, and a big hat. For the roundup Davis also had him buy a tarpaulin, a buffalo robe, and two blankets. Then they set out for the ranch in a buckboard pulled by two half-broken broncos that spent more time in the air than on the ground.

On the way Davis gave Bronson a pithy but positive lecture on what he could expect. "I'm not going to favor you," he said. "You've got to take your medicine with Con Humphrey's outfit, and he's about as tough a rawhide as ever led a circle. But he always gets there, and that's the only reason I keep him. It's lay close to old Con's flank, Kid, and keep your end up or turn in your string of horses. On the round-up no soldiering goes; sick or well, it's hit yourself in the flank with your hat and keep up with the bunch or be set afoot to pack your saddle; there's no room in the chuck wagon for a quitter's blankets, and no time to close herd sick ones. So for heaven's sake don't start out unless you have the guts to stand it."[22]

Bronson assured him that while he might be unhandy at the new work, the moment he found he was in the way he'd turn in his horses and leave.

"I'm tally branding this summer," Davis continued in a more kindly tone, "making a tally or inventory of all our cattle and horses for an accounting and settlement with my partner. The corrals are full of cattle and it will take all day tomorrow to run through the chutes and hair-brand. The next morning Con starts his outfit down Willow to round up the Pawnee Butte country. I'll pass you up to Con tonight, and what he makes of the new hand will depend on what he finds in it. We'll dump your blankets and tricks at the chuck wagon, and you can make down among the boys. Earlier you start the sooner you learn— and that, I guess, is what you're here for. Don't mind the boys. They'll rough you a lot, but most of it will be good-humored. If any get ugly, you'll have to call them down, that's all."[23]

There was a fire blazing at the end of the chuck wagon, with about sixteen cowboys sitting around it, eating beef, beans, and biscuits from tin plates, and drinking strong coffee from tin cups. They were all ages, from sixteen to sixty, but most were under thirty. While no life of greater privation and hardship existed than that of cowboys, no merrier lot ever lived, for they joked constantly about every condition of life from cradle to grave. Bronson helped himself to a plate of food, but he couldn't bring himself to eat much.

"Kid," drawled Tobacco Jake, "ef you reckons to tote that full grown gun all day tomorrow, yu better ile yer jints with sow belly an' fill up all th' holler places inside yu with beans an' biscuits; yu shore look like yu hadn't had no man's grub in a month."

Bronson admitted that he had been something of an invalid, but he had recuperated, even if his physical condition was not yet up to par.

"Look yere, Kid," Jake said, "ef yu cain't talk our langwidge, you jus make signs. What'n hell yu trying' to say, anyway?"

This sort of chaff went on and on, until Bronson began to feel hot under the collar, when he heard the friendly voice of Tex Fuller. "Fellers," Tex said quietly, "jest shet y'r yawp, pronto! Let the kid alone—it's me sayin' it. Course he ain't goin' to keep up with no leaders on th' circle, but I've got a fool idea he won't be so far behind we'll lose him none." Tex spoke softly, but everyone listened, and there were no more comments that night, only a few whispers and snickers.

The next day the great corrals were filled with range cattle, old and young and of all the colors characteristic of the old Longhorn stock of South Texas. There were also traces of other breeds, the dark red and greater bulk of the Durham cross, Herefords, and even a few Angus. All were wild, with blazing eyes and rattling horns, surging threateningly back and forth between the corral fences.

Along one side of the corral was a narrow branding chute long enough to hold twenty animals. At one end of the chute was a small pen; the other end opened onto the prairie. Men on foot drove cattle from the main corral into the small pen and then pushed them into the chute. Two or three men with hot irons quickly branded them, then turned them loose. Except for an hour off for the midday meal, this work continued all day.

The work was hard and perilous, but all the men except the ill-natured foreman remained playful and joking. Bronson received both mock sympathy for his weakness and real anxiety for his safety. If an angry beast charged his way, others pushed him aside and took his place. They even mopped his sweating face with bandannas. That night Bronson thoroughly enjoyed the beans and biscuits and easily slept on the lumpy mattress of buffalo grass. The next day the wagon crew moved out on roundup; Bronson soon learned that Davis had assigned him five unusually good horses to be entrusted to a tenderfoot.

Roundup boss Con Humphrey knew cattle and horses, but hated all humans, including himself. The cowhands could see merit in Humphrey's self-hate, for to know him was not to love him. The danger was in Humphrey's taking his hatred out on someone like Bronson, who might not be able to defend himself.

Bronson started out on circle with the others, which meant riding at top speed for half a day, pushing all of the cattle toward the center. It was a brutal way for a tenderfoot to harden his saddle muscles, for, as Bronson admitted, the old cow saddle gave him "harder cramps and tenderer spots in more parts of the anatomy than any punishment conceivable short of an inquisition rack."[24] By night every movement was agony, but his appetite and capacity for sleep astonished him. Within a week he was hardened to the work and confident of his ability to ride.

As Bronson's confidence grew he was determined to demonstrate what he had learned about handling bad horses, to convince the men that he no longer needed to be looked after. A big yellow-eyed, Roman-nosed, heavy muscled buckskin called Walking Bars was the worst outlaw in the whole ND outfit. The horse's name came from the motion of the walking bars, or beams, of side-wheel river boats. Bronson, through an uncontrollable surge of courage or foolhardiness, decided to start with the worst horse available.

Walking Bars was in the string of a slender, wiry little vaquero named José, whose skill enabled him to handle the big horse with disarming ease. Using an outlaw for cow work simply compounded one's problems, however, and José had grown tired of the constant battle. He was shocked beyond belief, therefore, when Bronson offered to swap the best horse in his string for the ornery buckskin.

"Madre de Dios! muchacho, he keela you, keela you sure," he exclaimed, but when he saw that Bronson was serious, he added, "but if you weesh, you heem have, *y que Dios te aguarda!* (and may God protect you!)."

At noon, when it was time to saddle fresh mounts, Bronson roped Walking Bars while the cowboys looked on in silence. After a hard battle Bronson worked his way up the rope and stuck a lump of sugar in the surprised horse's mouth, then easily bridled him. Unbelieving, the cowboys watched while the outlaw stood quietly.

Getting the saddle on required considerable diplomacy and caution, for Walking Bars was well known for his skill in whirling and kicking. When the saddle was on, one of the awed cowboys remarked, "Ya shorely has a medicine bag fo' outlaws hid about you."

When Bronson swung into the saddle and the horse walked off quietly, the cowboys shouted their approval, thereby breaking the spell. Walking Bars suddenly remembered that he had a reputation to uphold; he tucked his head between his front legs and hit the air, coming down with earth-jarring force. Bronson managed to hang on until the horse stopped, as if it suddenly remembered the sugar lump, then quietly trotted off after the other cow horses. Tex turned to another cowboy. "Lew," he asked, "does yu allow it's loco or sense an' sand th' Kid's sufferin' most from?"

Con Humphrey, probably because Bronson was the only one of the crew he didn't fear, roped Walking Bars and removed the hackamore that had been left on him permanently as a halter. It was impossible, Humphrey knew, to bridle the horse without the hackamore in place. Bronson would get himself killed or at least look ridiculous in the attempt to bridle Walking Bars.

José was the first to know what Humphrey had done. He found Bronson and told him to kill Humphrey, eagerly offering to help. They would have to "go on the scout" afterward, he said, meaning hide from the law. Bronson was trying to figure a way out of the difficulty without either killing Humphrey or letting him get away with it, when his friend Tex rode up. Tell Con if he ever fools with your horse again you'll have his hide and scales, Tex advised him. Ride in and stay real close to him, so if he reaches for his gun you can crack him good over the head. One of the Texas ranch codes was that no man, foreman or owner, could tamper with a cowboy's string, and Humphrey had openly violated that code. Some Texans would have killed him for it.

He would stay near, Tex said, but he would let Bronson make his play, " 'n ef he gets yu, Kid, it'll be th' last gun game he'll git to ante in, 'n then it'll be Tex fer the scout. But we'll make her a squar' play; I won't chip in 'fore yu're down."

With this assurance, Bronson rode close to Humphrey and warned him to leave his string alone or he'd have trouble. Humphrey's rage was almost beyond control when he heard a horse whinny. He looked around and saw Tex sitting on his horse about seventy-five yards away, his Winchester .44 partly raised. Tex might have been looking at the cattle, for his face was expressionless.

This sight was a great inspiration to Humphrey to bring his temper under control. He had only been funnin', he lied, and meant no harm. He would have the boys rope Walking Bars and replace the hackamore, he said, and rode away. "Allus knew he was a coyote," Tex told Bronson on his way back to the drag.

Humphrey was not through trying to bring Bronson down; he ordered him to drive a cow and calf to the ranch headquarters, at least twenty miles away, across the unfamiliar Iliff range. There was no trail and few landmarks, and the range was covered with cattle. It would have been difficult for two men, but Bronson had no choice.

Again Tex came to the rescue. Ease her along gently the whole way, he advised, so she will naturally think she has business there she's bound to tend to herself. By keeping calm and riding hard only when necessary to keep the cow from joining others, Bronson eased her along, trying to follow the landmarks Tex had described.

A heavy rain struck as they neared the ranch headquarters; the weary cow and calf became unmanageable. Bronson rode on to the ranch for a fresh horse. Davis saw him coming and wanted to know why he was there. When Bronson explained, Davis was furious. "Well, where is she, anyhow?" Bronson told him he'd left the cow and calf about two miles away when the storm struck. "Well, I guess you'd better get her," Davis told him.

Saddling a fresh horse, Bronson had closed a corral gate on the cow and calf by the time the sun set. Davis walked up as Bronson unsaddled. "Kid," he said, "you've sure won puncher spurs today." This feat and his mastering of Walking Bars gave Bronson a reputation in Wyoming that enabled him, an eastern tenderfoot, to hire a crew of Texas cowboys when he established a ranch of his own.[25]

Although there were wide differences of opinion concerning cowboys and their traits of character, on the range they were generally an admirable group. Their wages were invariably low; they were attracted not by the pay but the way of life. As a rule they were reserved around strangers, and they distrusted any man who talked a lot at the first meeting. Meanness, cowardice, dishonesty, and chronic complaining were not tolerated on the range or the trail.

Teddy Roosevelt, a Dakota rancher in the 1880s, observed that cowboys were smaller and less muscular than men who wielded ax or pick, but they were as hardy and self-reliant as any. Peril and hardship were part of their daily life. The struggle for survival on the range, Roosevelt noted, was sharp; the West was no place for softies.

"Some cowboys are Mexicans," Roosevelt added, "who generally do the actual work well enough." Roosevelt was expressing an unacknowledged bias of his own, for Mexican vaqueros were unsurpassed in roping and riding and handling cattle. Some Texans, Roosevelt continued, "among whom the intolerant caste spirit is very strong," did not employ many Mexicans. Others relied heavily on them. Mexicans were, Roosevelt admitted, the best ropers, but some Texans were not far behind them. A top hand could, without assistance, rope, throw, and tie a cow or steer in a remarkably short time.[26]

A contemporary of Roosevelt commented in the *Providence Journal* that cowboys were a strange mixture of good nature and recklessness. "You are as safe with them on the plains as with any men," he wrote, "so long as you do not impose upon them. They will even deny themselves for your comfort, and imperil their lives for your safety. But impose upon them, or arouse their ire, and your life is of no more value in their esteem than a coyote. Morally, as a class, they are . . . blasphemous, drunken, lecherous, utterly corrupt."[27]

Before he married one of Granville Stuart's daughters and moved up from cowboy to cowman, Teddy Blue Abbott was a typical cowboy, and he explained the range riders' attitudes toward women. In Miles City, he said, the cowboys would go to town and "marry" a girl for a week, to be with her day and night. They couldn't do that elsewhere, he noted, without risking arrest. "I suppose those things would shock a lot of respectable people. But we wasn't respectable and we didn't pretend to be, which was the only way we was different from some others."

Cowboys had their own strict code. "I never knew of but one case where a fellow cheated one of those girls," Abbott continued,

> and I'll bet he never tried it again. He came up the trail for one of the N Bar outfits . . . and he went with Cowboy Annie for a week. Then he got on his horse and rode away, owing her seventy dollars. First he went back to the Niobara, but the foreman of the outfit heard of it and fired him, then he went down in Texas, but they heard of it down there and fired him again. And the N Bar fellows took up a collection and paid what he owed, because they wouldn't have a thing like that standing against the name of the outfit.
>
> That shows you how we were about those things. As Mag Burns used to say, the cowpunchers treated them sporting women better than some men treat their wives.
>
> Well, they were women. We didn't know any others. And any man that would abuse one of them was a son of a gun. I remember one P.I. [pimp] beat up on his girl for not coming through with enough money . . . a fellow I know jumped him and half-killed him. The man hadn't done nothing to him. It was none of his business. It was just the idea of mistreating a woman.[28]

Edgar Rye, who also knew the old-time Texas cowboys, wrote, "All honor to the Texas cowboy, living or dead. With all his faults his virtues were many." Generosity, he said, was characteristic, despite the daily hardships, for "nowhere on the earth is true manhood put to a more severe test." Hospitality was another virtue, for there was always a "rough, cheerful sincerity about the cowboy's manner that made one feel at ease." In a cowboy camp, he added, "a stranger always received a hearty welcome."[29]

What were the open range, trail-driving cowboys really like? The consensus among those who actually knew them was that they were hard-working youths who reveled in life in the saddle, and who chose to follow it for a time despite the poor pay and hardships. Their virtues were loyalty, fearlessness, generosity, and constant good humor. Their vices were occasional drunken sprees and an unwillingness to live by the Puritan code of thrift. Their proudest boast was "We held the herd."

The so-called bad men of the cowtowns should not be confused with cowboys, although a few trail hands like Sam Bass did graduate to robbing trains and other shady activities. Most cowboys carried guns, for they felt half-naked without them, but they did not make a habit of using them on one another.

There may be a parallel between the romantic view of the cowboy and of the wild mustang. From a distance the wild horses, with arched necks and tossing manes, clearly gloried in their freedom and appeared to be the most superb animals on earth. Once caught and broken to the saddle, however, they were simply ordinary cow ponies. Like the wild horses, cowboys in action were quite different from cowboys out of their element.

Charles Goodnight, one of the major cowmen who had gotten his start as a trail boss, summed up his feelings about his trailing days and paid the cowboys perhaps their finest tribute. "Taken all in all," he said, "my life on the trail was the happiest part of it. I wish I could find words to describe the companionship and loyalty of the men toward each other. It is beyond imagination. The cowboy of the old days is the most misunderstood man on earth. Few people of the younger generation realize that the Western men—the cowboys—were as brave and chivalrous as it is possible to be. Bullies and tyrants were unknown among them. They kept their places around a herd under all circumstances and if they had to fight they were always ready."[30]

Cowboys sweeping gracefully around a herd made an inspiring sight, as John Clay admitted. Away from the range and on foot, the cowboy lost his aura. But there can be no doubt that the cowboy of the trail-driving era captivated Americans as no other folk hero before or since. When all else is said, this fact remains.

CHAPTER 7

Longhorns and Mustangs

"Wherever cattle were driven, it took the
Spanish horse to do the work."
Frank Collinson

WHEN Anglos migrated to to Texas in the early nineteenth century, there were thousands of Spanish cattle running wild all
across South Texas between the Nueces and the Rio Grande,
along the San Gabriel and San Saba rivers and other tributaries
of the upper Colorado. They could be found from the Louisiana
border to the upper Brazos, and they were equally at home on
the coastal plains and in the brush country.

The early descriptions of these wild cattle suggest some,
though not all, of the colors and other characteristics of the later
Texas Longhorns. Not all the cattle in the region were wild, for
some were kept under control on old Spanish ranches as well as
Anglo establishments. In 1832, Charles Sealsfield visited the
ranch of a Kentuckian named Neal, which was a few miles off
the Harrisburg-Austin road. While Sealsfield was visiting the
ranch, Neal and three Negro cowboys were rounding up twenty
or thirty steers to take to New Orleans. Sealsfield accompanied
them; they rode four or five miles and then, Sealsfield reported,
"We came in sight of a drove, splendid animals, standing very
high and of most symmetrical form. The horns of these cattle
are of unusual length and in the distance have more the appearance of stag's antlers than bull's horns. We approached the herd
first to within a quarter of a mile. They remained quiet. We rode
around them and in like manner got in the rear of a second and
third drove and then began to spread out so as to form a half
circle and drive the cattle toward the house." About this time
Sealsfield's mustang pitched him off. He was lost for several days
and as a result missed the rest of the roundup.[1]

During the rebellion against Mexico many cowmen were

105

forced to abandon their ranches, and their herds scattered. No doubt it was during this time that the development of the Long-horns began, for they were a mixture of Anglo and native, or Spanish, stock. It was a matter of survival of the strongest, with-out the guiding hands of cattle breeders and the matching of pedigrees. After independence had been won, ranchers or-ganized cow hunts to rebuild their herds.

In 1840, James Huckins saw many cattle along the San Ber-nard. "I have never seen cattle superior to those I find in this region," he wrote. "They are large and in good condition pre-senting horns of a very great size."[2] The San Marcos region was also stocked with wild cattle, but they were so shy and alert that only the most expert hunters could get a shot at them. The settlers' cattle were quick to join the wild ones at any opportu-nity, and thereby continued contributing to the development of the Longhorn.[3] Although the colors of these wild cattle were not stated, it seems likely that those nearest the settlements were already mixed with stock the Anglos introduced.

Farther from the settlements, near the sources of the San Gabriel and the Brushy and along the Leona, San Saba, Llano, and Little rivers, the wild cattle were still unmixed Spanish stock. An anonymous visitor in the 1840s called them a "singular" breed. They differed in form, color, and habits from all the varieties of domestic cattle in Texas. "They are invariably of a dark-brown color with a slight tinge of dusky yellow on the tip of the nose and on the belly. Their horns are remarkably large and stand out straight from the head. Although these cattle are gen-erally much larger than the domestic cattle, they are more fleet and nimble and when pursued often outstrip horses that easily outrun the buffalo. Unlike the buffalo, they seldom venture far out into the prairies, but are generally found in or near the forests that skirt the streams in that section. Their meat is of an excellent flavor and is preferred by the settlers to the meat of the domestic cattle. It is said that their fat is so hard and compact that it will not melt in the hottest days of summer."

Some men believed that these cattle were of a distinct breed indigenous to America. "But," according to this observer, "as these cattle are now found only in the vicinity of the old

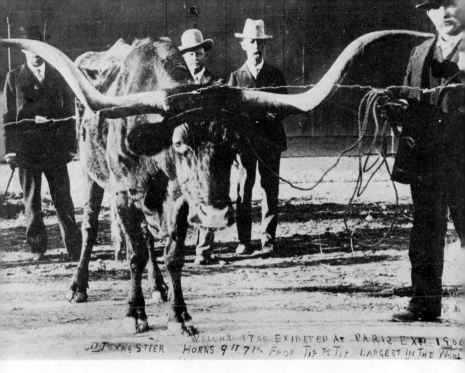

An old Texas Longhorn steer, with horns measuring nine feet seven inches from tip to tip. Steers' horns grew much longer than those of bulls or cows. Courtesy of the Oklahoma Historical Society

missions, it is much more probable that they are the descendants of the cattle introduced by the early Spanish adventurers." Attempts to domesticate them, the unknown writer added, were so far unsuccessful.[4]

Although the native cattle already had horns long enough to attract the attention of those seeing them for the first time, there is at least a slight possibility that this tendency was reinforced by the infusion of British long-horned cattle that had been imported into the United States at various times. In 1817 some of them were taken to Kentucky, and early Anglo Texans like the Mr. Neal mentioned above may have brought a number of these cattle with them. In 1821 a herd of British long-horned cattle was seen in Ohio.

The colors of the British longhorns were similar to those of many of the later Texas Longhorns—red, red roan, blue roan, yellow, and fawn color. Some had white on the back or belly.[5]

Whether or not British longhorns contributed to the development of the Texas stock, other British breeds did mix with the wild Spanish cattle to produce the Texas Longhorn of the post–Civil War era.

Texas Longhorns might be any of a great variety of colors and combinations of colors, most of them dull rather than bright. There were browns and blacks, solid or with white patches. Whites might be clear or peppered with red (sabinas). Pale red was common, and so were various shades of yellow and dun. Many were pintos, and some duns had dark lines down the back. Brindles and blue or red roans were also frequent. Although the Longhorn became a recognizable breed, it had not existed long enough for any one or two colors to become predominant through superior qualities for survival.

Despite its accidental creation and its ungainly appearance, the old Texas Longhorn was a unique, history-making animal, in this regard unrivaled by any other breed. The long-legged Longhorn was accustomed to ranging far for feed and water. This quality, together with its especially hard hoofs, made the Longhorn ideal for the long drive. The Longhorns' ability to gain weight on the way to market, and the fact that they stayed together and were less likely to scatter than other breeds, also enhanced their value as trail animals. Although they attained their maximum weight more slowly than others, in the days of free grass and open range that was not a serious flaw. With the coming of barbed wire and fenced pastures, however, it quickly became a factor that had to be considered.

On the trail Longhorns fell into position in the herd according to strength or other qualities, and maintained the same place day after day. The strongest cattle were always in the van; the weak or lame were always in the drag. A steer that was lame for several days would fall back into the drag, then resume its former place when its lameness ended.

A few steers instinctively assumed the role of leaders; others followed them without hesitation. When crossing rivers and at other times of trouble good lead steers were as valuable as extra cowboys. Lead steers such as Charles Goodnight's old Blue were so valuable they were used dozens of times and never sold. On

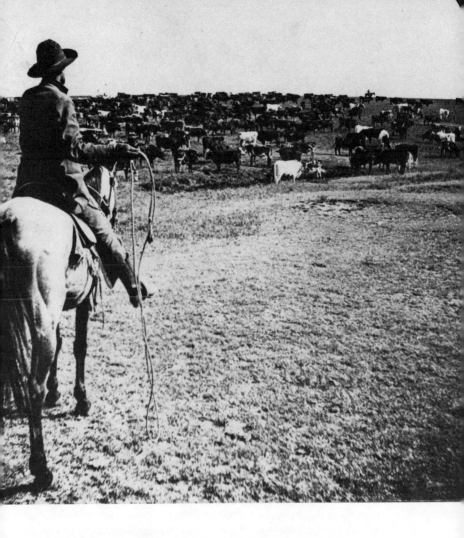

Holding herd on Sherman Ranch, Genessee, Kansas, 1902. The cattle are Longhorns crossed with Herefords and Durhams. Courtesy of the Amon Carter Museum of Western Art, Fort Worth

returning to Texas with the remudas and chuck wagons, these steers easily kept up with the cow ponies. Blue was finally retired to Goodnight's Palo Duro ranch, where he lived another twenty years. On the trail Blue and other veteran lead steers would come to the wagon at night for a handout of biscuits. Blue wore a bell that one of the men tied at night to prevent it from ringing.

In the morning Blue approached one of the point men so he could untie the bell.

Old Tom was another much traveled lead steer. He was large and his horns spread seven feet—each had a gold ring on it near the tip, rings that grateful cowboys had fashioned out of twenty-dollar gold pieces. Old Tom was a proud, natural leader; the cowboys could yell "gee" or "haw" to him, and he would turn in the right direction.[6]

In 1870, Bill Blocker had gathered a herd on the Pedernales when he saw a big, wild bay steer that caught his eye because it looked so proud and free. Blocker's herd was already set, but he decided the bay steer must join it. The steer was soon accustomed to the trail, and it assumed the lead. After ten days Blocker could ride alongside Pardner, as he named the steer, and rest a hand on one of its horns. Sad to say, Blocker was unable to take it back to Texas—this was its only trip up the trail.

Jack Potter's herd in West Texas was saved during a severe blizzard by his lead steer, "John Chisum." While other cattle drifted before the storm, "John Chisum" headed into it, for that was the way to Trempero Canyon and shelter. They came to a fork in a canyon; in the blinding snow Potter took the wrong fork. The steer refused to follow him, so he followed it, and soon was thankful that he had. The herd was saved, while thousands of cattle that had drifted before the storm were lost.

Longhorns reveled in their freedom, and many an old mossy horn bull or steer roped in the brush and yoked to an ox would lie down and die rather than enter a corral. Some became troublemakers on the trail, for they were ever restless and eager to escape, and their nervousness kept the other cattle jumpy and ready to run.

Ben Borroum of Del Rio was taking a herd north one spring; once across the Red River the lead steer began to sniff the wind as Longhorns did when there were buffalo in the vicinity. Soon all of the cattle were nervous, and when bedded down at night they did not let the air out of their lungs as they did when they intended to stay down. The herd ran twenty-two times that night, and no one got any sleep. The next morning a band of Comanches rode up and asked for a "wohaw." Borroum had a couple of cowboys rope the lead steer and take him away from the herd. Once that steer was gone there were no more runs the rest of the drive.[7]

One herd on the Goodnight-Loving Trail stampeded when a night guard's horse caught its hoof in the tree of a McClellan saddle, and the frightened animals ran over the chuck wagon and flattened it. They ran every night after that. John Chisum, who owned the herd and was riding with another of his herds ahead of it, came back after the cattle were bedded down. While riding slowly through the herd he pointed out a leggy, one-eyed pinto steer and ordered the cowboys to separate it from the herd and kill it. There were no more stampedes.[8]

Wherever they went, Longhorns made their presence felt. In 1876, either pranksters or idiots at Fort Benton, Montana, put a Longhorn steer aboard the steamer *Carroll* as a milk cow. Justifiably offended, the steer cleared the decks with a few sweeps of its horns, then "majestically walked on shore and solemnly devoured a quarter acre of *primolo adorato*. No milk on board the *Carroll* this trip."[9]

In 1883, J. L. Hill was with a herd of yearlings and two-year-olds near the North Platte. In the herd was a pot-bellied little dogie that had stayed in the drag all the way from Llano County. The cowboys named it Baby Mine. The trail passed around a rocky bluff overhanging the river; at one place it was so narrow the cattle had to go in single file. One of the larger steers hooked Baby Mine and knocked him over the bluff, sending him sliding down the rock to a fall of forty feet into the water. The drag rider, knowing he would miss the little dogie, said "Goodbye, Baby." But next morning Baby Mine was in his usual place at the end of the herd.[10]

"As trail cattle," Charles Goodnight said of the Longhorns, "their equal has never been known. Their hoofs are superior to those of any other cattle. They can go farther without water and endure more suffering than others."[11] Their meat was marbled, even on a diet of grass, and their hides were more valuable for leather than other cowhides.

Longhorns were also immune to the tick fever that was fatal to other cattle, and the epidemics that followed importations of

Longhorns were the main reason for the bias against them. Once they had been wintered in the North, however, they were free of the disease-carrying ticks.

Of the millions of Longhorns trailed north, less than 40 percent were shipped out immediately. Many were bought by feed lot operators; others were sold to fill beef contracts at Indian agencies. Probably the greatest number went to the new ranches opening all over the northern plains. Steers were held there for a year or two, then sold for beef, having gained several hundred pounds more than they would have gained in Texas. Longhorns fattened better on grass than Shorthorns or other beef cattle, but did not do as well as others on corn. Since corn-fed beef brought the highest prices, cowmen began buying Shorthorn, Hereford, or Angus bulls to cross with Longhorn cows. Such crosses produced excellent range cattle, for they retained enough of the Longhorns' hardiness and ability to forage while acquiring the rapid growth qualities of the other breeds. By the mid-1880s the Longhorn was disappearing from the northern ranges and even Texas. In 1885, D. W. Hinkle wrote Joseph Nimmo that "there are but few, very few, of the old long-horn Texans in the State. All show that good blood has been infused in them."[12]

The Longhorn, which had helped Texas rise from its economic nadir after the Civil War, seemed doomed to early and undeserved extinction as ranchers turned to the British breeds that reached maximum weight quickly. Frank Collinson, who followed many a Longhorn up the trail, wrote the most touching requiem to the vanishing breed.

"Some folks," he said, "pity the bull in the ring at Spanish or Mexican bullfights. I pitied the old Texas Longhorns that came to such a sad end, after weathering the trail so nobly. In my mind they were the real sports. They were among the wildest known cattle and made good beef. They also made good work animals and helped haul heavy loads across the Plains. They could get along without water longer than any other cattle. They had harder and better hoofs. I'm sorry that they are gone from the range."[13]

As a postscript to Collinson's remarks, in the 1920s Texan

Graves Peeler made a search for pure Longhorns and put together a small herd, barely in time to save the breed from total extinction. As the numbers gradually increased, the Texas Longhorn Breeders Association of America was established, and it created a Longhorn registry. By 1978 the association had more than five hundred members and its registry listed upwards of fifteen thousand Longhorns. Because of the qualities that made it valuable a century ago, the Longhorn is again making an impact on the beef cattle industry, and today it has a bright future as well as an illustrious past.

The Longhorn's counterpart in the trailing era was the mustang cow pony. As western writer Eugene Manlove Rhodes remarked to Harry Sinclair Drago, "The mustang and the Longhorn went together like ham and eggs."[14] Together the Longhorn and mustang gave character to a historic era; it would have been a vastly different story without them.

Early visitors to Texas had much to say about mustangs, not all of it in admiration. In 1832, Charles Sealsfield bought one on his visit to Texas. "These mustangs are small horses," he wrote,

> rarely above fourteen hands high, and are descended from the Spanish breed introduced by the original conquerors of the country. During the three centuries that have elapsed since the conquest of Mexico, they have increased and multiplied to an extraordinary extent and are to be found in vast droves in the Texas prairies, although they are now beginning to be somewhat scarcer. They are taken with the *lasso.* . . .
>
> The lasso is usually from twenty to thirty feet long, very flexible, and composed of strips of twisted ox-hide. One end is fastened to the saddle, and the other, which forms a running noose, held in the hand of the hunter who thus equipped rides out into the prairie. When he discovers a troop of wild horses, he maneuvers to get to the windward of them and then to approach as near as possible. If he is an experienced hand, the horses seldom escape him, and as soon as he is within twenty or thirty feet of them, he throws the noose with unerring aim over the neck of the one he has

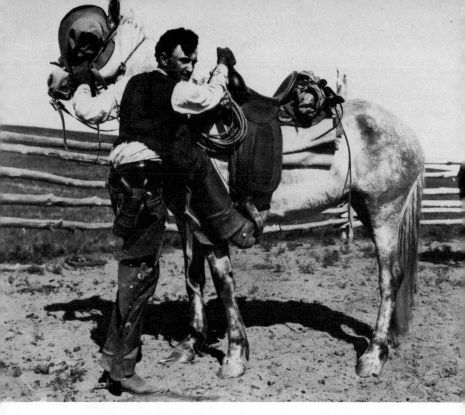

Mounting a bronc, probably a mustang cross. The horse had been ridden before; otherwise the cowboy would have blindfolded it. Photo by F. H. Corbin. The Montana Historical Society

selected for his prey. This done, he turns his own horse sharp round, gives him the spur, and gallops away, dragging his unfortunate captive after him breathless. . . . After a few yards, the mustang falls headlong to the ground and lies motionless and almost lifeless, sometimes badly hurt and disabled.

The breaking process was equally rough on the mustangs, for they were of little value. "The eyes of the unfortunate animal are covered with a bandage, and a tremendous bit, a pound weight or more, clapped into his mouth; the horse breaker puts on a pair of spurs six inches long and with rowels like penknives, and jumping on his back urges him to his very utmost speed. If the horse tries to rear or turns restive, one pull, and not a very hard one either, at the instrument of torture they call a bit is sufficient to tear his mouth to shreds and cause the blood to flow in streams."

The mustang was forced to run until exhausted, then was rested for a time and ridden hard again. "If he breaks down during this rude trial, he is either knocked on the head or driven away as useless; but if he holds out, he is marked with a hot iron and left to graze on the prairie. Henceforward, there is no particular difficulty in catching him when wanted. The wildness of the horse is completely punished out of him, but for it is substituted the most confirmed vice and malice that it is possible to conceive. These mustangs are unquestionably the most deceitful and spiteful of the equine race. They seem to be perpetually looking out for an opportunity of playing their master a trick, and very soon after I got possession of mine, I was nearly paying for him in a way that I had not calculated upon."

When Sealsfield rode near some mustangs on Neal's ranch, his own decided to join them. It ran away with him, then pitched him over its head. Sealsfield's experience on this occasion was one of the reasons for his low opinion of mustangs.[15]

Despite Sealsfield's dislike of mustangs, his contemporary, Colonel H. C. Brish, considered them superior to any others for cavalry mounts.[16] Many mustangs that were well treated by their owners became thoroughly dependable one-man horses.

Josiah Gregg, who traded with New Mexico and Chihuahua in the 1840s, also described the horses. "The New Mexicans," he wrote, "so justly celebrated for skillful horsemanship . . . leave the propagation of their horses exclusively to chance; converting their best and handsomest studs into saddle horses.

"The race of *horses* is identical with that which is found running wild on the prairies, familiarly known by the name of *mustang*. Although generally very small, they are quick, active, and spirited; and were they not commonly so much injured in the breaking they would perhaps be as hardy and long-lived as any other race in existence. Some of their *caballos de silla*, or saddle-horses, are so remarkably well trained, that they will stop suddenly upon the slightest check, charge up against a wall without shrinking, and even attempt to clamber up its sides."[17]

In 1849, W. Steinert, a German visitor to Texas, noted that American horses cost from $100 to $130. What he called pure Spanish horses were priced about the same, and were raised on ranches in Mexico. "The Mexican horse, which is very hardy and can make out on ordinary feed, can be bought for ten, twenty, thirty dollars or more," he wrote. "The mustangs cannot be used much because they rarely become entirely tame. You can buy them for five to ten dollars, but as a rule they run off if they have not been thoroughly trained. Catching and taming them is breakneck work, and it is performed mostly by Mexicans."[18] The Mexican horse Steinert mentioned was the same animal as the mustang except that it had been ranch-raised rather than caught from among wild herds.

Wherever cattle were raised there were also horse ranches, though many ranchers raised their own cow ponies. In 1847 Thomas A. Dwyer established a horse and mule ranch on the lower Nueces, crossing mustang mares with blooded stallions and jacks. "I well remember," he wrote, "seeing thousands and tens of thousands of wild horses running in immense herds all over the western country as far as the eye or telescope could sweep the horizon." The whole country seemed alive with them. He often had trouble controlling his pack mules, for the playful mustangs would keep circling around them on the run and gradually close in, then with a rush make off with the mules. "The supplies of wild cattle and horses then seemed so abundant as to be inexhaustible."[19] Many travelers reported that mustangs had circled them. Trail hands often had to drive them off to keep them from charging through herds and scattering the cattle.

In the 1880s Frederic Remington described the Texas cow pony as having "fine deer-like legs," a long body with a pronounced roach just forward of the coupling, and quite likely a "glass eye" and a pinto hide. "Any old cowboy will point him out as the only creature suitable for his purposes." Though difficult to break and small in size, "he can cover leagues of his native plains, bearing a disproportionately large man, with an ease to himself and his rider which is little short of miraculous."

One thing was certain, Remington added: "Of all the

monuments which the Spaniard has left to glorify his reign in America there will be none more worthy than his horse." Broncos had no equal in intelligence or stamina. "As a saddle animal the bronco has no superior," Remington concluded.[20]

The mustang cow pony, like the Longhorn, had a number of qualities that compensated for others it lacked, such as size and weight. Mustangs had "cow sense," hardiness, endurance, a remarkably good sense of direction, and a wild animal's alertness for signs of danger. In size they were only fourteen hands at best, and they weighed no more than nine hundred pounds on the average. They were adaptable and versatile, serving as roping, cutting, and night horses on ranches, and were used by the Pony Express, the Texas Rangers, and the U.S. Cavalry.[21]

The mustang may have been the original pitching or bucking horse, for pitching is believed to be an American horse trait. There has been much speculation about its origins; the most likely theory is that pumas or panthers, which attack their prey by springing on them slightly behind the shoulders, caused the animals to pitch in an effort to save themselves.[22]

Unlike cattle, wild horses never left their own familiar range voluntarily, for no matter how long and hard they were pursued, they always circled back to it. This trait made it possible for mustangers to "walk down" herds of mustangs by following them constantly in relays. A party of mustangers with access to a corral would camp on the mustangs' range. One man at a time would ride after the frightened animals and keep them in sight until his relief spelled him.

At first sight of a rider the mustangs were off and running, and they might travel sixty miles before turning back. By the third day of constant pursuit with no chance to rest or eat, they allowed the rider to approach fairly near. After a week or ten days the mustangs could be mixed with a tame herd or driven into a corral. Some mustangers attached long rawhide straps to a front leg of each animal just above the hoof, then turned them out of the corral. When they tried to run, they stepped on the strap with a hind hoof and threw themselves. Soon they were easily herded.

Frequently there were domesticated horses or mules running with the mustangs, and these, having only recently acquired their freedom, were more jealous of it than the mustangs. Mules were especially alert for the sight or smell of men, and when one or more of them were with a bunch of mustangs, that bunch was especially difficult to corral. It was impossible to slip up close to mules, and when attempts were made to walk them down, they proved inexhaustible.

On the prairies the strongest and best stallions retained most of the mares in their harems, though they had to fight off other stallions, especially during the mating season. Because of this the mustangs were by no means degenerate. The best of them made exceptional cow ponies despite their small size. Among the Mexicans small horses were preferred; their saying went "Praise the tall but saddle the small."[23]

In the 1860s there was little demand for horses in Kansas, so the trail hands drove the remudas back down the trail. When ranching spread in the North, however, northern cowmen soon realized that they needed both Texans and mustangs to handle their Longhorns. Thereafter remudas were sold at the end of the drives, and in addition an estimated million horses, mainly mustangs, were driven north and sold.

Many of the best cow ponies and cutting horses had formerly been wild mustangs. Some also became winners on the race track. In 1873, Miguel Antonio Otero, who lived near the Kansas-Colorado border, bought a two-year-old blue roan stallion from a party of New Mexico mustangers. He gelded the roan and named him Kiowa. Otero kept Kiowa for thirty years, during which time he never saw his equal for intelligence, speed, or stamina. He won many short races, one against a Thoroughbred stallion for one thousand dollars.[24] Sam Bass's Denton Mare was also said to have been caught by mustangers from a wild herd.

The mustangs' alertness, sense of direction, and cow sense made them valuable as night horses, for in a stampede at night about all a cowboy could do was give his cow pony its head and hang on. The well-trained night horses found their way over rough country on the darkest nights as they ran to overtake the lead steers.

There were many stories reflecting the intelligence of night horses. Some knew exactly when the two hours of night herding were over and would insist on returning to the wagon. Pinnacle Jake Snyder had an old black horse in his string he used for night herding, for it was gentle, wise, sure-footed in the dark, and it liked to work around cattle. He named it Dick Head after the Texas trail boss who sold it to him.

Even on the darkest nights, when Jake had no idea where the chuck wagon was, the horse would stop where he had dropped the picket rope. On one occasion Jake was with a crew driving nine hundred big, wild steers from Porcupine Creek, Wyoming, to Lusk for shipping to Chicago. The country was especially hilly, and it was necessary to bed the steers where other herds had been bedded recently, which added to their nervousness. When one of the relief riders was on his way to the herd, his horse stumbled, his saddle creaked, and the steers were on their feet and running.

Jake had already ridden the ten to midnight guard, but when he heard the familiar rumble of stampeding cattle he ran to his night horse, which met him at the end of the picket rope. Racing after the steers in rough, unfamiliar country was hazardous, and it was a long time before the cattle stopped running. Jake wearily dismounted, leaned against a rock, and slept. Some time later his horse pushed him roughly and woke him up. Jake hastily mounted and the horse was off on the run. Only then Jake learned that the cattle were drifting away and scattering. He managed to hold them together until morning.

During the morning the trail boss rode up, for he had followed the tracks. If Jake hadn't been on the best night horse, he told him, he would have gone over a bank and broken his neck—if he rode over the same country by daylight and saw how close he had come to death his hair would turn white. The strenuous chase after the cattle had used up the old horse beyond recovery. Jake turned him loose on the range and never rode him again.[25]

As ranching spread to West Texas and over the plains, ranchers considered mustangs a nuisance, for they ran off brood mares. When the big ranches were fenced, many mustangs were shot. At the same time mustangers were active, and most of the best mustangs were caught.

Thoroughbred stallions had been introduced into Texas in the 1830s, primarily for racing, but some of these as well as Morgan stallions were bred to native mares to produce fine saddle horses and cow ponies. Most of the racing, at least that which was advertised in the newspapers, was over mile tracks. In 1839, Sam Houston brought the famous Quarter Horse stallion Copper Bottom from Pennsylvania to Texas. In 1840 the first recorded quarter-mile race in Texas was held in Houston, although quarter-mile match races undoubtedly had been held before Anglos arrived in Texas.[26]

Other noted Quarter Horse stallions brought to Texas from Kentucky, Illinois, and Tennessee were Steel Dust, Monmouth, Shiloh, Dan Tucker, and Peter McCue. Many modern bloodlines trace back to them.

By the 1880s the best of the mustangs were gone from the prairies, and mustang blood, like that of the Longhorn, was rapidly being bred out of existence. In Texas the crosses were with Thoroughbreds, Morgans, and Quarter Horses. In the mountainous cattle regions of the North and Northwest larger horses were needed, and mustang mares were crossed with heavier stallions. In Oregon, Clydesdales were popular, and produced a useful, short-set, compact, and muscular horse with large bones and hairy legs—the "Oregon Lummox." In Montana and the Dakotas, Percheron stallions were widely used—their cross on mustang mares was the "Percheron Puddin-Foot." Since the range cattle to be handled were no longer wild and swift Texas Longhorns, the mustangs' speed and endurance were not as necessary as before.[27]

Some of the mustang and mustang-cross cow ponies were exceptional in many ways. Edgar Beecher Bronson, who in 1877 was the first to establish a ranch along the White River in the heart of Sioux country, rode one, the best cow pony he ever owned, to Cheyenne late in September. The horse was a dark red bay, short-backed and deep-barreled, with great blazing eyes and as alert as its mustang ancestors. Its favorite gait was a swift, daisy-clipping lope.

Before he set out on the 121-mile return trip to his ranch, Bronson learned that Dull Knife and the Northern Cheyennes had made their desperate effort to return to the North. Early that afternoon Bronson reached the last ranch between Cheyenne and his own, fifty miles north of Cheyenne. He had planned to spend the night there, but reports that a Cheyenne scouting party had been seen east of the ranch convinced him that travel by daylight was unsafe. He headed on that night, and shortly before sunup reached his own ranch. Between sun and sun his remarkable cow pony had covered 121 miles without quirt or spur.[28]

The mustang and Longhorn were contemporaries of the trailing era, and it is not surprising that when one disappeared the other soon followed. Although the Longhorn has made a rapid comeback since the 1920s, the mustang revival is more recent and not so far advanced, but it has begun. A mustang registry has been established, and the hardy little horses are being bred once more.

CHAPTER 8

The Trail Towns

"Everyone is aware of the amount of money
spent in this city by cattlemen and cowboys."

Fort Worth Democrat

BEFORE the Civil War, Baxter Springs, Kansas, and Sedalia, Missouri, had a brief reign as the principal end-of-trail towns. Both exhibited some of the rough characteristics of the later Kansas cowtowns, but they did not handle large numbers of huge herds and hundreds of trail hands like those that reached Abilene after 1867.

Abilene became a trail town overnight, but its decline was equally rapid. It began as an Overland Stage station which received rare but favorable notice in 1859 when Horace Greeley announced that it was there he ate the last square meal on his trip across the plains. That, and the fact that Abilene had a biblical name, were its sole claims to distinction. In 1867, when Joseph McCoy stopped there in his search for a suitable railhead for Texas cattle, he found only a dozen families living in simple cabins, a post office, a store, and a saloon or two. On September 5 of that year the first trainload of Texas cattle was shipped to Chicago from McCoy's pens.

That first season 35,000 cattle reached Abilene; the following year around 75,000 head arrived; in 1869 the number rose to 160,000. Not all were shipped to market, for many were sold to ranchers in Nebraska. By that time some of the regular residents of Abilene were concerned over the saloons, gambling houses, and dance halls that lined Texas Street. Their efforts to clean up the town were frustrated by the fact that peace officers had a short tenure when the boisterous trail hands were in town. When the Texans saw a stone jail being erected, they happily tore it down.

In 1870, Marshal Tom Smith tamed Abilene somewhat by

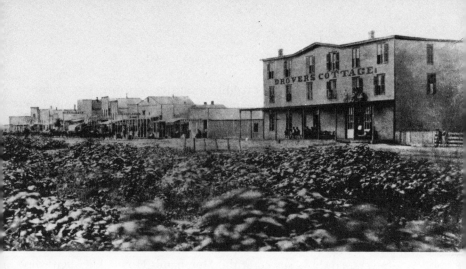

Ellsworth, Kansas, 1870s. Part of the Drovers Cottage was moved there from Abilene. Western History Collections, University of Oklahoma Library

posting an ordinance against carrying guns. Because Smith enforced the law with his fists rather than with guns, he gained some grudging respect from trail hands before he was murdered while helping the sheriff arrest a couple of killers.

Joseph McCoy, who had brought prosperity to Abilene, purchased cattle on credit in 1869 and lost heavily when the market fell. When the railroad reneged on its agreement to pay him one-eighth of the freight he processed to be shipped from Abilene, McCoy lost everything, even though the courts eventually ruled in his favor. He was able to pay off his debts and he remained closely connected with the cattle business, but he was never again a big operator.

Abilene became famous all over the West, so well known it was natural that people would suppose that it was a city of substance and size. A Texan rode into the center of the town and asked how far it was to Abilene. When told he was there, he replied, "Now, look here, stranger, you don't mean this here little scatterin trick is Abilene." He was told it was. "Well I'll swar I never seed such a little town have such a mighty big name." More important than its size, Abilene's cattle business produced three million dollars a year.[1]

Opposition to the sinful activities on Texas Street intensified, and the permanent residents insisted that the fleshpots be moved to the Devil's Addition outside of town. The saloons along Texas Street remained, and dissatisfaction continued to grow.

In 1870, Abilene had some five hundred residents—the transients who were after the cowboy trade vanished with the last herd of the season and returned before the first herds arrived in the spring. By the trailing season of 1871 Abilene was thoroughly prepared, with ten saloons, five general stores, two hotels, and two so-called hotels in which patrons did not necessarily spend the entire night. The Drover's Cottage, which McCoy no longer owned, catered to trail bosses and cattle buyers; cowboys stayed at the Merchant's Hotel. The men who drove most of the six hundred thousand cattle north swarmed into Abilene in such numbers the saloonkeepers, gamblers, and pimps rejoiced, but the rest of the people had seen enough of Texas cattle and their keepers.

That year was Abilene's most active, but it was also its last year as a trail town. By summer the Atchison, Topeka, and Santa Fe had extended its rails to Newton, near the Chisholm Trail south of Abilene. When the railroad brought Joseph McCoy there to supervise the building of loading pens, a collection of rude shacks was hastily erected. By mid-August 1871 the first trainload of cattle was shipped from Newton to Kansas City. Around forty thousand cattle passed through Newton that year, but its career as a trail town was short as well as violent. By 1873 its trailing days were over, for the Wichita and Southwestern Railroad had reached Wichita.

Early in 1872, before herds had started north, a circular printed in Abilene by the Farmers Protective Association of Dickinson County was circulated widely in Texas. It stated that members of the association "most respectfully request all who have contemplated driving cattle to Abilene the coming season to seek some other point for shipping, as the inhabitants of Dickinson will no longer submit to the evils of the trade."[2] McCoy and others launched a countercampaign to persuade Texans to bring their cattle to Abilene, but in vain.

The Kansas and Pacific Railroad, which had treated Abilene rather cavalierly and had actually tried to cheat McCoy, suddenly awakened to the fact that it was losing the lucrative cattle-hauling business to the rival Santa Fe Railroad. It decided to provide Texans a new railhead that was easily accessible and without the irritations they had suffered from the farmers surrounding Abilene. The new shipping point was Ellsworth, about seventy miles west of Abilene. The railroad hired Shanghai Pierce and Colonel W. E. Hunter to supervise the building of pens, and sent men to mark out a route from the Chisholm Trail to Ellsworth.[3]

The railroad also sent Shanghai Pierce to Texas to persuade cattlemen to send their herds to the new shipping point. With both Newton and Ellsworth offering inducements to trail men, Abilene was ignored. Many Abilene businessmen quickly loaded their wares on wagons, said good-by to deserted Texas Street, and headed for Ellsworth. The new owner of the Drover's Cottage even moved part of it to the new railhead. For a time Abilene was little more than a ghost town, but it soon became the center of a prosperous wheat-growing business. A stone marker was all that reminded people of the town's former days as "Abilene—The End of the Chisholm Trail."[4]

Ellsworth was an instant success as a trail town, for it took over much of the enormous trade that had previously gone to Abilene. From the start it could truthfully claim to be the leading cattle market of Kansas. In its first season, 1872, at least one hundred thousand cattle reached Ellsworth.

Aware of Abilene's troubles with lawlessness, Ellsworth established a police force and confined the "soiled dove" population to the Smoky Hill bottoms outside the town, a district soon known as Nauchville.[5] The police force concentrated on the town proper, leaving Nauchville wide open. Ellsworth's efforts to control violence were no more successful than those of other trail towns. Its police force proved corrupt and adept at cheating Texas cowboys with false arrests and illegal fines. Some men feared that the Texans' resentment would result in an uncontrollable eruption.

John Montgomery, editor of the *Reporter,* tried to avoid the impending blowup by suggesting raising money by licensing the "fair Cyprians" of Nauchville. "If it can't be rooted out," he

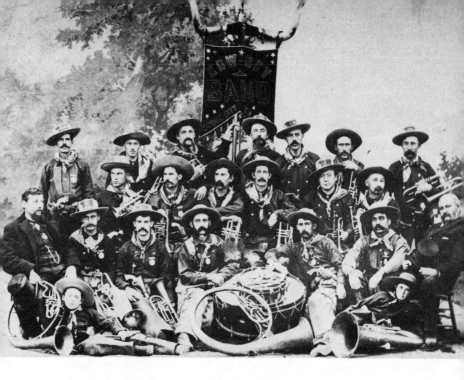

Dodge City's Cow-boy Band, which helped publicize the "Cowboy Capital." Courtesy of the Amon Carter Museum of Western Art, Fort Worth

wrote, "the vicious vocation should be made to contribute to the expense of maintaining law and order." Although respectable citizens were shocked at this suggestion, the town council agreed to it,[6] and the licenses provided Ellsworth's main source of revenue.

Ellsworth lasted only a few years as a railhead for Texas cattle, for competition among railroads resulted in the establishment of newer and more convenient outlets. Ellsworth's only big year was 1873, but when the financial panic began in September there were many herds in the area awaiting buyers who never came. Of the thousands of cattle that had to be wintered there that year, fewer than twenty thousand "made it through to grass." No herds arrived in 1874.

The extension of the Santa Fe's subsidiary line, the Wichita and Southwestern, to Wichita in 1872 brought four hundred thousand Texas cattle to that town in 1873. Joseph McCoy had completed the shipping pens in time for the 1872 season. It was at Wichita that the buying of cattle for the northern Indian reservations reached its peak. When the Wichita market opened, some of the merchants who had deserted Abilene for Ellsworth loaded their wagons once more and headed for the new cattle center.

By 1873 Wichita was clearly the major cattle market in Kansas. The town enlarged its shipping pens and built a toll bridge across the Arkansas at Douglas Avenue, which was also designated as the official route for driving cattle through town to the stockyards and shipping pens. Most of the dance halls and saloons were located in the quarter called Delano across the river from the rest of the town, but around the intersection of Douglas Avenue and Main Street saloons and brothels were plentiful.

Wichita had been the northern terminus of Jesse Chisholm's wagon road, for his trading post was near where the town was later built. As a result, in the years of Wichita's preeminence as a trail town—1872–76—the herds followed the original Chisholm Trail a greater distance than at any other time.

Those who bought cattle at Wichita or elsewhere were of three main categories: ranchers from the area from Colorado to the Dakotas in search of stock cattle, feed lot owners from corn belt states, and packing house agents who were after fat cattle. During Wichita's years as a trail town, cattle prices reached their highest level for the whole trailing era. A nine-hundred-pound steer that sold for eleven to fourteen dollars in Texas brought twenty to twenty-five dollars in Kansas, and ten dollars more in Chicago or St. Louis. The same animal might net seventy dollars or more in New York City.[7]

When Tobe Odem sold his herd at Dodge City in the spring of 1877, he told his cowboys their pay would continue until they got back to Goliad with their horses and the lead steer, Old Tom. When they reached Goliad, another herd would be ready. Then he invited them to town for "some fun and few drinks." Dodge City's reputation for wickedness, young cowboy Jesse Benton decided, was undeserved.

"Dodge City were a sight to see: saloons, gambling houses, dance halls on every corner," Benton remembered. There were

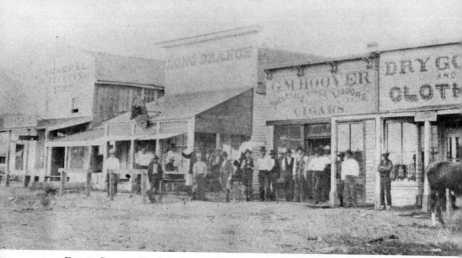

Front Street, Dodge City, 1875. Left of center is the Long Branch saloon. Courtesy of the Amon Carter Museum of Western Art, Fort Worth

around five hundred cowboys and buffalo hunters in town, "everybody there to have a good time and blow off from the long trail. I've read some of the most exaggerated things about Dodge City. But they are wrong." Most of the cowboys were good-hearted young fellows with money to spend; if they didn't have any, their boss would furnish it. And, he added, Dodge City knew how to treat them right.

"I walked up to the dance halls and looked in. What a sight to anyone, the prettiest gals from all over the world, dressed like a million dollars, was all there. If you did not come in to dance, they would grab you and pull you in, whether you wanted to dance or not. All the girls acted glad to see you. Round after round of drinks, then all would dance."

Odem bought all the drinks for his men; they didn't return to camp until daybreak. After breakfast they rolled up in their blankets, for no one thought of starting for Texas that day. The following day they didn't feel much better.[8]

By 1876 farms and fences had virtually cut off access to Wichita, and cowmen turned to Dodge City, which had handled some trail cattle from 1872 on. Dodge City would continue to be

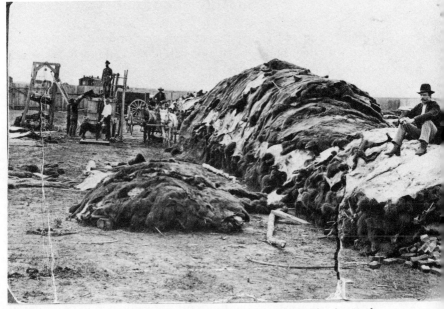

Rath and Wright's buffalo hide yard, Dodge City, 1874. Charles Rath sits on a pile said to contain forty thousand hides. Courtesy of the Amon Carter Museum of Western Art, Fort Worth

a major cattle center to 1885–86, the longest existence of any of the Kansas trail towns. This "Queen of the cowtowns," this "wickedest little city in America," this "Beautiful Bibulous Babylon of the Frontier" boasted a saloon for every fifty residents. Perhaps Dodge's earlier history as a center for buffalo hunters and shipping point for buffalo hides had a lasting influence on its character. The other Kansas trail towns all started full-blown as cowtowns.

Because of the profitable hide-shipping business, Dodge largely ignored the possibilities of handling cattle until 1875, although some herds had passed that way as early as 1872, when the Santa Fe tracks reached Dodge. Since there were no loading facilities, herds to be shipped were driven on to Great Bend or elsewhere.[9]

For nearly fifteen years Dodge City was considered the wildest town in the West. By 1875 cattle were regularly trailed there, and it was on its way to becoming the "Cowboy Capital" of the nation. Dodge continued to flourish until 1886, when the quarantines against Texas cattle put an end to the declining trailing business. In its heyday Dodge was the location of the original Boot Hill cemetery, resting place for dozens of men who died with their boots on. It also boasted the Cowboy Band, which helped publicize the city.

The continued spread of farmers and barbed wire pressed a greater and greater percentage of trail cattle on Dodge, but in the end the herds stopped coming. The 1884 quarantine law, which prohibited Texas cattle from crossing Kansas between March 1 and December 1, meant that any herds moving north thereafter would have to keep west of the Kansas line. Many herds made it through in 1884, but none did after that. Kansas cattle were still trailed to Dodge for shipment, but after the big freeze of 1886–87 the Cowboy Capital could no longer be considered an important cattle market.

The last of the Kansas cowtowns to figure prominently in the trailing era was Caldwell, the "Border Queen" on the Chisholm Trail just north of Indian Territory. Caldwell was settled in 1871, but it had no railroad. During the winter of 1873–74, however, when thousands of cattle had to be wintered on the plains, many herds were held near Caldwell, and it served as a supply center and also as the place cowboys went for a spree.

Even before the railroad reached it in 1880 Caldwell already had a reputation for violence and killings. The sight of a horse thief "idling his time away under a cottonwood tree" (at the end of a rope) was not unusual.[10] A marshal's term in office in Caldwell was about two weeks on the average. There was a saying, "In Caldwell you're lucky to be alive."[11]

When the railroad reached Caldwell, it gave the Chisholm Trail a slight but temporary advantage over the Western Trail to Dodge City, but the rapidly spreading farms were making it increasingly difficult to move herds without trouble with grangers, and 1884 was the Chisholm Trail's last year.

As the demand for stocker cattle or young steers blossomed in the North, most of the herds sold in Kansas were delivered to ranches in Wyoming, Montana, or the Dakotas. Ogallala, Nebraska, rose as a new cattle center, and many herds not sold in Kansas found buyers among cowmen assembled there. By the mid-1870s Cheyenne, Wyoming, was another important cattle center where many Texas herds were sold. Ogallala and

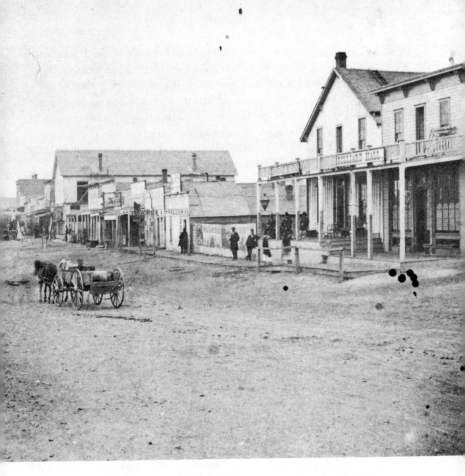

Dodge City in 1878. Left of the Billiard Hall is the Dodge House.
Courtesy of the Amon Carter Museum of Western Art, Fort Worth

Cheyenne became as important to Texas cattlemen as the Kansas railheads had been. Cheyenne was, in addition, headquarters for all the cattlemen of the North and Northwest. In 1877, Miles City, Montana, became the cattle center for that region.

The town that benefited most and longest from the Chisholm Trail was Fort Worth. In 1865, as a result of the exodus caused by the Civil War, Fort Worth had more houses than people, for the inhabitants of all ages numbered no more than 250. The empty town made, as newcomer K. M. Van Zandt remarked, "a gloomy picture." The town had a blacksmith shop, a flour mill, and a cobbler's shop, but lacked such vital institutions as a post office and a saloon.[12] As the Longhorn was the economic salvation of Texas, the Chisholm Trail was the savior of Fort Worth, which owed its favorable location on the cattle trail to accident. At least in the early days it was the last place for making purchases before reaching central Kansas.

Before its revival Fort Worth was not impressive. "We went by Waco, Cleburne, and Fort Worth," George Saunders wrote of his first trip up the trail. "Between the last named places the country was somewhat level and untimbered. . . . When we reached Fort Worth we crossed the Trinity River under the bluff, where the present street car line to the stockyards crosses the river. Fort Worth was then but a very small place, consisting of only a few stores, and there was only one house in that part of town where the stockyards are now located. We held our herd here two days.[13]

Other men on the early drives noted that Fort Worth was a small village with few stores, but as the purchases of supplies for trail herds infused new life into the town, the population doubled between 1865 and 1868. It continued to grow because of rumors that a railroad line would soon be extended there.

When Colonel John Wien Forney visited Texas in 1871, Fort Worth's population had grown to upwards of twelve hundred. It was, Forney noted, beautifully situated on a broad plateau. "Fort Worth is a city set on a hill, and as the point of junction between two branches of the Texas and Pacific, is particularly enviable, inasmuch as from this locality the Grand Trunk line to the Pacific will be projected and pushed. . . . During the last year 500,000 head of cattle were driven through Fort Worth on their way to Missouri and Kansas, and as we left the town we met a single drove containing 1250 head."[14]

In anticipation of the coming of the railroad others flocked to Fort Worth, doubling the population again in 1873. Around four hundred thousand cattle had been trailed to Kansas that year, but the financial panic beginning in September left thousands of cattle unsold. What hurt Fort Worth even more was that railroad construction everywhere was suspended. The city's population immediately declined to about one thousand, and "grass literally grew in the streets. This was not a metaphor to indicate stagnation, but a doleful fact" said the editor of the *Democrat*.[15] Former Fort Worth lawyer Robert E. Gowart informed the *Dallas Herald* that Fort Worth was such a drowsy place he saw a panther asleep in the street near the courthouse. To Dallasites, Fort Worth was thereafter Panther City.

Like Abilene's city fathers, Fort Worth officials had to cope with the problems caused by overly exuberant cowboys as well as gamblers, pimps, and prostitutes. In 1873 they passed a number of ordinances prohibiting gambling, prostitution, and the wearing of guns. Because it was soon clear that these regulations were harmful to business, however, the orders were suspended and Fort Worth was again known as a "tolerant" town.[16]

Most of the gambling dens and dance halls were confined to Hell's Half Acre around the intersection of Rusk (later Commerce) and Twelfth streets, and in this district Fort Worth was considered wide open. Like other trail towns that attracted lawless elements, Fort Worth needed some fearless man to keep the peace, and for a time Marshal "Long Hair" Jim Courtright filled the job effectively. When he was hired, his duties were made explicit—he was to keep the peace, not clean up the town.

In 1876, Fort Worth residents turned out, boy and man, to complete construction of the Texas and Pacific track to the city limits. The first train reached the city on July 19, and the expected boom began. By January 1877 all dwellings were filled and an estimated one thousand people lived in tents around the city limits. Fort Worth residents, now confident of their city's future, happily named everything "Panther."

Although some cattle were shipped out of Texas by the various railroads, such shipments posed no immediate threat to the trailing business. It was still far less expensive to trail cattle to Kansas than to ship them by rail.

In 1878, Fort Worth launched a cleaning-up program, and word soon spread among cowboys that a visit to the town likely meant a stopover in the jail. Trail crews now shunned it. In April citizens and businessmen placed an ad in the *Fort Worth Democrat* calling attention to the cost of strict enforcement of laws against drinking, gambling, and other cowboy amusements.

"The cattle season beginning, we think more freedom ought to be allowed as everyone is aware of the amount of money spent in this city by cattlemen and cowboys, thus making every trade and business prosper. We notice especially this year that contrary to their usual custom, almost all of them remain in their camps a few miles from the city and give as the cause the stringent enforcement of the law closing all places of amusement that attract them."[17]

The city council yielded to public pressure, to the great dissatisfaction of Marshal Courtright. As merchants recovered their trade with trail men, the *Democrat* noted that the dance halls were "in full blast again."[18]

By 1880, when the Missouri-Kansas-Texas Railroad reached Fort Worth, the town had a population of 6,663. A year and a half later the Santa Fe also laid tracks through the town, so it had ample rail facilities for serving as a trade and cattle center. It was evident that the city needed to expand its economic base, for the Chisholm Trail would eventually be obliterated by the spread of farms and the increasing use of barbed wire by ranchers.

Former Confederate captain B. B. Paddock, who began editing the *Fort Worth Democrat* in 1872, constantly prodded local businessmen into promoting the city and chided them mercilessly when they let opportunities pass. In the spring of 1875 he had written: "This city is on the nearest and best route. . . . Fencing will be a serious obstacle to herdsmen in many places. This route also allows owners and herdsmen a better opportunity of securing supplies than is afforded by any other route."[19] By 1875 cattle buyers were already coming to Fort Worth to contract for herds moving up the Chisholm Trail.

Looking ahead to the day when the northern trails would be closed, Paddock predicted that Fort Worth would become a center for the meat-packing industry. He chastised the Texas and Pacific Railroad and others for making no effort to develop the shipping of live cattle by offering reasonable freight rates. He pointed out that to ship two thousand head, or one hundred carloads, of cattle from Dallas to St. Louis cost $11,500. The same herd could be driven to Ellsworth, Kansas, for only $1,000; and it cost only $7,500 more to ship them from Ellsworth to St. Louis—a total of $8,500, or $3,000 less than shipping directly from Texas. Eventually the railroads would begin to compete for the cattle business by lowering their freight charges.

Fort Worth continued to grow. In 1877 construction began on the courthouse and the three-story El Paso Hotel, and a slaughterhouse shipped its first carload of refrigerated beef to St. Louis in March. Even though some herds were following the new Western Trail by way of Fort Griffin to Dodge City, many still came up the Chisholm Trail, and the owners bought provisions and equipment at Forth Worth. The cowboys kept the Tivoli Hall, Trinity Saloon, and the various dance halls busy. That same year the Texas and Pacific Railroad shipped more than fifty-one thousand live cattle from Fort Worth.[20]

Although herds continued to pass through or near Fort Worth in the spring of 1878, many turned off the Chisholm Trail at Belton, owing to the blandishments of agents the Fort Griffin merchants sent there to persuade trail bosses to use the Western Trail. Paddock reprimanded Forth Worth merchants for supinely allowing so much business to be siphoned off by rivals from Fort Griffin. "That our merchants should have lost sight of the importance of having a representative to offset the influence of Fort Griffin's enterprise at Belton," he wrote "is singular indeed."

When it was known that only 100,000 cattle had followed the Chisholm Trail, while 150,000 had taken the route past Fort Griffin, Paddock renewed his attack: "Had our businessmen been equally active in securing this immense drive, the season drive would not have fallen short of 200,000. Experience is a dear teacher. We hope that their eyes will be opened to their best interest next year."[21] The Fort Worth merchants responded by sending their own agent to Belton to persuade trail bosses to stay on the Chisholm Trail. This effort succeeded, for by late June of 1879 more than 135,000 cattle had passed by Fort Worth, while a little over 100,000 had gone up the Western Trail.

By the early 1880s trailing cattle to or through Kansas was

becoming so difficult that Texas cowmen launched a campaign to have a national cattle trail set aside from Texas to Montana. Northern ranches were now well stocked, and northern cowmen refused to encourage competition from Texas. The project was never approved.

Because of cordial relations already existing between the businessmen of Fort Worth and the cattlemen of northern and western Texas, "Cow Town" remained a cowmen's headquarters even after the Chisholm Trail was only a memory. As the trailing era ended, the railroads began competing for the cattle traffic, and Fort Worth's position as a rail center enabled it to continue to play an important role in the beef cattle business. This role was enhanced by the coming of the packing houses.

In April 1875 the editor of the *Fort Worth Democrat* had written, "There is no reason why Fort Worth should not become the great cattle center of Texas, where both buyer and seller meet for the transaction of an immense business in Texas beef. Fort Worth promises every advantage required in doing a very heavy beef packing business. With an abundance of pure water, ample herding grounds and soon to have shipping facilities by rail to all markets of the East and North, it would seem an admirable point for packing beef."

It was not until 1890, when the Fort Worth Dressed Meat and Packing Company was established, that this advice was followed. In the next few years Swift and Armour opened packing plants in the city. These plants and the business they brought were at least partly responsible for the city's increase in population from around twenty-seven thousand in 1900 to more than seventy-three thousand in 1910.[22]

Trail towns had profited from the trailing business for from several years to a decade or longer. Some declined drastically in population when the herds stopped coming. Although this often meant a distinct improvement in the quality of the local citizenry, it also meant a substantial loss of income. In the more forward-looking or fortunate towns, like Wichita and Fort Worth, other economic activities were quickly developed, and these towns continued to grow on the foundations the trailing era had provided.

CHAPTER 9

Trailing Contractors and Ranching Syndicates

"When everybody is wanting to sell, I buy;
when everybody is wanting to buy, I sell."
George W. Littlefield

WHEN the Chisholm Trail opened, many ranchers had a few hundred steers to sell but no way to get them to market; those who had several thousand could not afford to take their cowboys away from ranch work for several months. All were short of funds. Almost immediately, however, men devised ways to gather herds and get them to Abilene without a large cash outlay. A number of arrangements and combinations of plans were made to the mutual profit of cattle raisers and those who delivered their beeves to market.

One method was payment of a flat fee of $1.00 or $1.50 a head to a contractor who delivered the cattle and sold them for the owners. In this case the owners retained title to the cattle and took the risks, but they also stood to profit when the price was high. For his fee the contractor furnished crew, cook, wagon, trail boss, provisions, and horses. This saved the ranchers not only substantial cash outlays before their cattle were sold but also responsibility for organizing and conducting the drive. Cattle lost on the way were charged to the contractor, who naturally encouraged strays to join his herds. In some cases cattlemen provided for the expenses of the drive and paid the contractor a smaller fee.

The contract-trailing business, with its promise of fair profits with small risks or larger profits with greater risks, attracted many men. So important was their role in moving cattle to market that in any given year trailing contractors were in charge of the vast majority of the herds on the trail. Contractors made whatever arrangements the circumstances permitted. George W. Littlefield bought cattle on credit for others, a special type of contracting.

Some, like Dillard R. Fant of Goliad, devoted themselves exclusively to trailing cattle for others; over the years Fant handled about two hundred thousand head. Others, like John T. Lytle, were primarily trailing contractors but also purchased cattle for speculation when conditions seemed promising. In this way they made a guaranteed profit and occasionally added to it substantially when the market was favorable. Lytle and his partners—McDaniel, Schreiner, and Light—were among the major trailing contractors, handling around six hundred thousand head, or perhaps 15 percent of all the cattle trailed out of Texas.

Family firms were also successful trailing contractors, among them George Webb Slaughter and his six sons, Coggins and Parks Cattle Company, Blocker Brothers, Pryor Brothers, Snyder Brothers, and several others. Slaughter began in 1868 by trailing his own marketable beeves and training his sons. In less than a decade the Slaughters trailed and sold cattle worth nearly half a million dollars. Moses and Samuel Coggins had run small ranches before the Civil War, but in 1868 went into the cattle business seriously. They raised and trailed their own cattle and contracted to deliver others for their neighbors. By 1873 they were able to purchase all of the cattle they took to market, thereby greatly increasing their potential profits. They were especially active in stocking new ranches from New Mexico to Montana, and in obtaining government contracts for supplying beef to Indian reservations.[1]

Blocker Brothers of Blanco County was another successful family firm of trailing contractors and ranchers, although two of the four brothers—Ab and Jenks—remained employees rather than partners. At the outset the Blockers delivered cattle for others; thereafter they secured orders from northern buyers and then purchased Texas cattle to fill them. As this business grew they hired W. H. Jennings to buy cattle for them, then made him a partner.

Before their trailing business became so large they had to

hire a number of crews, the Snyder brothers were their own trail bosses. They began by buying cattle on credit and trailing them to Abilene. Over the years Snyder cattle were driven to New Mexico, Colorado, Nebraska, Wyoming, and Montana, where they helped stock the ranches springing up over the northern grasslands.

Another successful family firm was Pryor Brothers Cattle Company of Mason County. Ike T. Pryor drove his first herd all the way to Ogallala in 1876. It was made up of 1,250 steers under contract and 250 of his own. By wise use of his profits Pryor became a major trailing contractor by 1880, when he sent 12,000 head up the trail, mainly cattle he had purchased. On those he owned he made a profit of from three to five dollars a head; on those under contract he made at most one or two dollars.

In 1881, Ike Pryor formed a partnership with his brother and expanded the business. In the spring of 1884 they contracted to deliver forty-five thousand head of South Texas Longhorns, which they moved in one enormous drive of fifteen herds. For this major movement of cattle Pryor Brothers hired 15 trail bosses, 15 cooks, and 160 trail hands. They supplied fifteen chuck wagons, and more than one thousand horses.

The huge drive started off badly, for every herd had scattered during the first week. The cattle were rounded up and pushed up the trail, and the overall loss was only 3 percent. For years afterward Pryor received payments for steers bearing his road brand that had mixed with other herds. In the 1884 season Pryor Brothers made a net profit of $130,000, which enabled them to lease enough rangeland in Colorado to fatten twenty thousand head a year. They lost heavily in the winter of 1886–87, but Ike Pryor remained in the cattle business, recovered his losses, and died a millionaire.[2]

Charles Goodnight and others entered the cattle business as trailing contractors, then used their profits to become cattlemen. In 1866, Goodnight and Oliver Loving contracted to supply beeves to Fort Sumner, New Mexico, and pioneered the Goodnight-Loving Trail there. Although Loving died of wounds received from the Comanches, Goodnight established a ranch at

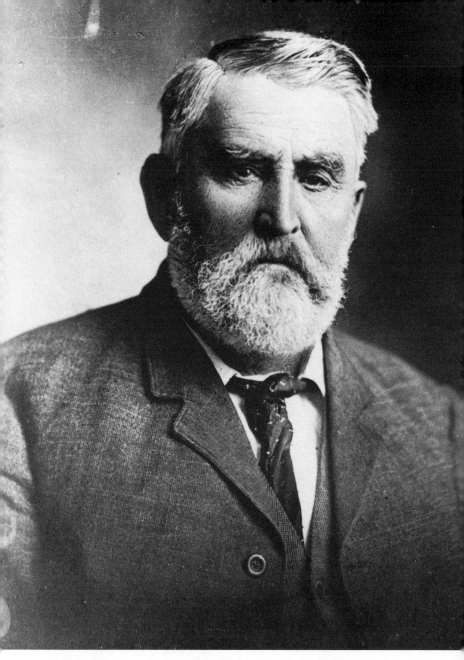

Charles Goodnight, Texas cowman and trail driver. Western History Collections, University of Oklahoma Library the Bosque Grande on the Pecos. He arranged with John Chisum to deliver cattle to the Bosque Grande at one dollar a head over Texas prices. Chisum lost two entire herds to Indians, but he and Goodnight developed a profitable relationship; Chisum drove cattle to New Mexico, and Goodnight trailed them on to Colorado. They divided the profits, enabling both men to expand their ranching activities.[3]

As the trailing business expanded, the contractors' methods became more systematic. The Slaughters and Blockers could rely on family members to manage herds and supervise sales. All of the brothers served as trail bosses at first, but when either firm had a dozen or more herds on the trail it was necessary for each brother to oversee a number of outfits at once. Blocker Brothers handled an impressive share of the trail cattle, between three hundred thousand and five hundred thousand, or 7 to 10 percent of all the cattle driven north from Texas. The reason the figures can only be estimated for most trailing contractors is that they kept the barest minimum of records. In the words of Jimmy Skaggs, they were "hip-pocket businessmen."[4]

At the height of the trailing era about a dozen major contractors were responsible for three-fourths of the trail herds. These men were essential to the growth of the cattle industry, for they were the organizers who provided the necessary links between the cattle raisers in Texas and the cattle buyers.

Mark Withers, whose family moved from Missouri to Texas, was one of the most active of the independent trailing men. He made his first drive in 1859 at the age of thirteen, from Lockhart to Fredericksburg, both in Texas. In 1862 he helped trail a herd from Lockhart to Shreveport for the Confederate Army; in 1868, with eight men and a cook, he drove six hundred big steers to Abilene. He bought the steers on credit for ten dollars a head, held them near Abilene to fatten, and sold them in the fall for twenty-five dollars; his expenses were four dollars per steer, which gave him a profit of eleven dollars a head. That same summer Withers took part in Joseph McCoy's wild west show to attract cattle buyers to Abilene. Withers followed the trail from 1868 to 1887, most of the time driving cattle he had purchased.

Another famous Texas trail man was R. G. (Dick) Head, also

from Missouri. At the age of thirteen he helped drive a herd for the Confederate Army, then enlisted three years later. After the war he trailed cattle for Colonel J. J. Myers, and soon had full charge of Myers's trailing business, which meant supervising a dozen herds on the trail at the same time.

In 1875 Head became general manager for Ellison, Dewees, and Bishop, trailing contractors who moved from thirty thousand to fifty thousand cattle a season. Head and Bishop were partners from 1878 to 1883; the next three years Head was general manager for the British-owned Prairie Cattle Company, which operated three large ranches. In 1886 he became president of the International Range Association, and owned an interest in ranches in Texas and New Mexico.

Hundreds of men trailed cattle from Texas during the two decades the trails remained open. Some succeeded and became fairly wealthy; others lost their investments because of troubles with Indians or outlaws, or because of price fluctuations or the lack of buyers. Some men were able to finance the wintering of their herds and were fortunate enough to sell them profitably the following season. Others lost nearly all of their cattle because of severe weather. Among those who trailed cattle for a living, as in other businesses, what counted most was efficiency. Men who had the knowledge and ability to supervise the successful movement of ten or fifteen herds in a season were the ones who became wealthy.

The services the trailing contractors provided were less costly than shipping by railroad by four or five dollars a head, which could mean as much as fifteen thousand dollars more in profits on a single herd. If weather and other conditions were favorable, the cattle usually gained weight on the trail. Cattle shipped by rail, on the other hand, lost weight and frequently were injured.

Trail men estimated that it cost sixty cents a head to move cattle 1,500 miles; a federal survey of 1886 put the figure at seventy-five cents.[5] In 1884 the breakdown of trailing expenses was thirty dollars a month each for nine riders and a cook, and one hundred dollars for a trail boss, for a total of four hundred dollars. Adding one hundred dollars for provisions, the total cost, after the initial outlay for wagons and horses, was five hundred dollars to move three thousand cattle 450 to 500 miles. Until the railroads revised their rate schedules and made them competitive, trailing was much less expensive than shipping. As long as the trails remained open, the trailing contractors played a vital role in the range cattle business.

Another product of the trail drives and the cattle boom was the syndicate, domestic or foreign, that went into the cattle business on a grand scale and provided the funds for rapid expansion. Much of the capital that launched the syndicates came from Britain. A great many Britishers also came to the cattle country, some eager to be cowboys, others determined to become ranchers or ranch managers. John Clay and Murdo Mackenzie, both Scots, were two of the most successful ranch managers. Mackenzie, for years the boss of the Matador, was one of the best-known cowmen in the country.

When easterners and Britons began buying cattle and range rights, ranch managers were in great demand, but only men of superior qualities. Isaac Ellwood, owner of the Frying Pan Ranch, expressed the desires of many: "I want a man who knows something of land and water problems, can make a good bargain in cattle sales and is able to manage cowhands." He was advised to settle for someone "who can get along with your men and is reasonably honest. If you receive this he will be worth his pay." As Ellwood advised his son William, "The major success of a ranch, my friends in Texas tell me, is due to its choosing a good manager."[6]

Managing one of the huge ranches was no simple matter. "It was not an easy job," wrote Nebraska cowman John Bratt, "to handle two hundred or more cowboys with nearly a dozen different outfits and one thousand to twelve hundred horses, keeping the work moving intelligently, finding camping places for each outfit and see that all, even the lone representative, had equal share and a square deal, but I had a reputation for doing it."

The main reason for the flurry of investment in ranching syndicates was the widespread delusion about easy wealth to be made in the open range, free grass, cattle industry. Encouraging the expectations of certain and substantial profits that helped spark the wild speculation in cattle in the 1880s was the publication in 1881 of James S. Brisbin's *The Beef Bonanza; or, How to Get Rich on the Plains.* A U.S. general who had served for years on the plains, Brisbin spoke with authority, and he verified the rumors and stories of fabulous profits to be made that had circulated throughout the East and in Britain.

Emphasizing the relative decline in cattle breeding, Brisbin concluded that "for at least ten years yet the stock growers need have no fear of overstocking the beef markets."[7] It was, according to Brisbin, ridiculously easy to sit back and let one's profits accumulate on free grass and open range. To raise a three-year-old steer worth twenty-five to thirty dollars cost only six to ten dollars. Hundreds of investors leaped at the opportunity; few of them ever saw a return on their money. And while it may have been true that there was no immediate fear of glutting the market, there was a real danger of overstocking the range.

Even before Brisbin's book appeared many easterners had invested in western range cattle companies. All no doubt expected to make handsome profits, but there were plenty of other get-rich-quick schemes available. Many were intrigued by the reports of friends who had already bought stock in some cattle company; others had already put money into western mining or railroad ventures. For a time investing in the range cattle business was considered smart.

Until the main influx of eastern and British capital, the partnership was the usual type of large ranch organization. Easterners such as banker Augustus Kountze and his brothers might enter an agreement, or "association," with a western cattleman such as Shanghai Pierce of South Texas. In 1885 the Kountzes agreed to furnish the capital to purchase two hundred thousand acres and twelve thousand yearlings selected by Pierce, who would receive one-sixth of the profits from cattle sales. Although relations between the conservative Kountzes and the colorful Pierce were stormy, the arrangement proved profitable to all concerned.[8] Other easterners entered similar agreements with individual cowmen, but not always with happy results.

Like the Kountze-Pierce partnership, most of these were

marred by misunderstandings caused by unreasonably high expectations on the one hand, and a growing irritation with those who provided the funds on the other. Often the eastern partners, totally unfamiliar with the cattle ranges, tried to lay down conditions that could only outrage the cowmen. James T. Gardner of Albany, New York, for example, wrote his partner, George McClellan, "Be sure to hire sober men; I shudder at the thought of our cattle running around the plains cared for by some fuzzy minded cowboy."[9] As more and more investors turned to the beef cattle business, the partnership was superseded by the syndicate, with its board of directors and multitude of stockholders.

One of the major difficulties of syndicate ranching was maintaining satisfactory communications between managers and their employers, for neither understood or appreciated the problems of the other. Some managers wrote infrequently and told their distant superiors as little as possible; others wrote lengthy, rambling letters. Neither practice was what was desired, but, as one manager glumly noted, they were damned for whatever they did or didn't do.

Managers also prepared annual reports, presumably to keep stockholders informed on range conditions and prospects for sales. The manager's annual report was almost a new branch of American literature, if semifiction could be considered new, for it was skillfully written to beguile and please far-off directors and shareholders. Bad news was artfully disguised or omitted. Managers did what they believed was expected of them; it seemed clear they were called on to produce good news. After the cattle boom collapsed, annual reports became dull and factual, for shareholders wanted no more double talk or fairy tales.[10]

Syndicate ranches, especially foreign-owned ones, experienced labor troubles that had not been characteristic of cowman-cowboy relations in the past. The basic problem was that the average cowboy could not respect absentee owners, especially British aristocrats who looked on cowboys as their retainers and, when they visited their ranches, expected a show of deference and humility.

Typical of the incidents resulting from this attitude, which provoked deep resentment among cowboys, was the Englishman Moreton Frewen's visit to one of the Wyoming ranches in which he had invested. Ranch manager Hank Devoe met him as he rode up; Frewen handed him the reins and ordered him to unsaddle his horse. Devoe informed him that he was nobody's servant.

"I own an interest in this ranch and I will have you fired," Frewen told him. Devoe replied that he couldn't fire him, for he had already quit.[11]

William A. Baillie-Grohman had a warning for other Englishmen who planned to run ranches in the West: "It is 'to do as others do.' That marked feature of America, social equality, which, while it has often a way of expressing itself in a very extravagant and disagreeable fashion, is undoubtedly a main factor in the unusually rapid growth of the Great West, must never be forgotten by the English settler. A man out West is a man, and let him be the poorest cowboy he will assert his right of perfect equality with the best of the land, betraying a stubbornness it is vain and unwise to combat. This is an old truth. . . . In connection with the cattle business it is . . . of tenfold importance: in no vocation is popularity more essential than in this, for let a man receive once the name of being possessed by unsociable pride, and there will not be a man in the country who, while he otherwise would gladly share his last pipe of tobacco or cup of coffee with him, will not then be ready and willing to spite or injure him."[12]

Some of the ranches with absentee owners were pilfered by their own employees as well as by their neighbors. It was well known that such ranches had a smaller calf production and many more mavericks than others. Small ranchers resented being virtually crowded off the overstocked ranges, and they didn't hesitate to kill even branded strays from big ranches for food, or to brand any mavericks they found. Some cowboys paid saloon debts or provided for their mistresses by marking calves with their brands or even altering brands. The Sweetwater, Wyoming, ranch that John Clay managed used a 71̸ (71 quarter circle) brand. The owner of a nearby road ranch and saloon adopted the rocking chair brand (⚞), which could easily be made out of the ⚞ quarter circle.[13]

Although there was occasional hostility between big and small ranchers, some of the big ones treated the small ones fairly and maintained cordial relations with them. During the round-ups these small ranchers were "dinner reps" when the wagon and crew were in their area. They got their cattle rounded up and branded, had a few square meals, and usually carried home a big piece of beef the cook gave them.

Concerning ranch management in the North, Colonel Samuel Gordon of the *Yellowstone Journal* noted later, "As a majority of the 'companies' and individuals knew nothing of the business, it was essential that there be at the head of each outfit a manager or superintendent to take charge of the technical part of it. These managers were usually cowboys who had become 'top-hands' on the southwestern ranges and were absolutely competent to run herds, but were rarely good financial managers."

Some company ranches, he continued, had competent businessmen as managers, men who were out of place on the range. "Looking backward, it is hard to guess which method was most disastrous; the manager with 'cow sense' but no idea of the value of money, or the thrifty financier who didn't know a branding iron from a poker. They were bad combinations, each of them."[14]

Despite the investors' great expectations from their managers, few managers were well paid—ninety dollars a month was probably close to the average. Exceptions were Dick Head of the Prairie Land and Cattle Company, Murdo Mackenzie of the Matador, and John Clay. But most were less fortunate; as one protested to the distant owner, "You expect us to spend nights on the range, using sod as a bed, drinking brackish water, while you enjoy good food and a soft bed, all for the smallest money."[15] Curiously, most investors saw no connection between adequate pay and managerial effectiveness. The managers' only alternative was to ask frequently for loans, which investors dared not refuse or insist on being repaid.

The sudden influx of nesters, or homesteaders, who

preempted some of the best land and cut off access to water, forced all ranchers to buy at least enough land to give them control of the water. Faced with the unexpected need to buy thousands of acres, many investors had to overextend their credit, even though some had never received a single dividend from the money they had invested in cattle. But in order to protect their investments, the big ranches had to buy land; often it meant sending good money after bad. Forced to acquire land for survival, some cattlemen did not hesitate to fence in huge sections of the public domain.

In 1879 fencing became a serious concern in the North as the Swan Land and Cattle Company, the Anglo-American Cattle Company, and other large outfits fenced vast areas of federal or railroad land, in some cases enclosing homesteads as well. Because of complaints, in 1883 the secretary of the interior authorized settlers to destroy illegal fences that blocked their way to land they wanted to homestead. In 1885 Congress outlawed such enclosures of the public domain, and President Cleveland ordered the fences removed.[16]

One of the most successful of the syndicate ranches, the Matador, was established in 1879 and branded its first calf crop 50M, reflecting the fifty-thousand-dollar capitalization. Later this brand was used only on horses. In 1882 Scottish investors bought the Matador, made it a joint-stock company, and increased its holdings to more than a million acres.

Although the Matador's cattle had been purchased according to the customary tally book count, and it paid for many more than it received, under the astute management of Scot Murdo Mackenzie the ranch prospered. At the outset the Matador sold young cattle to northern ranchers, who profited by grazing them for two years and then selling them for beef. In 1892, Mackenzie arranged for Western Ranches to graze two thousand head of Matador two-year-old steers along the Little Missouri. This introduced a new phase of cattle raising that enabled the Matador to profit not only by breeding cattle but also by maturing them in the North and marketing them. The company acquired its own range in Montana; because trailing was still less expensive than shipping by rail, the Matador trailed its own herds north until

1896.[17] Other big ranches in Texas adopted the same practice.

The Prairie Land and Cattle Company, the "mother of the British companies," was organized in Edinburgh in 1880–81. The western range cattle industry had been presented to Scottish investors as simply a matter of buying young cattle, fattening them on free grass, and selling them. So obvious a way to wealth attracted investors by the hundreds. The new company bought ranches in Colorado, New Mexico, and Texas. Its early profits, however, especially the first year's sensational dividend of slightly more than 20 percent, were from the sale of recently purchased cattle, not from natural increase.

For a few years during the 1880s there were scores of ranching companies organized on the tenuous foundations of blind faith and great expectations. There was something satisfying about investing in cattle ranches, inviting friends to visit the ranch headquarters, and wining and dining them at the Cheyenne Club. But, as Britisher William A. Baillie-Grohman mourned, "In no business is a man so dependent upon his neighbors, so open to petty annoyances, and so helplessly exposed to vindictive injury to his property as in stock raising out West."[18]

The years 1882, 1883, and 1884 were deceptively successful for the rapidly expanding western range cattle business, for prices remained high and there were plenty of eager buyers. In 1885, however, managers suddenly reported that the ranges were overstocked. When two extraordinarily severe winters followed, the Prairie Company, like most of the others, was hard hit. But although many went out of business, it survived until 1917.[19]

The XIT Ranch was established in 1882 when the Texas legislature offered three million acres in the Panhandle in exchange for building a new capitol (larger than any other state possessed) to replace the one that had burned down. The contract went to the Capitol Syndicate, John V. and Charles B. Farwell and Associates, of Chicago. At its greatest extent the XIT was about two hundred miles long and from twenty to forty miles wide, for the Farwells added fifty thousand acres to the original three million. Ab Blocker, who delivered the ranch's first herd, suggested the XIT brand as one that rustlers could not easily alter. Since the XIT included all or parts of ten counties, to many the brand meant "Ten in Texas."

The Farwells ran the XIT with efficiency and success. They eventually fenced the entire ranch, a job which required six thousand miles of barbed wire. The ranch employed 150 cowboys and ran 150,000 cattle. The Farwells, learning that the northern ranges were superior for fattening cattle, acquired a finishing range of about a million acres in Montana. They trailed young steers to it each year, and ran as many as 30,000 head on their Montana range. By 1906 all of the XIT's indebtedness had been paid off.[20]

John Clay represented Scottish syndicates that owned ranches in California, Wyoming, and Kansas during the peak years of investment in range cattle. In those years, when there were more potential buyers than sellers, cattle were bought on tally book records of roundups and of the number of calves branded rather than on actual range counts of the cattle sold. These book count deals, Clay discovered, were invariably disasters, for the tally books might show twice as many cattle as were actually on the range. But buyers optimistically paid for the book counts; men who insisted on actual counts were ignored as long as there were others less cautious with money to spend. The winter of 1884–85 was severe, and many Wyoming ranchers gloomily discussed their losses in Luke Murrin's saloon in Cheyenne. "Cheer up boys," he told them, "whatever happens the books won't freeze."[21]

Among the cattle kings of Wyoming was Alexander Swan, who began ranching in 1873. With his partner, Joseph Frank, he owned thousands of cattle on a vast range extending from near Ogallala, Nebraska, to Fort Steele, Wyoming, and from the Union Pacific Railroad to the Platte River. The principal Swan range was from the Chug and Sybille creeks westward over the mountains to the Laramie plains. Such an enormous range could make a man feel godlike, and that misfortune befell Alec Swan.

Swan was, nevertheless, a pioneer in the upgrading of Wyoming range cattle. In 1877 he began bringing Hereford bulls from Illinois and Iowa, and in 1883 imported purebred

Hereford cows and bulls from England. As a result of his efforts, in some years Swan cattle sold for twice as much as cattle from other ranches.[22]

When Swan and Frank asked John Clay to make a report on the Swan holdings to be used in organizing the Swan Land and Cattle Company in Scotland in the spring of 1883, Clay refused unless there was to be an actual count of the cattle. The subject was quickly dropped, and Clay's services were not required. Because Swan had a great following of sycophants, investors in his company did not demand a range count of his cattle. Swan was carried away with his own power, and when he fell he dragged his friends and employees down with him; none of those he had helped in the past was willing to lend him a hand. As Clay remarked, "His rise was meteoric, his fall terrific, and in 1887 when he failed, it was the forerunner of many disasters."[23] Swan's failure shook the whole range cattle industry to its very foundations. In March 1888 Clay was named manager of the Swan Company, and he labored for more than eight years to enable the company to survive. Under his management it recovered somewhat, but by 1910 it had sold its cattle and turned to raising sheep.[24]

Among the eastern cattle barons were Harvard classmates Hubert Teschemacher and Fred de Billier, who in the late 1870s bought three ranches in Wyoming. Although they made satisfactory profits in 1881, the division of managerial duties and the poor keeping of financial records jeopardized their success. In 1882, Richard Trimble, another Harvard classmate, joined the firm, increasing the division of management responsibilities. The firm survived the bad winter of 1886–87, but it foundered and failed soon after.[25]

Many cowmen of the northern and central plains were ruined by the winter of 1886–87, since few had shown any foresight and most had overstocked their ranges. Many easterners and Britishers lost all interest in the range cattle business when they discovered that it was by no means an avenue to easy wealth. As John Clay summed it up, "The gains of the open range business were swallowed up by losses. From the inception of the open range business in the West and Northwest from say

1870 to 1888, it is doubtful if a single cent was made if you average up the business as a whole."[26]

Most of the big syndicates that survived the winter of 1886–87 were liquidated between 1900 and 1920, although a few, like the Matador, continued to stay in business. In most cases the emphasis shifted from cattle to sheep, agriculture, land sales, oil leases, or other activities. The tremendous investments in the range cattle business had enabled it to expand rapidly in the 1880s; if the investments had been made on more realistic foundations, it seems unlikely that the era of the big ranches would have ended so quickly.

CHAPTER 10

The Spread and Collapse of the Cattle Kingdom

"The gains of the open range business were
swallowed up by losses."

John Clay

THE spread of the cattle kingdom from the Rio Grande to
Canada was rapid in the late 1870s and early 1880s, for cattlemen followed in the tracks of the retreating buffalo and plains
tribes. A story that was widely circulated at the time concerned
freighter E. S. Newman, who in the winter of 1864–65 was
caught on the Laramie plains at the onset of winter. He left his
oxen to starve, but found them fat when he returned in March.
By this incident Newman learned that cattle could not only survive winters on the northern plains but actually gain weight at
the same time. The Newman brothers became major cattlemen,
with two ranches in Wyoming and others in Nebraska, Indian
Territory, and West Texas.[1]

Many men had, in fact, long known that cattle thrived in the
region, as the buffalo had before them. As early as 1830 William
Sublette, Jedediah Smith, and others had taken a few cattle into
the Wind River valley, and three years later Rocky Mountain Fur
Company men had brought cattle from Missouri to the Green
River rendezvous. In 1843, John C. Frémont saw cattle in the
Platte valley of Colorado where the trading post called Fort
Lupton was later built. A band of Mormon pioneers introduced
the first breeding cattle into Wyoming in 1847, and in 1852 army
sutler Seth E. Ward of Fort Laramie wintered hundreds of oxen
in the Chugwater valley.[2]

As soon as the Oregon Trail was opened in the 1840s, cattle,
both oxen and breeding stock, traveled acrosss the plains to
Oregon. In 1849, Richard Grant, formerly of the Hudson's Bay

153

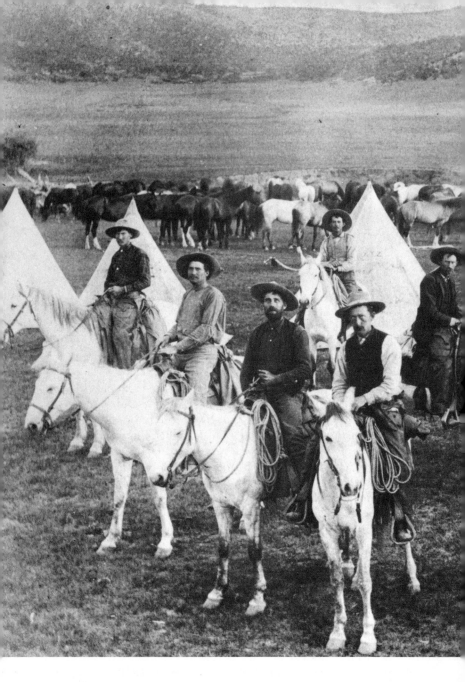

Roundup crew, tents, chuck wagon, and remuda. Tents and cook's awning indicate they were on a northern range. Courtesy of the Amon Carter Museum of Western Art, Fort Worth

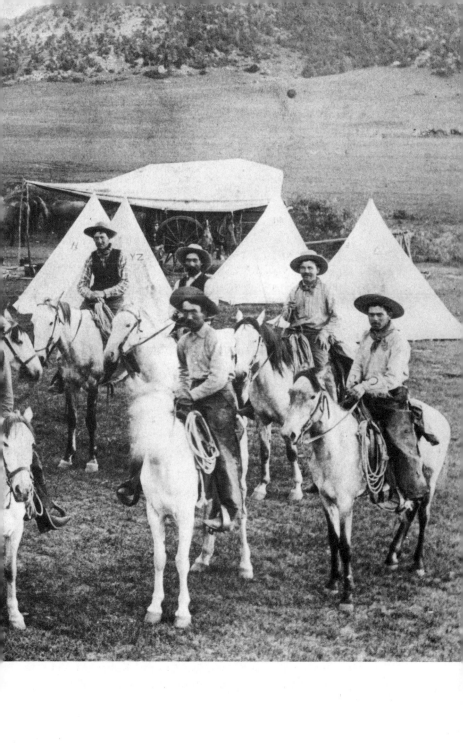

Company, began raising cattle at his trading post in the Jefferson valley of Montana. Within a few years other men were bringing cattle to the Bitterroot valley for fattening and sale to settlements along the Columbia River. During the 1850s others brought cattle to the same region as well as to the future site of Missoula.

When Granville Stuart took sixty head to Montana in 1858 he found a number of small herds already there. By 1863, he noted, the cattle industry was well established in the Alder Gulch mining area. As further evidence of the importance of cattle raising, in 1864 Montana's first territorial legislature passed a law regulating marks and brands.[3]

In 1866, Nelson Story went from Montana to North Texas and for ten thousand dollars bought around one thousand cattle, mostly cows with calves thrown in. With twenty-five cowboys he pointed the herd north, overcoming one obstacle after another all the way to Montana. The summer was unusually wet on the plains, and most of the rivers were over their banks. The cattle, Story complained, swam as much as they walked. Toll collectors harrassed him in Indian Territory, and bands of armed men threatened him in Kansas.

When Story and his cattle finally reached Fort Phil Kearny on the Bozeman Trail, Colonel H. B. Carrington ordered them to go no farther. The trail led through the last hunting grounds of the Teton Sioux, and Red Cloud's Oglalas were determined to preserve them against invasion by whites. Story's men were armed with new Remington breech-loading rifles, however; they ignored Carrington's order and continued at night up the trail. They got through with only one brush with the Sioux and the loss of one man. Story kept his breeding stock, bought others, and established a ranch near Bozeman.[4] In 1869, W. D. Jeffers brought one thousand Texas cattle to the Madison valley in a drive that took six months. In the next two years he brought up three thousand more Texas cattle.[5] In 1871 many cattle were trailed from Texas to Montana and settled on ranches in the Sun valley, along the Missouri River, and in the Big Hole country.[6]

Montana's major cattleman was Conrad Kohrs, who got his start by operating butcher shops in mining camps, a job that kept him constantly searching for cattle. In 1866 he bought John Grant's ranch and cattle in the Deer Lodge valley, although the land had not been surveyed and Grant had no title. Kohrs continued building up his herds with Texas Longhorns and Shorthorns from Missouri. Later he brought purebred Hereford bulls to his ranch and experimented with crossbreeding.[7]

John W. Iliff, for a time the leading cattleman of the whole Northwest, arrived at the Cherry Creek mining region of Colorado in 1859, the same year that John Dawson brought a herd to the Cherry Creek camps. Iliff began buying oxen and fattening them to sell as beef to the miners. By 1865 he was fully occupied with raising cattle, and began buying selected parcels of land to obtain control of the limited water supply over a vast range running one hundred miles east and west and upwards of sixty miles north and south. He bought Texas cattle from Charles Goodnight and imported Shorthorn bulls from Illinois and Iowa. By the time of his death in 1878 his land and cattle were worth a million dollars.[8]

Pioneer cattlemen of the Great Plains found the grass exceptionally nutritious. As Iliff noted, "I have engaged in the stock business in Colorado and Wyoming for the past fourteen years. During all that time I have grazed stock in nearly all the valleys of these territories, both summer and winter . . . no feed or shelter is required. I consider the summer-cured grass of these plains and valleys as superior to any hay."[9]

Another early cattleman, R. C. Keith of North Platte, Nebraska, began raising cattle in 1867 with a few "American" cows. In both 1869 and 1870 he bought one thousand Texas cattle. By 1875 he had sold sixty-three thousand dollars' worth of cattle and had a herd of more than five thousand valued at nearly one hundred thousand dollars.[10]

Although many parts of the plains remained unsafe for men and cattle as long as both buffalo and plains warriors roamed freely over them, cattle raising had spread fairly widely along the borders of the Sioux country by the mid-1860s. In the summer of 1865 a Dr. Corey followed the Loup Fork of the Platte northwest of Omaha to the Niobrara and the base of the Black Hills, then returned along the Big Horns and down the

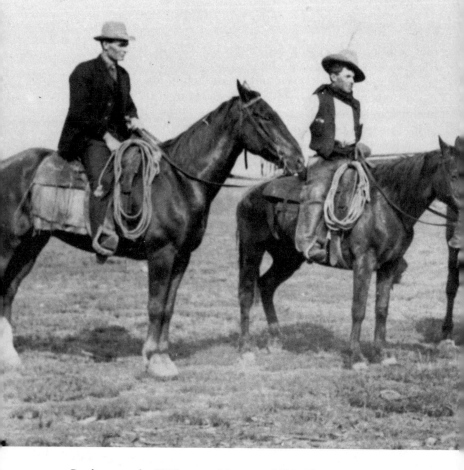

Cowboys on the XIT range, Montana, 1905. Photo by John L. Breum. The Montana Historical Society

Platte. On the way he saw numerous herds of cattle, sheep, and horses. "Old mountaineers, hunters, and trappers all told me," he reported, "that the winter grazing was fine and uninterrupted by snow. I have been familiar with the winter grazing in that country for six winters, and I am sure the stock will winter on the native grass without shelter."[11]

It was not the discovery that the grass supporting millions of buffalo would also support cattle that led to the explosive spread of cattle ranches in the northern and central plains. Until the

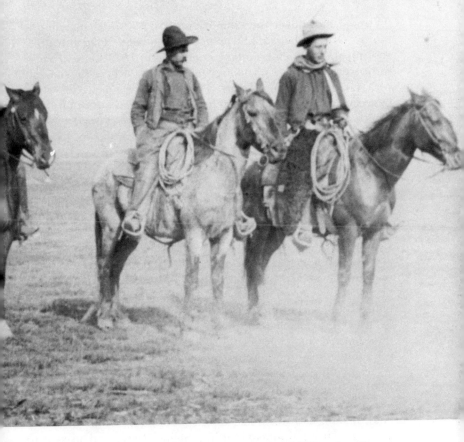

virtual extermination of the buffalo in the 1870s, the Sioux, Cheyennes, Comanches, and Kiowas could not be controlled, and men who valued their hair had to wait on buffalo hunters and the U.S. Cavalry. The new military posts on the plains and in the mining camps provided steady markets, and as the buffalo disappeared the thousands of reservation Indians also had to be fed beef.

Even before the great flood of cattle from Texas to Wyoming and Montana began, herds were driven to those regions from Oregon and Utah. Oregon's first cattle were those Ewing Young trailed from California to the Willamette valley in 1836; two years later the Hudson's Bay Company brought in two thousand more over the same route. In 1843 the major migration to Oregon began, and many good-quality "Pilgrim cattle" accompanied the emigrants.[12] Beginning in 1875 some of these cattle were trailed to Wyoming and Montana, where they mixed with Longhorns from Texas. The peak year was 1880, when between 150,000 and 200,000 head were driven out of Oregon. Thereafter Oregon had fewer surplus cattle to export.[13]

Among the early Colorado and Kansas cattlemen, in addition to John Iliff, were Joseph P. Farmer, John Hittson, William K. Schaeffer, and Charles Goodnight. Farmer came from Ireland, arriving in 1861 in Colorado, where he bought land that gave him control of water along the West Bijou, a tributary of the Platte. Starting with a few Texas cattle and Shorthorn bulls, by careful management he built up a herd and, at the same time, a stable of blooded horses.

Hittson had first settled in Palo Pinto County, Texas, and at one time owned one hundred thousand head. But chronic Indian troubles caused him to shift to Colorado, where he bought a half section of land on the middle Bijou that effectively controlled the only available water in that area. In 1873 he drove eleven thousand of his Texas cattle there, and in the following year brought up twenty thousand more.

Schaeffer earned money to become a rancher by trailing a herd of steers from Texas to Nevada. Although the drive lasted a year and a half, he sold the cattle for fifty-two dollars a head in gold, making it a profitable venture. He bought four thousand acres in central Kansas along the Saline River, and used it to winter twenty-five hundred cattle each year. He owned no stock cattle, but bought and fattened Texas steers, making substantial profits and greatly reducing the risk of losses. In a typical year he bought twenty-five hundred steers for twenty dollars a head, or fifty thousand dollars. It cost him two dollars a head to hold them until time to sell, and about ten thousand dollars in interest on his loan. Camp supplies and other items for his men might cost an additional $2,500, making his total investment $67,500. He sold the cattle for $93,750, or a net gain of $26,250.[14]

Charles Goodnight and Oliver Loving were among the first cowmen to drive Texas cattle to New Mexico and Colorado.

After Loving's death, Goodnight turned to ranching rather than trailing; in 1868 he bought rangeland southwest of Pueblo, Colorado, and a few years later acquired another large tract of land near Trinidad. Later he established a ranch in Palo Duro Canyon, Texas.

Although there was an irrepressible delusion that the rangeland and grass of the Great Plains were inexhaustible, as early as 1876 J. M. Wilson of the Colorado Cattle Growers Association expressed doubts. In the January meeting of the association he said, "The belief seems to prevail with those who have not watched and noted its steady decline, that our range is unlimited, and that all that is necessary is to come with horses, cattle and sheep, no matter how many, and turn them loose, and all will do well." Colorado's rangeland was extensive, he admitted, but "that it is unlimited, and cannot be overstocked, is simply nonsense, and the sooner we realize the truth the better for ourselves and the better for the country."[15] It would be only a decade before Wilson was proved to be painfully correct.

In the North there was more conflict between the big spreads and the little ranches than in Texas, although the "Fence War" was largely an attack of small ranchers on large ones. The cattlemen's association that met in Jacksboro, Texas, in 1883, the year the war began, passed a resolution to the effect that the state legislature should enact laws protecting property rights against wanton destruction. All property taxed by the government, the resolution continued, "is entitled to the same protection, no matter to whom belonging, and whether the property be used for agricultural or grazing purposes." And there should be gates wherever public roads passed through the pastures.[16]

South Dakota small rancher Bruce Siberts maintained that there was open hostility between big and small ranches in that region. One of his steers got in with Hash Knife cattle and was shipped with them to Chicago and sold by the Wyoming Stock Growers Association, which put the proceeds from the sale of the steer into its stray account. Even though Siberts presented proof of ownership, he was refused the money.

Later when he accompanied a shipment of cattle to Chicago,

Siberts called on Clay Robinson of the Wyoming association, who told him he would have to bring suit to collect his money. Siberts vowed he would collect it on the range in his own way. Robinson, Siberts recalled, didn't like it and "talked pretty mean to me." He never heard of a little rancher being reimbursed for cows he lost in a big roundup, but he suspected that the policy cost the big ranchers more than they gained. Their cattle were widely scattered, and it was easy to kill strays from distant ranches.[17]

Some ranchers, such as Print Olive and his brothers, brutally eliminated little ranchers in Texas as well as in the North. Wherever the Olives ranged their cattle no small rancher was safe, and many who occupied land the Olives wanted in both Texas and Nebraska disappeared, either driven out or murdered.

The big ranches of Wyoming continued to suffer heavy losses to rustlers. In 1892 a group of frustrated ranchers hired some Texas gunmen and invaded Johnson County to deal justice to some of the more notorious cattle thieves. They were soon outnumbered and surrounded by irate residents of the county; troops from Fort McKinney apprehended the cattlemen and took them to Cheyenne, where they were eventually released. Undoubtedly there was right as well as wrong on both sides. What heightened the conflict in the North was the fact that most of the struggle was for control of lands the federal government owned, not private holdings. In Texas, once barbed wire was accepted, cattlemen large and small quickly acquired title to the land they used or quit ranching. For this reason there was little resentment against Texas ranchers who decided to run sheep as well as cattle on their own lands.

In Wyoming it was partly resentment against easterners and Britons who established huge ranches that stimulated cattle stealing, for it was never more widespread than in that time and area. Edgar Beecher Bronson was one who overcame the Texans' dislike for "No'therners," and was able to hire a loyal crew. "While all the best punchers were Texans," Bronson wrote, "the elders themselves were ex-Confederate soldiers."[18] Even when stock association inspectors arrested men who had stolen cattle in their possession, it was nearly impossible to secure convictions from local juries, whose sympathies were with the "little men." When, for example, a Colorado stock inspector arrested a man who had five Pony Cattle Company calves in his barn, witnesses solemnly testified that it was quite common for calves to leave their mothers and break into barns. The thief was acquitted. The inspector angrily and unwisely remarked that this was what was to be expected when a cow thief jury and a cow thief judge tried a cow thief. The judge heard about the remark and fined him twenty-five dollars.[19]

Since fewer than half of the cattle sent up the trails from Texas were immediately shipped out by rail, the others went to stock new ranches or to Indian agencies, army posts, or feed lots. Credit was vital to the cattle business. Cowmen who could not sell their cattle were obliged to hold them on the range over the winter, which usually meant borrowing money for current expenses. In 1873, for example, when the financial panic drove away potential buyers, Texas cowmen in Kansas borrowed a million and a half dollars. Credit would become increasingly important in the cattle boom of the 1880s. As Gene Gressley has pointed out, the "Western range cattle industry during the last two decades of the nineteenth century was operated basically on borrowed capital."[20]

As new ranches sprang up over the northern plains, Texas cattle, horses, and cowboys were much in demand. Some Texas cowmen also settled in the North, but there was a greater influx from the East and from Britain. No matter where the owners were from, they all soon learned that for handling wild cattle on the open range they needed at least a nucleus of Texans. Early settlers in Montana and the Dakotas remarked that they could not step outside their cabins and spit without hitting a Texan.[21]

As a result, Texas cowboys gave their stamp to the entire range cattle industry east of the Rockies. Their style differed considerably from that of the California vaqueros and the Oregonians who copied it. For a time dally and tie-fast roping styles mingled in the Northwest, but the tie-fast custom of the more numerous Texas cowboys eventually predominated.

No one questioned the fact that Texans knew cattle and

horses as no other men, but off the range their knowledge was extremely limited before they broadened their experience by going up the trail. Texans were known in the North by the unflattering term of "Rawhides," since rawhide, or "Mexican iron," was the plastic mending or binding material for all things—in this sense the forerunner of baling wire.

Texans referred to men from farming regions as "short-horns," and to non-Texas northern cowboys as "sagebrush men" or "God-damn knock-kneed Oregonians." Teddy Blue Abbott, who settled in Montana before large numbers of Texans arrived, enjoyed telling "Texas" or "Rawhide" jokes about the newcomers.

One reason so many Texans remained in the North after delivering herds to ranchers in Wyoming and elsewhere was that Texas outfits fed their men as cheaply as possible. In the North there were wealthy easterners and Britons who enjoyed being cattle barons. They loved to bring friends to visit their ranches, especially during roundups. They liked to "rough it" with the men, but in comfort and style; the result was that diet and working conditions in the North were vastly superior to what they were in Texas. Even tents and cots were supplied for round-up and trail crews. Although a few old-time Texas cowboys grumbled at such evidence of physical and moral decay, they soon saw the advantages.

Few Texas cowboys had ever seen white flour or sugar in the early days, for cornmeal and sorghum took the places of wheat flour and sugar. A favorite "Rawhide" joke was of a Texas cowboy who rode into a Montana roundup camp at mealtime. When he poured a cup of coffee someone handed him a sugar bowl. "No thanks," he said, "I don't take salt in my coffee."[22]

Texas cattle reached the Cheyenne region as early as 1867 or 1868, and they continued to arrive. By 1874 there were an estimated ninety thousand cattle in Wyoming Territory; six years later the number had increased to more than five hundred thousand. The first beef shipment east from Wyoming was in 1870. A Wyoming stock growers' association was organized at Cheyenne in 1871, six years before the first one was organized in Texas.[23]

The cattle available in Wyoming in the late 1870s were of several grades. Cheapest were the "gaunt, leggy, wild long-horn stock of straight Spanish breed come out of the chapparal along the lower reaches of the Rio Grande; the dearest, the thick-loined, deep-quartered, dark red half-breed short-horn Oregonians, descended from some of the best Missouri and Illinois strains, trailed by emigrants across the plains in the early 50s. Between these two extremes were two intermediate grades, the Middle Texas and Utahs."[24]

Although British syndicates bought up most of the Texas Panhandle, even more Britons flocked to Wyoming, Montana, and the Dakotas, where vast quantities of open range grassland had only recently been opened to occupancy by cattlemen. Wealthy men enjoyed the prestige of owning huge herds and controlling an immense acreage; for many youths, including remittance men, it was glamorous and adventuresome to become cowboys.

Wealthy easterners and eastern college students were also attracted to the cattle country, for popular magazines frequently carried articles on the cattle kingdom and the men who ruled it. Many, like Theodore Roosevelt and Edgar Beecher Bronson, hoped to improve their health in the West.

One of the by-products of this influx of wealthy and educated men from the East and the British Isles was the establishment of the exclusive Cheyenne Club. There was nothing like it elsewhere in the cattle country, which perhaps was fortunate, for the members were more concerned with social graces than with calf crops. As John Clay observed, one might meet men all over the world who "gloried in the fact that they were members of this unique place."[25]

The Cheyenne Club set the social tone for the northern ranchers. Club members wore tuxedos for dinners and soirees; cowboys uncharitably labeled them "Herefords." Some members tried to maintain the same atmosphere at their ranch headquarters. At the Swan Ranch, for example, guests were served champagne at all meals. Ranchers like the Swans dazzled their guests by taking them to the Cheyenne Club. "Here with the flash of youth on their brows in the late seventies and early eighties came Britishers and Bostonians, New Yorkers and Ohians, not forgetting Canucks and Chicagoans, a motley group full of ginger and snap, with more energy than business sense. . . . There was an atmosphere of success among its members. They spent money freely, for all along the line there was a swelling song of victory."[26]

Some Wyoming ranchers were seduced by the Cheyenne Club's high-toned atmosphere and tried to uphold it by maintaining costly establishments in town as well as at ranch headquarters. Well-stocked bars and lavish entertainment did nothing to upgrade herds. Visiting their ranches only occasionally, and accompanied at such times by throngs of admirers, these men invited disaster, and disaster accepted.

The Cheyenne Club was, however, also the business center. Scientist Clarence King stopped at the club on his way to the Pacific coast. By the time he departed he was involved in a partnership with N. R. Davis and in several other cattle schemes. It was to N. R. Davis that Edgar Beecher Bronson went with a letter of introduction from King.

The Cheyenne Club was also headquarters for remittance men from England and wayward eastern scions whose families banished them to the West in hope of "redemption or at least retribution."[27] Owen Wister, when touring the West, called the Cheyenne Club "the pearl of the prairies." But the club was as out of place in the West as some of its misfit members; it gradually lost its glitter and eventually had to close its doors.

The flood of British capital into the cattle industry caused uneasiness throughout the United States. What raised fear and resentment was alien ownership of large tracts of land—by 1883 twenty-one of the major American cattle companies were incorporated in Britain. Scottish investment in the western cattle industry was around twenty-five million dollars; British companies owned or controlled at least twenty million acres of rangeland.

Opposition to this alien invasion was expressed in various state governments as well as in Congress. Governor James Hogg of Texas predicted that the huge British holdings in his state would be divided among "inferior foreign tenants" who would give political power to the aristocratic landlords.[28] States such as

Texas which tried to legislate against alien ownership of property saw their efforts blocked by the courts as unconstitutional.

While eastern and British men and capital were heading for Cheyenne or elsewhere in the cattle kingdom, thousands of cattle plodded up the trail toward the same ranges. Men with trail herds were still likely to encounter opposition whenever they exposed local cattle to the ravages of tick fever. In 1869 some Colorado farmers had tried to turn back a Goodnight herd; Goodnight's cattle came from central Texas, however, and they were free of the disease. Apparently the farmers refused to accept Goodnight's explanations. Finally he ran out of patience, loaded his shotgun, and ordered his men to get Winchesters from the chuck wagon. They rode up to the men blocking the herd. "I've monkeyed as long as I want to with you sons of bitches," Goodnight informed them. The roadblock was immediately lifted.[29]

In the 1880s, as all the trails were closed except through the Panhandle, Goodnight and other ranchers of that area established a "Winchester quarantine" of their own against herds from South Texas. Tick fever was the main reason for their action, but they admitted that cattle from other parts of Texas were also competitors.[30]

By 1882 there were signs that even the route to and past Dodge City was closing, for farmers who had settled north of the town were protesting against herds crossing their lands. A year later armed men were demanding payment from trail bosses for allowing their herds to pass through and to use the water holes. Trail bosses had no choice but to pay for water.

In the spring of 1885 the protest was so strong that the Kansas legislature virtually prohibited Texas cattle from crossing the state. Ranchers who had spent money upgrading their cattle were especially opposed to risking devastating losses from tick fever such as had occurred in 1884, one of the worst years.

When word spread that herds moving up from Texas would reach the Canadian River early in June 1885, ranchers' associations met and decided they must fight to protect their cattle. The herds left the old trail at the Texas border and turned west through the Neutral Strip toward Colorado. Cowmen of the

Cherokee Strip and Kansas, as well as some "bad men" from Dodge City, rode south to intercept them. They nervously set up a "war camp" on a creek southwest of Camp Supply, about fifty miles north of the Texas herds along the Canadian.

One morning there was great excitement over a rumor that seventy-five Texans were on their way to wipe out the defenders. All were ready to concede defeat and head north. John Clay and another man agreed to ride south and check on the supposed invasion. At Wolf Creek they came to a line camp, where some cowboys had just returned from visiting the herds and trail crews along the Canadian. They reported that there had been great excitement over rumors that Kansas cowmen were on the way to drive them back into Texas.

There was no battle. The Kansans had a good laugh and went home. John R. Blocker, who had herds on the Canadian, wired Washington, and cavalry troops were detailed to see that the herds got through unmolested. As the Kansans had feared, however, hundreds of their cattle died of tick fever.[31]

Because of the variety of possibilities for calamities such as this, the range cattle business was one in which losses could be staggering. The Snyder brothers, for example, were once among the wealthiest of western cowmen—in 1884 they turned down an offer of one million dollars for their land and cattle. After the severe winter of 1885 they were in debt an equal amount.[32]

In the rapid expansion of the 1880s many ranchers carried heavy debts. One Texan glumly remarked that he was living on "the interest on what I owe." Ike Pryor recalled a South Texas rancher who asked a lawyer to examine his will. The lawyer was surprised that he had named six bankers as pallbearers, and asked if he would not rather have friends in that role. "No, Judge, that's all right," the rancher replied. "Those fellows have carried me so long they might as well finish the job."[33]

One of the signs of impending disaster was the reckless way men invested in cattle raising without knowing anything about it. Don Lovell, Andy Adams's cowman in *The Outlet*, commented in 1884 after seeing a rank amateur mismanaging a trail herd: "Boys, there goes a warning that the days of the trail are numbered. To make a success of any business, a little common sense is necessary. Nine tenths of the investing in cattle today in the Northwest is being done by inexperienced men. No other line of business could prosper in such incompetent hands, and it's foolish to think that cattle companies and individuals, nearly all tenderfeet at the business, can succeed. They may for a time,—there are accidents in every calling,—but when the tide turns, there won't be one man or company in ten survive. I only wish they would as it means life and expansion for the cattle interests in Texas. . . . But there's a day of reckoning ahead, and there's many a cowman in this Northwest country who will never see his money again. Now the government demand is a healthy one; it needs the cattle for Indian and military purposes; but this crazy investment, especially in *she* stuff, I wouldn't risk a dollar in it."[34]

Northern ranch managers consistently wrote optimistic reports to stockholders or owners, playing down winter losses as "probably one or two percent." Experienced cowmen in Montana considered 10 percent a normal annual mortality. After herds purchased on tally book counts had been ranged in the North four or five years, owners were beginning to inquire why beef shipments were not larger.[35]

The year 1885 was the high point of the range cattle industry on the Great Plains, for profits were high and optimism unbounded. Although the Great Plains ranges were already overstocked, in August President Grover Cleveland ordered cattlemen to remove their cattle from the Cheyenne-Arapaho Reservation in Indian Territory. This forced two hundred thousand more cattle onto overcrowded ranges just before winter set in. The winter was severe in the central plains, and by spring 85 percent of these cattle had died.

The summer of 1886 was unusually dry over much of the Great Plains, and there was little grass to be found. Despite this, more and more cattle were driven up from Texas or east from Oregon and Washington onto ranges already overgrazed. In July, South Dakota rancher Theodore Roosevelt commented that well-managed ranches were making fair profits, but there were now too many men in the cattle business, and the day of excessive gains was past. He noted the effects of the drought and of too many cattle, for he had not seen a "green thing" anywhere.

On August 1 the *Glendive Times* of Montana observed that cattle prices were depressed and most cattlemen were reluctant to ship their stock until the market improved, "but the condition of the ranges does not encourage this desire to hold their cattle." The *Helena Independent* added another note of caution in September, because of the lack of moisture and scarcity of grass. It concluded that "much depends upon the coming winter." Observant men saw only ominous signs. The fall rains were light; the remaining beavers piled up unusually large supplies of saplings for their winter food supply. Ducks and geese headed south much earlier than in other years, and range cattle grew longer coats than usual.[36] Snow fell several times in November, and Teddy Blue Abbott saw white arctic owls for the first time. "The Indians said they were a bad sign, heap snow coming, very cold, and they sure hit it right," Abbott recalled.[37]

Heavy snow began falling on Christmas Eve, and it continued to fall off and on for most of the next two months. Late in January the warm breeze called the Chinook melted the snow on the surface; then temperatures plunged below zero. "The snow crusted," said Abbott, "and it was hell without the heat."[38] The blanket of ice over the snow was impenetrable; cattle died by the thousands, many of thirst.

Future cowboy artist Charlie Russell was working on the OH Ranch of Jesse Phelps. When one of his partners wrote Phelps asking about range conditions, Russell drew a humped up, starving cow, calling it "Waiting for a Chinook." Someone changed the title to "The Last of Five Thousand"; it helped launch Russell's career in art. Phelps tore up the letter he was writing and sent only the drawing for a reply.[39] In the spring the Montana Stockgrowers Association summed up the situation as "a drouth without parallel; a market without a bottom; and a winter, the severest ever known in Montana."[40]

Cattlemen were stunned; none could fathom the extent of his losses until the spring roundup, and even then men kept hoping their cows had drifted south before the storms and would show up in some distant roundup. Roosevelt returned to his ranch to determine his losses. "Well," he wrote Henry Cabot Lodge, "we have had a perfect smashup all through the cattle country of the northwest. The losses are crippling. For the first time I have been utterly unable to enjoy a visit to my ranch."[41] As John Clay concluded, "It hit the just and the unjust. It was the protest of nature against greed, mismanagement, and that happy-go-lucky sentiment which permeates frontier life."[42]

In the spring Granville Stuart sent Teddy Blue Abbott as his representative on roundups to the south, but a big drive on Timber Creek netted only one lean steer. The roundup boss sardonically asked all of the reps present if they didn't want to cut the herd for their brands.[43] On one range where there had been forty thousand cattle in the fall, the roundup crew found seven thousand.

In July, Abbott and others were working the range around Box Elder Creek in hot weather and the heavy stench of dead cattle. "There was one old fellow working with us who had some cattle on the range," Abbott recalled later; "I don't remember his name. But I'll never forget the way he stopped, with sweat pouring off his face, and looked up at the sun, sober as a judge, and said: 'Where the hell was you last January?' "[44]

Granville Stuart's losses were reckoned at about 66 percent; others suffered even heavier losses, for of the cattle brought up from the south the previous summer, only 10 percent survived. "A business that had been fascinating to me before," Stuart remarked, "suddenly became distasteful. I wanted no more of it. I never wanted to own again an animal that I could not feed and shelter."[45]

Through the spring of 1887 cattlemen north and south were in a state of gloomy apprehension, and when they finally realized the appalling extent of their losses, some threw up their hands and quit. As early as January the huge Dolores Land and Cattle Company of Texas went under. Even worse news was in store, for in May Swan brothers failed. Since Alec Swan was widely admired and idolized as a financial wizard, news that his company was being reorganized was as shocking as if some deity had announced that his heaven was in receivership.

There is, however, another side to the Big Die-up, as Colonel Samuel Gordon of the *Yellowstone Journal* pointed out many years later. "It is comforting," he wrote, "to reflect on the number of reputations that were saved by the 'hard winter' of 1886–87. It *was* a hard winter—the latter end of it—and the worst of it came when the cattle were weak and thin and unable to stand grief, but it never killed half the cattle that were charged to it. It came as a God-sent deliverance to the managers who had for four or five years past been reporting 'One percent losses,' and they seized the opportunity bravely, and comprehensively charged off in one lump the accumulated mortality of four or five years. Sixty percent loss was the popular estimate. Some had to run it up higher to get even, and it is told of one truthful manager in an adjoining county that he reported a loss of 125%, 50% steers and 75% cows. The actual loss in cattle was probably thirty to fifty percent, according to localities and conditions."[46]

The Big Die-up of 1886–87 did not result in a wholesale exodus of eastern and British capital, as has often been implied, although many men did abandon any connection with the cattle business. Some investors had become unhappy even before the disastrous winter, for it had already become clear that the anticipated easy profits would never materialize. Many investors retained their stock in cattle companies, but new investments were slow to come. Companies with adequate capital and able managers survived and soon recovered. In western Montana ranchers had put up hay for winter feeding for several years, and their losses were much lower than those of central and eastern Montana.[47]

One man who quickly took advantage of the situation was the Frenchman Pierre Wibaux of South Dakota, who had access to funds from France at the time investments from the East and Britain had virtually dried up. In the spring of 1887 Wibaux began buying up remnants of herds at twenty dollars a head. That fall he sold the beeves only, at a profit of forty to forty-five dollars on each animal. He continued buying up entire brands, and by 1890 owned forty thousand cattle and branded ten thousand calves. Because of the shortage of cattle, prices remained high for several years, to the considerable advantage of men like Wibaux who had beeves to sell.[48]

Conrad Kohrs lost heavily in the Big Die-up, but he recovered quickly. He borrowed one hundred thousand dollars and purchased about nine thousand steers in Idaho, all that were available. In 1889 he bought more cattle in Idaho and Oregon, making a profit of fifteen dollars a head. His best year was 1891, when his profits averaged $62.50 a head and total sales amounted to $290,000.[49]

The Big Die-up marked the end of an era by hastening the end of the cattle boom. That phenomenon would have ended in any event because of overstocking, overproduction, and poor management. In coming years quality took precedence over quantity in the cattle business, which meant owning and fencing ranges, upgrading herds, and providing winter forage. The cattle industry recovered fairly quickly, but the day of the open range was not yet over in Montana. "Before the end of the eighties, there were more cattle on Montana ranges than ever."[50]

The problem of overcrowding by cattle and sheep on the eastern Montana ranges again became serious in the 1890s, for the number of ranchers who depended on the public domain for most of their pasture but owned or leased land to produce hay for winter increased considerably after the hard winter. In the 1890s the size of herds in the region declined, as small ranchers gradually replaced the open range cowmen. The damage had been done, however, for the best grasses had been cropped too closely, and in some places had died out, to be replaced by poorer grasses or sagebrush. As Robert S. Fletcher has observed, "Overstocking had become a cruel reality in the last years and a hastening agent in the movement toward a new era."[51]

Whenever cattle prices were low, cowmen usually blamed the meatpackers, whom they viewed as monopolists determined to ruin cattleraisers. The solution seemed to be to fight the packers with their own major weapon—monopoly. Edward M. McGillin of Cleveland, who invested heavily in the range cattle industry, was one of the leaders of the movement. Early in 1887 he presented members of the International Range Association with a plan for a beef trust incorporated at one hundred million dollars.

The purpose of the huge trust was to "arrange, manage, sell every animal from the time it was dropped a calf until it was beef." The American Cattle Trust created in the spring of 1887 was patterned after the Standard Oil Trust. Its board of directors included prominent western cattlemen as well as eastern financiers: R. G. Head of New Mexico, John T. Lytle and C. C. Slaughter of Texas, and Francis E. Warren and Thomas Sturgis of Wyoming. Sturgis was elected chairman of the board.

The American Cattle Trust was launched with enthusiasm and expectations, but it was torn by dissension between eastern and western trustees, and many cattlemen refused to join. In 1889 it was on the verge of bankruptcy, for its efforts to secure markets in the East had been defeated by Swift and Armour. By the summer of 1890 it was no more, but it had taught cattlemen and investors one valuable lesson: their only hope of curbing the meat-packing industry was through political action.[52]

With the end of the range cattle boom, western ranching changed drastically from what it had been in the era of open range and free grass. Genuine cowmen, for whom raising beef cattle was the only acceptable way of life, adapted to the new conditions and continued. Even those who had lost everything could not abandon the life they loved; many swallowed their pride and worked for others on ranges where they had once grazed their own cattle. In a letter to barbed wire maker Isaac Ellwood asking for a job as manager of his Frying Pan Ranch, Dudley Snyder added, "Please don't think for a moment I would feel humiliated in managing your business after having owned the greater part of it."[53]

The cattle kingdom and trailing era lasted little more than twenty years, but in many ways these were the most memorable two decades in the nation's history. Then everything changed. Fenced pastures ended the open range and cut up the trails. The nervous Longhorns, the first truly American cattle, disappeared; placid Herefords, Angus, and other imported breeds that matured quickly, took their places. Muscular Quarter Horses, which had originated in colonial Virginia, displaced the little mustang cow ponies. Trail bosses and their crews had no place in the new order; the cowboys who succeeded them dug post holes, strung wire, and repaired windmills. Cattle cars superseded trail drives. There were no more great open range roundups, no mavericks. Ranchers even learned to eat their own beef.

The passing of the old West was mourned by many, but it was not forgotten. Over the years it has, as C. L. Sonnichsen noted, come to fill our basic need for a "heroic past." We have made the nameless hired men on horseback our Galahads and Gawains, the chuck wagon our Round Table. The old West is still with us, for we need it more than ever.

Notes

INTRODUCTION

1. W. H. Hutchinson, "The Cowboy and Karl Marx," *Pacific Historian* 20 (Summer 1976): 119.

2. Oscar Edward Anderson, Jr., *Refrigeration in America: A History of a New Technology and Its Impact* (Princeton: Princeton University Press, 1953), pp. 47–61; Mary Whately Clarke, *A Century of Cow Business: A History of the Texas and Southwestern Cattle Raisers Association* (Fort Worth: Texas and Southwestern Cattle Raisers Association, 1976), pp. 86–89.

3. Henry D. and Frances T. McCallum, *The Wire That Fenced the West* (Norman: University of Oklahoma Press, 1965), pp. 68–70.

4. Gene M. Gressley, ed., "Harvard Man Out West: The Letters of Richard Trimble, 1882–1887," *Montana, the Magazine of Western History* 10 (Winter 1960): 20n; Wayne Gard, "The Fence-Cutters," *Southwestern Historical Quarterly* 51 (July 1947): 1–15.

5. Richard Irving Dodge, *Our Wild Indians: Thirty-three Years' Personal Experience among the Red Men of the Great West* (Hartford: A. D. Worthington and Co., 1886), pp. 608–9.

6. Wayne Gard, "Retracing the Chisholm Trail," *Southwestern Historical Quarterly* 60 (July 1956): 61; John R. Lunsford, "E. B. Baggett Speaks of Chisholm Trail," *Frontier Times* 8 (December 1930): 127.

7. Gard, "Retracing the Chisholm Trail," p. 55; Richard Harding Davis, *The West from a Car-Window* (New York: Harper and Brothers, 1892), p. 136.

8. W. J. Morris, "Over the Old Chisholm Trail," *Frontier Times* 2 (April 1925): 41–43. Morris was actually describing the Western Trail to Dodge City. Charles Moreau Harger, in "Cattle-Trails of the Prairies," *Scribner's Magazine* 11 (June 1892): 734, states that the Chisholm Trail was named for John Chisholm, "an eccentric frontier stockman, the first to drive a herd over it."

9. Gard, "Retracing the Chisholm Trail," p. 53; Wayne Gard, *The Chisholm Trail* (Norman: University of Oklahoma Press, 1954), p. vi.

10. C. L. Sonnichsen, *From Hopalong to Hud* (College Station: Texas A & M Press, 1978), pp. 8, 16–18. See also Joe B. Frantz and Julian Ernest Choate, Jr., *The American Cowboy: The Myth and the Reality*

(Norman: University of Oklahoma Press, 1955), and William W. Savage, Jr., "The Cowboy Myth," *Red River Valley Historical Review* 2 (Spring 1975): 162–71. Reflecting the universal interest in the American West are the Westerners International corrals of Norway, Sweden, West Germany, Denmark, France, Britain, Japan, and Mexico.

Chapter i

1. Gilbert J. Jordan, Jr., tr. and ed., "W. Steinert's View of Texas in 1849," pt.5, *Southwestern Historical Quarterly* 81 (July 1977): 46. See also "The First Cattle Ranch in Texas," *Frontier Times* 13 (March 1936): 304–8.

2. Rupert Norval Richardson, *The Frontier of Northwest Texas, 1846 to 1876* (Glendale, Calif.; Arthur H. Clark Co., 1963), p. 155.

3. Michael Doran, "Antebellum Cattle Herding in the Indian Territory," *Geographical Review* 66 (January 1976): 48–54.

4. Grant M. and Herbert O. Brayer, *American Cattle Trails, 1540–1900* (Bayside, N.Y.: Western Range Cattle Industry Study in Cooperation with the American Pioneer Trails Society, 1952), p. 28.

5. In 1832, when Charles Sealsfield visited Neal's ranch, Neal was preparing to drive twenty or thirty steers to New Orleans.

6. J. Frank Dobie, "Tom Candy Ponting's Drive of Texas Cattle to Illinois," *Cattleman* 35 (January 1949): 34–55; George Squires Herrington, "An Early Cattle Drive from Texas to Illinois," *Southwestern Historical Quarterly* 55 (October 1951): 267–69.

7. Joseph G. McCoy, *Historic Sketches of the Cattle Trade of the West and Southwest* (Columbus, Ohio: Long's College Book Co., 1951), p. 88; Thomas Ulvan Taylor, *The Chisholm Trail and Other Routes* (San Antonio: Naylor Co., 1936), pp. 4, 7–9.

8. Richardson, *Frontier of Northwest Texas,* p. 253.

9. Ibid., pp. 262–63.

10. Ramon Adams, *The Best of the American Cowboy* (Norman: University of Oklahoma Press, 1957), p. 138.

11. Will S. James, *27 Years a Maverick; or, Life on a Texas Range* (Austin: Steck-Vaughn Co., 1968), p. 67.

12. Ibid., p. 73.

13. Ibid., pp. 74–76.

14. Michael S. Kennedy, ed., *Cowboys and Cattlemen* (New York: Hastings House, 1964), pp. 103–8.

15. William Curry Holden, *A Ranching Saga: The Lives of William Electious Halsell and Ewing Halsell,* 2 vols. (San Antonio: Trinity Univer-

sity Press, 1976), 1:63; Taylor, *The Chisholm Trail*, pp. 90, 98.

16. Louis Pelzer, *The Cattleman's Frontier: A Record of the Trans-Mississippi Cattle Industry from Oxen Trains to Packing Companies, 1850–1890* (Glendale, Calif.: Arthur H. Clark Co., 1936), pp. 38–40.

17. McCoy, *Historic Sketches*, p. 102. The following direct quotation is from the same source, p. 65.

18. Holden, *A Ranching Saga*, p. 64. See also, E. P. Earhart, "Up the Cattle Trail in 1867," *Frontier Times* 8 (February 1931): 194–95.

19. McCoy, *Historic Sketches*, pp. 185–88.

CHAPTER 2

1. Ernest Staples Osgood, *The Day of the Cattleman* (Minneapolis: University of Minnesota Press, 1954), p. 29.

2. J. Frank Dobie, *A Vaquero of the Brush Country* (New York: Grosset and Dunlap, 1929), pp. 198–99.

3. E. C. ("Teddy Blue") Abbott and Helena Huntington Smith, *We Pointed Them North* (Norman: University of Oklahoma Press, 1954), p. 61.

4. Richardson, *Frontier of Northwest Texas*, pp. 153–263.

5. See Clarke, *A Century of the Cow Business;* Lewis Nordyke, *Great Roundup: The Story of the Texas and Southwestern Cowmen* (New York: Morrow, 1955); and "Old Cowman Tells of a Big Steal," *Frontier Times* 3 (June 1926): 36–37.

6. McCoy, *Historic Sketches*, p. 145.

7. Ibid., p. 146.

8. Orland L. Sims, *Cowpokes, Nesters, and So Forth* (Austin: Encino Press, 1970), p. 58.

9. Emily Jones Shelton, "Lizzie Johnson: A Cattle Queen of Texas," *Southwestern Historical Quarterly* 50 (April 1947): 349–60.

10. Gene M. Gressley, *Bankers and Cattlemen* (Lincoln: University of Nebraska Press, 1966), pp. 174–77.

11. Joyce Gibson Roach, *The Cowgirls* (Houston: Cordovan Corporation, 1977).

CHAPTER 3

1. W. J. Morris, "Over the Old Chisholm Trail, p. 42.

2. Abbott and Smith, *We Pointed Them North*, p. 62.

3. James G. Bell, "A Log of the Texas-California Cattle Trail, 1854," ed. J. Evetts Haley *Southwestern Historical Quarterly* 35 (April 1932): 304.

4. Dobie, *Vaquero,* pp. 91–92.

5. Ibid., p. 93; Jesse James Benton, *Cow by the Tail* (Boston: Houghton Mifflin Co., 1943), p. 45.

6. Andy Adams, *The Log of a Cowboy: A Narrative of the Old Trail Days* (Lincoln: University of Nebraska Press, 1964), p. 231.

7. Abbott and Smith, *We Pointed Them North,* p. 67.

8. Gard, *The Chisholm Trail,* p. 243.

9. J. Frank Dobie, *The Longhorns* (Boston: Little, Brown Co., 1941), p. 97.

10. Taylor, *The Chisholm Trail,* pp. 181–82; J. Marvin Hunter, ed., *The Trail Drivers of Texas,* 2 vols. (New York: Argosy-Antiquarian, 1963), 2: 636.

11. Dobie, *Vaquero,* p. 262.

12. Dobie, *The Longhorns,* p. 111; Abbott and Smith, *We Pointed Them North,* p. 83.

13. Ibid., p. 68.

14. Benton, *Cow by the Tail,* pp. 4–49.

15. Ibid., pp. 49–53.

16. Hunter, *Trail Drivers,* 1:67; Jack Potter, "Up the Trail (and Back) in '82," *Montana, the Magazine of Western History* 11 (October 1961): 64.

17. Abbott and Smith, *We Pointed Them North,* p. 62. The following quotation from Jesse Benton is from *Cow by the Tail,* p. 70.

18. James, *27 Years a Maverick,* pp. 89–90.

19. Ibid., p. 91.

20. Benton, *Cow by the Tail,* pp. 69–70.

21. Randolph B. Marcy, *The Prairie Traveler* (Williamstown, Mass.: Corner House Publishers, 1968), pp. 118–20.

22. Ramon Adams, *The Old Time Cowhand* (New York: Macmillan Co., 1961), p. 105.

23. Sims, *Cowpokes,* p. 48; Will James, *Lone Cowboy* (New York: Charles Scribner's Sons, 1930), p. 178; Fred Fellows, "Illustrated Study of Western Saddles," *Montana, the Magazine of Western History* 16 (January 1966): 57–83.

24. Jane Pattie, "The Justin Boot: Standard of the West," *Quarter Horse Journal* 29 (September 1977): 127; "The Justin Boot," *Montana, the Magazine of Western History* 11 (January 1961): 86.

25. Walt Coburn, *Pioneer Cattleman in Montana: The Story of the Circle C. Ranch* (Norman: University of Oklahoma Press, 1968), p. 130. Stetson hats were available in the West at least by 1871. Levis were shipped to Texas soon after the Civil War. Bull Durham tobacco and

cigarette papers were also available about the same time. Foster-Harris, *The Look of the Old West* (New York: Bonanza Books, 1955), pp. 105, 112–13, 204.

26. Coburn, *Pioneer Cattleman,* p. 137. The term *cowpuncher* seems to have originated at the railroad loading chutes, where men prodded cattle with long poles. The term was used mainly in the North.

27. McCoy, *Historic Sketches,* p. 139.

28. Hunter, *Trail Drivers,* 1:118.

CHAPTER 4

1. Adams, *Log of a Cowboy,* p. 29. See also Charles Goodnight, "Managing a Trail Herd in the Early Days," *Frontier Times* 6 (November 1929): 250–52.

2. James Henry Cook, *Longhorn Cowboy* (New York: G.P. Putnam's Sons, 1942), p. 101.

3. Cordia Sloan Duke and Joe B. Frantz, *6000 Miles of Fence: Life on the XIT Ranch of Texas* (Austin: University of Texas Press, 1961), p. 81.

4. Abbott and Smith, *We Pointed Them North,* p. 94.

5. Hunter, *Trail Drivers,* 1:314–15.

6. Baylis John Fletcher, *Up the Trail in '79* (Norman: University of Oklahoma Press, 1968), p. 8.

7. Ibid., p. 53.

8. Adams, *Best of the Cowboy,* p. 221.

9. Fletcher, *Up the Trail,* p. 8.

10. Dobie, *Vaquero,* p. 179.

11. J. Frank Dobie, "Ab Blocker: Trail Boss," *Arizona and the West* 6 (Summer 1964): 99.

12. Frank Dalton, "Military Escort for a Trail Herd," *Cattleman* 32 (June 1944): 13–14; Hunter, *Trail Drivers,* 2:704.

13. Hunter, *Trail Drivers,* 1:471.

14. Chris Emmett, *Shanghai Pierce: A Fair Likeness* (Norman: University of Oklahoma Press, 1953), p. 125.

15. Hunter, *Trail Drivers,* 1:128–29.

16. Ibid., pp. 73–75.

17. Adams, *Best of the Cowboy,* p. 225.

CHAPTER 5

1. Walker D. Wyman, *Nothing but Prairie and Sky: Life on the Dakota*

Range in the Early Days (Norman: University of Oklahoma Press, 1954), p. 57.

2. J. Evetts Haley, *Charles Goodnight, Cowman and Plainsman* (Norman: University of Oklahoma Press, 1949), pp. 121–22.

3. Sims, *Cowpokes*, p. 63.

4. Brayer, *American Cattle Trails*, p. 86.

5. Haley, *Charles Goodnight*, p. 93.

6. Fletcher, *Up the Trail*, p. 46.

7. Hunter, *Trail Drivers*, 1:165.

8. Bob Kennon, *From the Pecos to the Powder: A Cowboy's Autobiography*, as told to Ramon F. Adams (Norman: University of Oklahoma Press, 1965), p. 61.

9. Charles A. Siringo, *A Texas Cowboy* (New York: William Sloane Associates, 1950), pp. 77–78.

10. Kennon, *From the Pecos to the Powder*, p. 84.

11. Ibid., p. 87.

12. A. B. Snyder, *Pinnacle Jake*, as told to Nellie Snyder Yost (Lincoln: University of Nebraska Press, 1951), p. 88.

13. Nordyke, *Great Roundup*, p. 62.

14. Sims, *Cowpokes*, p. 63.

15. Brayer, *American Cattle Trails*, p. 110.

16. Courtesy of William F. Bragg, Jr., of Casper, Wyoming.

CHAPTER 6

1. Lewis Atherton, *The Cattle Kings* (Lincoln: University of Nebraska Press, 1972), pp. 5–29; idem, "Cattleman and Cowboy; Fact and Fancy," *Montana, the Magazine of Western History* 11 (October 1961): 2–17.

2. Wyman, *Nothing but Prairie and Sky*, pp. 100–101.

3. John Clay, *My Life on the Range* (Norman: University of Oklahoma Press, 1962), p. 82.

4. Ibid., pp. 122–24.

5. Edward Douglas Branch, *The Cowboy and His Interpreters* (New York: D. Appleton and Co., 1926), pp. 11–12.

6. Mack Williams, *In Old Fort Worth: The Story of a City and Its People as Published in the News-Tribune in 1976 and 1977* (Fort Worth: Williams, 1977), pp. 7–8.

7. Frank S. Hastings, *A Ranchman's Recollections: An Autobiography* (Chicago: Breeder's Gazette, 1921), p. 118.

8. Abbott and Smith, *We Pointed Them North*, pp. 211–12.

9. Adams, *Best of the Cowboy*, pp. 4–5.

10. Ibid., p. 108.

11. Dodge, *Our Wild Indians,* pp. 609, 611.

12. Clifford P. Westermeier, *Man, Beast, Dust: The Story of Rodeo* (n.p.: World Press, 1947), p. 39.

13. See James Henry Cook, *Longhorn Cowboy,* ed. Howard R. Driggs (New York: G. P. Putnam's Sons, 1942); Frank Collinson, *Life in the Saddle,* ed. Mary Whately Clarke (Norman: University of Oklahoma Press, 1963); Baylis John Fletcher, *Up the Trail in '79* (Norman: University of Oklahoma Press, 1968); and E. E. MacConnell, *XIT Buck* (Tucson: University of Arizona Press, 1968).

14. Frazier Hunt, *The Long Trail from Texas: The Story of Ad Spaugh, Cattleman* (New York: Doubleday, Doran and Co., 1940).

15. This and the following quotations, including the tale of the silk hat, are from James, *27 Years a Maverick,* pp. 33–56.

16. O. W. Nolen, "Shanghai Pierce," *Cattleman* 31 (December 1944): 31.

17. Abbott and Smith, *We Pointed Them North,* p. 29.

18. Ibid., pp. 60–61. The following quotation is from the same source, p. 4.

19. Cook, *Longhorn Cowboy,* p. 35.

20. Ibid., pp. 113–14.

21. Kennedy, *Cowboys and Cattlemen,* pp. 115–28.

22. Edgar Beecher Bronson, *Reminiscences of a Ranchman* (Lincoln: University of Nebraska Press, 1962), p. 27.

23. Ibid., pp. 27–28.

24. Ibid., p. 41.

25. Ibid., pp. 46–73.

26. Theodore Roosevelt, *Ranch Life and Hunting Trail* (Ann Arbor: University Microfilms, 1966), p. 62.

27. Quoted from the *Cheyenne Daily Leader,* October 3, 1882, in Westermeier, *Story of Rodeo,* p. 40n.

28. Abbott and Smith, *We Pointed Them North,* pp. 107–9.

29. Edgar Rye, *The Quirt and the Spur: Vanishing Shadows of the Texas Frontier* (Chicago: W. B. Conkey Co., 1909), pp. 271–75.

30. Charles Goodnight, "Managing a Trail Herd," p. 252; see also *History of Montana, 1739–1885* (Chicago: Warner, Beers and Co., 1885), pp. 445–46.

CHAPTER 7

1. John Q. Anderson, ed., *Tales of Frontier Texas, 1830–1860* (Dallas: Southern Methodist University Press, 1966), p. 20.

2. Dobie, *The Longhorns,* p. 35.

3. John J. Linn, *Reminiscences of Fifty Years in Texas* (Austin: Steck Co., 1935), p. 338.

4. Anderson, *Tales of Frontier Texas,* pp. 63–64.

5. Lewis F. Allen, *American Cattle: Their History, Breeding and Management* (New York: Taintor Brothers Co., 1868), pp. 75–84.

6. Benton, *Cow by the Tail,* pp. 65–66.

7. Harry Sinclair Drago, *Red River Valley: The Mainstream of Frontier History from the Louisiana Bayous to the Texas Panhandle* (New York: Clarkson N. Potter, 1962), pp. 181–82.

8. Dobie, *The Longhorns,* pp. 181–4.

9. *Fort Benton Record,* June 23, 1876, in *Montana, the Magazine of Western History* 3 (Autumn 1953): 31.

10. J. L. Hill, *The End of the Cattle Trail* (Austin: Pemberton Press, 1969), pp. 66–67. *Dogie,* from *doughgut,* meant a pot-bellied orphan calf.

11. Gard, "Retracing the Chisholm Trail," p. 55.

12 Joseph Nimmo, Jr., *Report in Regard to the Range and Ranch Cattle Business of the United States* (New York: Arno Press, 1972), pp. 95, 144.

13. Collinson, *Life in the Saddle,* p. 42.

14. Drago, *Red River Valley,* p. 203.

15. Anderson, *Tales of Frontier Texas,* pp. 16–22.

16. Walker D. Wyman, *The Wild Horse of the West* (Caldwell, Idaho: Caxton Printers, 1945), p. 116.

17. Josiah Gregg, *Commerce of the Prairies* (Norman: University of Oklahoma Press, 1954), pp. 126–27.

18. Jordan, "Steinert's View of Texas," p. 46.

19. J. Frank Dobie, *The Mustangs* (New York: Bantam Books, 1954), pp. 82–83.

20. Frederic Remington, "Horses of the Plains," *Century Magazine* 37 (November 1888–April 1889): 335–42.

21. J. Frank Dobie, "The Spanish Cow Pony," *Saturday Evening Post* 207 (November 24, 1934): 13, 65–66.

22. Dobie, *Mustangs,* pp. 293–94. *Pitching* was the term used in the Southwest; *bucking* was used in the North.

23. Ibid., p. 48.

24. Ibid., pp. 161–62.

25. Snyder, *Pinnacle Jake,* pp. 24–32.

26. Malcolm D. McLean, *Fine Texas Horses: Their Pedigrees and Performance, 1830–1845* (Fort Worth: Texas Christian University Press, 1966), p. 82.

27. Wyman, *Wild Horse of the West,* p. 104.
28. Bronson, *Reminiscences,* pp. 153–56.

CHAPTER 8

1. McCoy, *Historic Sketches,* pp. 202–5.
2. Harry Sinclair Drago, *Great American Cattle Trails* (New York: Bramhall House, 1965), p. 140.
3. Ibid., pp. 140–41.
4. Ibid., p. 144.
5. Ibid, pp. 146–47.
6. Ibid., p. 148.
7. Robert R. Dykstra, *The Cattle Towns* (New York: Alfred A. Knopf, 1968), pp. 75–76.
8. Benton, *Cow by the Tail,* pp. 53–57.
9. Stanley Vestal, *Queen of the Cowtowns: Dodge City, "The Wickedest Little City in America," 1872–1886* (Lincoln: University of Nebraska Press, 1972), pp. 3, 86.
10. Harry Sinclair Drago, *Wild, Woolly and Wicked: The History of the Kansas Cow Towns and the Texas Cattle Trail* (New York: Clarkson N. Potter, 1960), p. 235.
11. Ibid., p. 255.
12. Khleber Miller Van Zandt, *Force without Fanfare,* ed. Sandra L. Myres (Fort Worth: Texas Christian University Press, 1968), p. 113.
13. Hunter, *Trail Drivers,* 1:431–32; Taylor, *The Chisholm Trail,* p. 62.
14. Leonard Sanders and Ronnie C. Tyler, *How Fort Worth Became the Texasmost City* (Fort Worth: Amon Carter Museum of Western Art, 1973), p. 36.
15. Ibid., p. 38.
16. Ibid., p. 65.
17. Ibid., p. 68.
18. Ibid.
19. Gard, *The Chisholm Trail,* pp. 217–18.
20. Ibid., p. 234.
21. Ibid., p. 238.
22. Sanders and Tyler, *Fort Worth,* p. 107.

CHAPTER 9

1. Jimmy Skaggs, *The Cattle-Trailing Industry between Supply and*

Demand, 1886–1890 (Lawrence: University of Kansas Press, 1973), pp. 41–44.

2. Ibid., pp. 54–57.

3. Ibid., p. 6.

4. Ibid., p. 1.

5. Ibid., p. 88.

6. Gressley, *Bankers and Cattlemen,* pp. 70, 119. The following direct quotation is from the same source, p. 119.

7. James S. Brisbin, *The Beef Bonanza; or, How to Get Rich on the Plains* (Norman: University of Oklahoma Press, 1959), p. 15.

8. Emmett, *Shanghai Pierce,* pp. 97–109, 154–57, 169–74, 185–90; Gressley, *Bankers and Cattlemen,* p. 77.

9. Gressley, *Bankers and Cattlemen,* p. 71.

10. Ibid., pp. 112–14.

11. Nellie Snyder Yost, ed., *Boss Cowman: The Recollections of Ed Lemmon, 1857–1946* (Lincoln: University of Nebraska Press, 1969), p. 168.

12. William A. Baillie-Grohman, "Cattle Ranches in the Far West," *Library Magazine of American and Foreign Thought* 6 (December 1880): 131.

13. John Clay, *My Life on the Range* (Norman: University of Oklahoma Press, 1962), p. 83.

14. Robert Henry Fletcher, *Free Grass to Fences: The Montana Cattle Range Story* (New York: University Publishers, 1960), pp. 90–91.

15. Gressley, *Bankers and Cattlemen,* p. 135.

16. Gressley, "Harvard Man Out West," p. 20n.

17. William Pearce, *The Matador Land and Cattle Company* (Norman: University of Oklahoma Press, 1964), p. 30.

18. Edward Everett Dale, *The Range Cattle Industry: Ranching on the Great Plains from 1865–1925* (Norman: University of Oklahoma Press, 1960), p. 58n.

19. Clay, *My Life on the Range,* pp. 127–35.

20. E. E. MacConnell, *XIT Buck* (Tucson: University of Arizona Press, 1968), pp. 172–75; Joe B. Frantz, "Texas' Largest Ranch—in Montana: The XIT," *Montana, the Magazine of Western History* 11 (October 1961): 46–56.

21. Clay, *My Life on the Range,* p. 114.

22. Harmon Ross Motherhead, *The Swan Land and Cattle Company, Ltd.* (Norman: University of Oklahoma Press, 1971), pp. 160, 165.

23. Clay, *My Life on the Range,* p. 50.

24. Ibid., pp. 202–4.

25. Gressley, "Harvard Man Out West," pp. 14–16.

26. Clay, *My Life on the Range,* p. 174.

CHAPTER 10

1. Robert H. Burns, "The Newman Brothers: Forgotten Cattle Kings of the Northern Plains," *Montana, the Magazine of Western History* 11 (October 1961): 28–36; Joseph Nimmo, Jr., "The American Cow-Boy," *Harper's New Monthly Magazine* 73 (November 1886): 880–84.

2. Maurice Frink, W. Turrentine Jackson, and Agnes Wright Spring, *When Grass Was King* (Boulder: University of Colorado Press, 1956), p. 36.

3. Granville Stuart, *Pioneering in Montana: The Making of a State, 1864–1887* (Lincoln: University of Nebraska Press, 1977), p. 98; Frink, Jackson, and Spring, *When Grass Was King,* p. 37.

4. Kennedy, *Cowboys and Cattlemen,* pp. 103–8.

5. Fletcher, *Free Grass to Fences,* p. 29.

6. Conrad Kohrs, *An Autobiography* (Deer Lodge, Montana: Plateau Press, 1977), p. 55.

7. Ibid., pp. 43–55; Larry Gill, "From Butcher Boy to Beef King: The Gold Camp Days of Conrad Kohrs," *Montana, the Magazine of Western History* 8 (Spring 1958): 40–55. Today the Kohrs Ranch in Deer Lodge valley is a national park.

8. Frink, Jackson, and Spring, *When Grass Was King,* pp. 336–55.

9. Brisbin, *Beef Bonanza,* pp. 73–74.

10. Ibid., pp. 25–26.

11. Ibid., p. 73.

12. Brayer, *American Cattle Trails,* pp. 33–37.

13. Ibid., pp. 71–76.

14. McCoy, *Historic Sketches,* pp. 342–68.

15. Frink, Jackson, and Spring, *When Grass Was King,* pp. 406–7.

16. Nordyke, *Great Roundup,* p. 90.

17. Wyman, *Nothing but Prairie and Sky,* pp. 58–59.

18. Bronson, *Reminiscences,* p. 75.

19. William MacLeod Raine and Will C. Barnes, *Cattle* (New York: Doubleday, 1930), pp. 233–41.

20. Gressley, *Bankers and Cattlemen,* p. 145.

21. Nordyke, *Great Roundup,* p. 101.

22. Abbott and Smith, *We Pointed Them North,* pp. 137–38.

23. Harold E. Briggs, "The Development and Decline of Open

Range Ranching in the Northwest," *Mississippi Valley Historical Review* 20 (March 1934): 521–22.

24. Bronson, *Reminiscences,* p. 78.

25. Clay, *My Life on the Range,* pp. 72–78.

26. Ibid., p. 53.

27. Gressley, *Bankers and Cattlemen,* p. 68.

28. Roger V. Clements, "British Investment and American Legislative Restrictions in the Trans-Mississippi West, 1880–1900," *Mississippi Valley Historical Review* 42 (September 1955): 207–15.

29. Atherton, *The Cattle Kings,* p. 45.

30. Nordyke, *Great Roundup,* p. 130.

31. Clay, *My Life on the Range,* pp. 177–79.

32. Nordyke, *Great Roundup,* p. 164.

33. Ibid., pp. 168, 185.

34. Andy Adams, *The Outlet* (Upper Saddle River, N.J.: Literature House, 1970), pp. 175–76.

35. Fletcher, *Free Grass to Fences,* p. 91.

36. Kennedy, *Cowboys and Cattlemen,* pp. 156–57.

37. Abbott and Smith, *We Pointed Them North,* p. 175.

38. Ibid., p. 176.

39. Nordyke, *Great Roundup,* pp. 161–62; Wallis Huidekoper, "The Story Behind Charlie Russell's Masterpiece: 'Waiting for a Chinook,' " *Montana, the Magazine of Western History* 4 (Summer 1954): 37–39.

40. Fletcher, *Free Grass to Fences,* p. 92.

41. Kennedy, *Cowboys and Cattlemen,* p. 165.

42. Clay, *My Life on the Range,* p. 200.

43. Abbott and Smith, *We Pointed Them North,* p. 184.

44. Ibid., p. 185.

45. Stuart, *Pioneering in Montana,* pp. 236–37.

46. Quoted in Fletcher, *Free Grass to Fences,* p. 91.

47. Ibid., p. 89.

48. Kennedy, *Cowboys and Cattlemen,* p. 66

49. Kohrs, *Autobiography,* pp. 87–93,

50. Fletcher, *Free Grass to Fences,* p. 93.

51. Robert S. Fletcher, "The End of the Open Range in Eastern Montana," *Mississippi Valley Historical Review* 16 (September 1929): 202–11.

52. Gressley, *Bankers and Cattlemen,* pp. 255–56.

53. Ibid., p. 95.

Bibliography

Books

Abbott, E. C. ("Teddy Blue"), and Smith, Helena Huntington. *We Pointed Them North.* Norman: University of Oklahoma Press, 1954.

Adams, Andy. *The Log of a Cowboy: A Narrative of the Old Trail Days.* 1903. Rpt. Lincoln: University of Nebraska Press, 1964.

———. *The Outlet.* 1905. Rpt. Upper Saddle River, N.J.: Literature House, 1970.

Adams, Ramon F. *The Best of the American Cowboy.* Norman: University of Oklahoma Press, 1957.

———. *Come and Get It.* Norman: University of Oklahoma Press, 1952.

———. *The Old Time Cowhand.* New York: Macmillan Co., 1961.

Allen, Lewis F. *American Cattle: Their History, Breeding and Management.* New York: Taintor Brothers Co., 1868.

Anderson, John Q., ed. *Tales of Frontier Texas, 1830–1860.* Dallas: Southern Methodist University Press, 1966.

Anderson, Oscar Edward, Jr. *Refrigeration in America: A History of a New Technology and Its Impact.* Princeton: Princeton University Press, 1953.

Atherton, Lewis. *The Cattle Kings.* Lincoln: University of Nebraska Press, 1972.

Barnes, Will C. *Apaches and Longhorns: The Reminiscences of Will C. Barnes.* Los Angeles: Ward Ritchie Press, 1941.

Benton, Jesse James. *Cow by the Tail.* Boston: Houghton Mifflin Co., 1943.

Branch, Edward Douglas. *The Cowboy and His Interpreters.* New York: D. Appleton and Co., 1926.

Brayer, Grant M. and Herbert O. *American Cattle Trails, 1540–1900.* Bayside, N.Y.: Western Range Cattle Industry Study in Cooperation with the American Pioneer Trails Society, 1952.

Brisbin, James S. *The Beef Bonanza; or, How to Get Rich on the Plains.* 1881. Rpt. Norman: University of Oklahoma Press, 1959.

Bronson, Edgar Beecher, 1910. Rpt. *Reminiscences of a Ranchman.* Lincoln: University of Nebraska Press, 1962.

Carpenter, Will Tom. *Lucky 7: A Cowman's Autobiography.* Austin: University of Texas Press, 1957.

Clarke, Mary Whately. *A Century of Cow Business: A History of the Texas and Southwestern Cattle Raisers Association.* Fort Worth: Texas and Southwestern Cattle Raisers Association, 1976.

Clay, John. *My Life on the Range.* 1924. Rpt. Norman: University of Oklahoma Press, 1962.

Coburn, Walt. *Pioneer Cattleman in Montana: The Story of the Circle C Ranch.* Norman: University of Oklahoma Press, 1968.

Collinson, Frank. *Life in the Saddle.* Edited by Mary Whately Clarke. Norman: University of Oklahoma Press, 1963.

Cook, Harold J. *Tales of the 04 Ranch: Recollections of Harold J. Cook, 1887–1909.* Lincoln: University of Nebraska Press, 1968.

Cook, James Henry. *Fifty Years on the Old Frontier.* New Haven: Yale University Press, 1923.

———. *Longhorn Cowboy.* Edited by Howard R. Driggs. New York: G. P. Putnam's Sons, 1942.

Dale, Edward Everett. *Cow Country.* Norman: University of Oklahoma Press, 1942.

———. *The Range Cattle Industry: Ranching on the Great Plains from 1865 to 1925.* Norman: University of Oklahoma Press, 1960.

Davis, Richard Harding. *The West from a Car-Window.* New York: Harper and Bros., 1892.

Degler, Carl N. *The Age of Economic Revolution, 1876–1900.* Glenview, Ill.: Scott, Foresman, 1967.

Dobie, J. Frank. *Cow People.* Boston: Little, Brown Co., 1964.

———. *The Longhorns.* Boston: Little, Brown Co., 1941.

———. *The Mustangs.* 1934. Rpt. New York: Bantam Books, 1954.

———. *A Vaquero of the Brush Country.* New York: Grosset and Dunlap, 1929.

Dodge, Richard Irving. *Our Wild Indians: Thirty-three Years' Personal Experience among Red Men of the Great West.* Hartford: A. D. Worthington and Co., 1886.

Douglas, C. L. *The Cattle Kings of Texas.* Fort Worth: Branch-Smith, 1968.

Drago, Harry Sinclair. *Great American Cattle Trails.* New York: Bramhall House, 1965.

———. *Red River Valley: The Mainstream of Frontier History from the Louisiana Bayous to the Texas Panhandle.* New York: Clarkson N. Potter, 1962.

———. *Wild, Woolly and Wicked: The History of the Kansas Cow Towns and the Texas Cattle Trail.* New York: Clarkson N. Potter, 1960.

Duke, Cordia Sloan, and Frantz, Joe B., *6000 Miles of Fence: Life on the XIT Ranch of Texas.* Austin: University of Texas Press, 1961.

Dykstra, Robert R. *The Cattle Towns.* New York: Alfred A. Knopf, 1968.

Emmett, Chris. *Shanghai Pierce: A Fair Likeness.* Norman: University of Oklahoma Press, 1953.

Flanagan, Sue. *Trailing the Longhorns a Century Later.* Austin: Madrona Press, 1974.

Fletcher, Baylis John. *Up the Trail in '79.* Norman: University of Oklahoma Press, 1968.

Fletcher, Robert Henry. *Free Grass to Fences: The Montana Cattle Range Story.* New York: University Publishers, 1960.

Foster-Harris. *The Look of the Old West.* New York: Bonanza Books, 1955.

Frantz, Joe B., and Choate, Julian Ernest, Jr. *The American Cowboy: The Myth and the Reality.* Norman: University of Oklahoma Press, 1955.

Frink, Maurice; Jackson, W. Turrentine; and Spring, Agnes Wright. *When Grass Was King.* Boulder: University of Colorado Press, 1956.

Gard, Wayne. *The Chisholm Trail.* Norman: University of Oklahoma Press, 1954.

———. *Reminiscences of Range Life.* Austin: Steck-Vaughn Co., 1970.

Gipson, Frederick B. *Cowhand: The Story of a Working Cowboy.* New York: Harper and Bros., 1948.

Gray, Frank S. *Pioneering in Southwest Texas: True Stories of Early Day Experiences in Edwards and Adjoining Counties.* Edited by Marvin Hunter. Austin: Steck Co., 1949.

Gregg, Josiah. *Commerce of the Prairies.* 1844. Rpt. Norman: University of Oklahoma Press, 1954.

Gressley, Gene M. *Bankers and Cattlemen.* 1966. Rpt. Lincoln: University of Nebraska Press, 1971.

Haley, J. Evetts. *Charles Goodnight, Cowman and Plainsman.* Norman: University of Oklahoma Press, 1949.

———. *George W. Littlefield, Texan.* Norman: University of Oklahoma Press, 1943.

Halsell, Harry H. *Cowboys and Cattleland.* Nashville: Parthenon Press, 1937.

Hamner, Laura V. *Short Grass and Longhorns.* Norman: University of Oklahoma Press, 1943.

Hastings, Frank S. *A Ranchman's Recollections: An Autobiography.* Chicago: Breeder's Gazette, 1921.

Hill, J. L. *The End of the Cattle Trail.* 1924. Rpt. Austin: Pemberton Press, 1969.

History of Montana, 1739–1885. Chicago: Warner, Beers and Co., 1885.

Holden, William Curry. *A Ranching Saga: The Lives of William Electious Halsell and Ewing Halsell.* 2 vols. San Antonio: Trinity University Press, 1976.

Hudson, Wilson M. *Andy Adams: His Life and Writings.* Dallas: Southern Methodist University Press, 1964.

Hunt, Frazier. *The Long Trail from Texas: The Story of Ad Spaugh, Cattleman.* New York: Doubleday, Doran and Co., 1940.

Hunter, J. Marvin, ed. *The Trail Drivers of Texas.* 2 vols. 1925. Rpt. New York: Argosy-Antiquarian, 1963.

James, Will. *Cowboys North and South.* New York: Charles Scribner's Sons, 1926.

————. *Lone Cowboy.* New York: Charles Scribner's Sons, 1930.

James, Will S. *27 Years a Maverick; or, Life on a Texas Range.* 1893. Rpt. Austin: Steck-Vaughn Co., 1968.

Jones, John Oliver. *A Cowman's Memoirs.* Fort Worth: Texas Christian University Press, 1953.

Kennedy, Michael S., ed. *Cowboys and Cattlemen.* New York: Hastings House, 1964.

Kennon, Bob. *From the Pecos to the Powder: A Cowboy's Autobiography.* As told to Ramon F. Adams. Norman: University of Oklahoma Press, 1965.

Knight, Oliver. *Fort Worth: Outpost on the Trinity.* Norman: University of Oklahoma Press, 1953.

Kohrs, Conrad. *An Autobiography.* Deer Lodge, Montana: Plateau Press, 1977.

Linn, John J. *Reminiscences of Fifty Years in Texas.* 1883. Rpt. Austin: Steck Co., 1935.

McCallum, Henry D. and Frances T. *The Wire That Fenced the West.* Norman: University of Oklahoma Press, 1965.

MacConnell, E. E. *XIT Buck.* Tucson: University of Arizona Press, 1968.

McCoy, Joseph G. *Historic Sketches of the Cattle Trade of the West and Southwest.* 1874. Rpt. Columbus, Ohio: Long's College Book Co., 1951.

McLean, Malcolm D. *Fine Texas Horses: Their Pedigrees and Performance, 1830–1845.* Fort Worth: Texas Christian University Press, 1966.

Marcy, Randolph B. *The Prairie Traveler.* 1859. Rpt. Williamstown, Mass.: Corner House Publishers, 1968.

Motherhead, Harmon Ross. *The Swan Land and Cattle Company, Ltd.* Norman: University of Oklahoma Press, 1971.

Nimmo, Joseph, Jr. *Report in Regard to the Range and Ranch Cattle Business of the United States.* 1885. Rpt. New York: Arno Press, 1972.

Nordyke, Lewis. *Great Roundup: The Story of the Texas and Southwestern Cowmen.* New York: Morrow, 1955.

Olmsted, Frederick Law. *A Journey through Texas; or, A Saddle-Trip on the Southwestern Frontier.* New York: Dix and Edwards, 1857.

Osgood, Ernest Staples. *The Day of the Cattleman.* Minneapolis: University of Minnesota Press, 1954.

Pearce, William. *The Matador Land and Cattle Company.* Norman: University of Oklahoma Press, 1964.

Pelzer, Louis. *The Cattleman's Frontier: A Record of the Trans-Mississippi Cattle Industry from Oxen Trains to Packing Companies, 1850–1890.* Glendale, Calif.: Arthur H. Clark Co., 1936.

Preece, Harold. *Lone Star Man: Ira Aten, Last of the Old Texas Rangers.* New York: Hastings House, 1960.

Raine, William MacLeod, and Barnes, Will C. *Cattle.* New York: Doubleday, 1930.

Richardson, Rupert Norval. *The Frontier of Northwest Texas, 1846 to 1876.* Glendale, Calif.: Arthur H. Clark Co., 1963.

Richthofen, Walter Baron von. 1885. Rpt. *Cattle-Raising on the Plains of North America.* Norman: University of Oklahoma Press, 1964.

Rickey, Don, Jr. *$10 Horse, $40 Saddle: Cowboy Clothing, Arms, Tools and Horse Gear of the 1880's.* Fort Collins, Colo.: Old Army Press, 1976.

Ridings, Sam P. *The Chisholm Trail: A History of the World's Greatest Cattle Trail.* Guthrie, Okla.: Coop Publishers, 1936.

Roach, Joyce Gibson. *The Cowgirls.* Houston: Cordovan Corporation, 1977.

Rollins, Philip Ashton. *The Cowboy: His Characteristics, His Equipment, and His Part in the Development of the West.* New York: Charles Scribner's Sons, 1926.

Roosevelt, Theodore. *Ranch Life and Hunting Trail.* Ann Arbor, Mich.: University Microfilms, 1966.

Rye, Edgar. *The Quirt and the Spur: Vanishing Shadows of the Texas Frontier.* Chicago: W. B. Conkey Co., 1909.

Sanders, Leonard, and Tyler, Ronnie C. *How Fort Worth Became the Texasmost City.* Fort Worth: Amon Carter Museum of Western Art, 1973.

Sandoz, Mari. *The Cattlemen, from the Rio Grande across the Far Marias.* New York: Hastings House, 1958.

Savage, William W., Jr., ed. *Cowboy Life: Reconstructing an American Myth.* Norman: University of Oklahoma Press, 1975.

Sims, Orland L. *Cowpokes, Nesters, and so Forth.* Austin: Encino Press, 1970.

Siringo, Charles A. *A Texas Cowboy; or, Fifteen Years on the Hurricane Deck of a Spanish Pony.* 1886. Rpt. New York: William Sloane Assoc., 1950.

Skaggs, Jimmy. *The Cattle-Trailing Industry: Between Supply and Demand, 1866–1890.* Lawrence: University of Kansas Press, 1973.

Smith, Helena Huntington. *The War on the Powder River.* Lincoln: University of Nebraska Press, 1967.

Snyder, A. B. *Pinnacle Jake.* As told to Nellie Snyder Yost. Lincoln: University of Nebraska Press, 1951.

Sonnichsen, C. L. *Cowboys and Cattle Kings.* Norman: University of Oklahoma Press, 1950.

———. *From Hopalong to Hud.* College Station: Texas A & M University Press, 1978.

Stone, William Hale. *Twenty-Four Years a Cowboy and Ranchman in Southern Texas and Old Mexico.* Norman: University of Oklahoma Press, 1959.

Streeter, Floyd Benjamin. *Prairie Trails and Cow Towns: The Opening of the Old West.* New York: Devin Adair, 1963.

Stuart, Granville. *Pioneering in Montana: The Making of a State, 1864–1887.* 1925. Rpt. Lincoln: University of Nebraska Press, 1977.

Taylor, Thomas Ulvan. *The Chisholm Trail and Other Routes.* San Antonio: Naylor Co., 1936.

Van Zandt, Khleber Miller. *Force without Fanfare.* Edited by Sandra L. Myres. Fort Worth: Texas Christian University Press, 1968.

Verckler, Stewart P. *Cowtown-Abilene: The Story of Abilene, Kansas, 1867–1875.* New York: Carlton Press, 1961.

Vestal, Stanley. *Queen of Cowtowns: Dodge City, "The Wickedest Little City in America," 1872–1886.* 1952. Rpt. Lincoln: University of Nebraska Press, 1972.

Ward, Don, ed. *Bits of Silver: Vignettes of the Old West.* New York: Hastings House, 1961.

Ward, Fay E. *The Cowboy at Work.* New York: Hastings House, 1958.

Westermeier, Clifford P. *Man, Beast, Dust: The Story of Rodeo.* N.P.: World Press, 1947.

Williams, Mack. *In Old Fort Worth: The Story of a City and Its People as Published in the News-Tribune in 1976 and 1977.* Fort Worth: Williams, 1977.

Wyman, Walker D. *Nothing but Prairie and Sky: Life on the Dakota Range in the Early Days.* Norman: University of Oklahoma Press, 1954.

———. *The Wild Horse of the West.* Caldwell, Idaho: Caxton Printers, 1945.

Yost, Nellie Snyder., ed. *Boss Cowman: The Recollections of Ed Lemmon, 1857–1946.* Lincoln: University of Nebraska Press, 1969.

ARTICLES

Armitage, George T. "Prelude to the Last Great Roundup: The Dying Days of the Great 79." *Montana, the Magazine of Western History* 11 (October 1961): 66–75.

Ashton, John. "Texas Cattle Trade in 1870." *Cattleman* 38 (July 1951): 21, 74–75.

Atherton, Lewis. "Cattleman and Cowboy: Fact and Fancy," *Montana, the Magazine of Western History* 11 (October 1961): 2–17.

Baillie-Grohman, William A. "Cattle Ranches in the Far West." *Library Magazine of American and Foreign Thoughts* 6 (December 1880): 112–31. Reprinted from the *Fortnightly Review* n.s. 28 (July–December 1880): 438–57.

"Barbed Wire Has Its Place in History." *Frontier Times* 16 (September 1939): 534–35.

Bell, James G. "A Log of the Texas-California Cattle Trail, 1854." Edited by J. Evetts Haley. *Southwestern Historical Quarterly* 35 (January 1932): 208–37; (April 1932): 290–311.

Briggs, Harold E. "The Development and Decline of Open Range Ranching in the Northwest." *Mississippi Valley Historical Review* 20 (March 1934): 521–36.

Brown, Mark H. "New Focus on the Sioux War: Barrier to the Cattlemen." *Montana, the Magazine of Western History* 11 (October 1961): 76–85.

Burns, Robert H. "The Newman Brothers: Forgotten Cattle Kings of the Northern Plains." *Montana, the Magazine of Western History* 11 (October 1961): 28–36.

"Chisholm Cattle Trails in Texas Preserved by Writers." *Frontier Times* 7 (September 1930): 554–55.

Clements, Roger V. "British Investment and American Legislative Restrictions in the Trans-Mississippi West, 1880–1900." *Mississippi Valley Historical Review* 42 (September 1955): 207–28.

Dalton, Frank. "Military Escort for a Trail Herd." *Cattleman* 32 (July 1944): 13–14.

Dobie, J. Frank. "Ab Blocker: Trail Boss." *Arizona and the West* 6 (Summer 1964): 97–103.

———. "The First Cattle in Texas and the Southwest Progenitors of the Longhorns." *Southwestern Historical Quarterly* 42 (January 1939): 171–97.

———. "The Spanish Cow Pony." *Saturday Evening Post* 207 (November 24, 1934): 12–13, 64–66.

———. "Tom Candy Ponting's Drive of Texas Cattle to Illinois." *Cattleman* 35 (January 1949): 34–45.

Doran, Michael. "Antebellum Cattle Herding in the Indian Territory." *Geographical Review* 66 (January 1976): 48–58.

"A Drive from Texas to North Dakota." *Frontier Times* 3 (April 1926): 1–4.

Earhart, E. P. "Up the Cattle Trail in 1867." *Frontier Times* 8 (February 1931): 194–95.

"Early Texas Cattle Industry." *Frontier Times* 5 (September 1928): 476–81.

Fellows, Fred. "Illustrated Study of Western Saddles." *Montana, the Magazine of Western History* 16 (January 1966): 57–83.

"The First Cattle Ranch in Texas." *Frontier Times* 13 (March 1936): 304–8.

Fletcher, Robert H. "The Day of the Cattleman Dawned Early—in Montana." *Montana, the Magazine of Western History* 11 (October 1961): 22–28.

Fletcher, Robert S. "The End of the Open Range in Eastern Montana." *Mississippi Valley Historical Review* 16 (September 1929): 188–211.

Frantz, Joe B. "Texas' Largest Ranch—in Montana: The XIT." *Montana, the Magazine of Western History* 11 (October 1961): 46–56.

Gard, Wayne. "The Fence-Cutters." *Southwestern Historical Quarterly* 51 (July 1947): 1–15.

———. "The Impact of the Cattle Trails." *Southwestern Historical Quarterly* 71 (July 1967): 1–6.

———. "Retracing the Chisholm Trail." *Southwestern Historical Quarterly* 60 (July 1956): 53–68.

Gibson, Arrell M. "The Cowboy in Indian Territory." *Red River Valley Historical Review* 2 (Spring 1975): 147–61.

Gill, Larry. "From Butcher Boy to Beef King: The Gold Camp Days of Conrad Kohrs." *Montana, the Magazine of Western History* 8 (Spring 1958): 40–55.

Gillett, James B. "Beef Gathering in '71 Was Thrilling." *Frontier Times* 3 (April 1926): 6–7.

Goodnight, Charles. "Managing a Trail Herd in the Early Days." *Frontier Times* 6 (November 1929): 250–52.

"Goodnight Sets Out upon 'New Adventure.' " *Frontier Times* 5 (October 1927): 28–30.

Gressley, Gene M., ed. "Harvard Man Out West: The Letters of Richard Trimble, 1882–1887." *Montana, the Magazine of Western History* 10 (Winter 1960): 14–23.

Grove, Fred. "The Old Chisholm Trail." *Oklahoma Today,* Autumn 1966, pp. 24–27.

Guice, John D. "Cattle Raisers of the Old Southwest: A Reinterpretation." *Western Historical Quarterly* 8 (April 1977): 167–88.

Haley, J. Evetts. "And Then Came Barbed Wire to Change History's Course." *Cattleman* 13 (March 1927): 78–83.

Halsell, H. H. "My Chronicle of the Old West." *Cattleman* 38 (August 1957): 98–102.

Harger, Charles Moreau. "Cattle-Trails of the Prairies." *Scribner's Magazine* 11 (June 1892): 732–42.

Hayter, Earl W. "Barbed Wire Fencing—A Prairie Invention." *Agricultural History* 13 (October 1939): 189–207.

Herrington, George Squires. "An Early Cattle Drive from Texas to Illinois." *Southwestern Historical Quarterly* 55 (October 1951): 267–69.

"Hige Nail, an Early Trail Driver." *Frontier Times* 4 (November 1926): 16.

Hollon, Gene. "Captain Charles Schreiner, the Father of the Hill Country." *Southwestern Historical Quarterly* 48 (October 1944): 145–68.

Holt, Roy D. "Fence Cutting War." *Cattleman* 61 (July 1974): 124–26.

———. "From Trail to Rail in Texas Cattle Industry." *Cattleman* 18 (March 1932): 50–59.

———. "Introducing Barbed Wire to Texas Stockmen." *Cattleman* 17 (July 1930): 26–31.

———. "The Introduction of Barbed Wire Into Texas and the Fence Cutting War." *West Texas Historical Association Year Book* 6 (June 1930): 65–79.

Houston, Dunn. "A Drive from Texas to North Dakota." *Frontier Times* 3 (April 1926): 1–4.

Huffman, Adolph. "A Long Dry Drive on the Cattle Trail." *Frontier Times* 8 (May 1940): 335–36.

Huidekoper, Wallis. "The Story Behind Charlie Russell's Masterpiece: 'Waiting for a Chinook.' " *Montana, the Magazine of Western History* 4 (Summer 1954): 37–39.

Hunter, J. Marvin. "George Saunders' First Trip." *Frontier Times* 5 (May 1928): 321–24.

Hutchinson, W. H. "The Cowboy and Karl Marx." *Pacific Historian* 20 (Summer 1976): 111–22.

"Introducing Barbed Wire in Texas." *Frontier Times* 9 (November 1931): 90–92.

Jordan, Gilbert J., tr. and ed. "W. Steinert's View of Texas in 1849," pt. 5. *Southwestern Historical Quarterly* 81 (July 1977): 45–77.

Jordan, Philip D. "The Pistol Packin' Cowboy: From Bullet to Burial." *Red River Valley Historical Review* 2 (Spring 1975): 65–91.

Jordan, Terry G. "Windmills in Texas." *Agricultural History* 37, no. 2 (1961): 80–85.

"The Justin Boot." *Montana, the Magazine of Western History* 11 (January 1961): 86–88.

Keese, J. Pomeroy. "Beef." *Harper's New Monthly Magazine* 69 (July 1884): 292–301.

Kennedy, Michael, ed. "Judith Basin Top Hand: Reminiscences of William Burnett, an Early Montana Cattleman." *Montana, the Magazine of Western History* 3 (Spring 1953): 18–23.

Lunsford, John R. "E. B. Baggett Speaks of Chisholm Trail." *Frontier Times* 8 (December 1930): 127–28.

McCaleb, J. L. "A Texas Boy's First Experience on the Trail." *Frontier Times* 5 (October 1927): 10–13.

Morris, W. J. "Over the Old Chisholm Trail." *Frontier Times* 2 (April 1925): 41–43.

Nimmo, Joseph, Jr. "The American Cow-Boy." *Harper's New Monthly Magazine* 73 (November 1886): 880–84.

Nolen, O. W. "Shanghai Pierce." *Cattleman* 31 (December 1944): 31.

Nunn, Annie Dyer. "Over the Goodnight and Loving Trail." *Frontier Times* 2 (November 1924): 4–7.

"Old Cowman Tells of a Big Steal." *Frontier Times* 3 (June 1926): 36–37.

"An Old Time Cattle Inspector." *Frontier Times* 3 (March 1926): 44–45.

Padgitt, James T. "Colonel William H. Day: Texas Ranchman." *Southwestern Historical Quarterly* 53 (April 1950): 347–66.

Pattie, Jane. "The Justin Boot: Standard of the West." *Quarter Horse Journal* 29 (September 1977): 124–32.

Potter, Jack. "Up the Trail (and Back) in '82." *Montana, the Magazine of Western History* 11 (October 1961): 57–65.

Remington, Frederic. "Horses of the Plains." *Century Magazine* 37 (November 1888–April 1889): 332–43.

Richardson, Ernest M. "John Bull in the Cowmen's West: Moreton Frewen, Cattle King with a Monocle." *Montana, the Magazine of Western History* 11 (October 1961): 37–45.

Russell, Don. "The Cowboy: From Black Hat to White." *Red River Valley Historical Review* 2 (Spring 1975): 13–23.

Sanders, A. Collatt. "Adventures on the Old Cattle Trail." *Frontier Times* 3 (July 1926): 1–3.

Savage, William W., Jr. "The Cowboy Myth." *Red River Valley Historical Review* 2 (Spring 1975): 162–71.

Shelton, Emily Jones. "Lizzie Johnson: A Cattle Queen of Texas." *Southwestern Historical Quarterly* 50 (April 1947): 349–66.

Sinclair, F. H. (Neckyoke Jones). "Down the Trail with a Range Rider." *Montana, the Magazine of Western History* 16 (Summer 1966): 56–64.

Stephens, R. M. "Recollections of a Texas Cowpuncher." *Frontier Times* 2 (July 1925): 11.

Streeter, Floyd Benjamin. "The National Cattle Trail." *Cattleman* 38 (June 1951): 26–27, 59–74.

Taylor, T. U. "Original Chisholm Trail." *Frontier Times* 8 (February 1931): 195–99.

"A Vivid Story of Trail Driving Days." *Frontier Times* 2 (July 1925): 20–23.

Welsh, Donald H. "Cosmopolitan Cattle King: Pierre Wibaux and the W Bar Ranch." *Montana, the Magazine of Western History* 5 (Spring 1955): 1–15.

Westermeier, Clifford P. "Cowboy Sexuality: A Historical No-No?" *Red River Valley Historical Review* 2 (Spring 1975): 93–113.

Wilkeson, Frank. "Cattle Raising on the Plains." *Harper's Monthly Magazine* 72 (1886): 285–96.

Wilson, Glen O. "Old Red River Station." *Southwestern Historical Quarterly* 61 (January 1958): 350–58.

Index

British capital